Primary FRCA:

450 MTFs and SBAs

Primary FRCA:

450 MTFs and SBAs

Kariem El-Boghdadly MBBS BSc (Hons) FRCA
Specialty Registrar in Anaesthesia,
South East School of Anaesthesia, London, UK

Imran Ahmad MBBS FRCA
Consultant Anaesthetist, Guy's and
St Thomas' NHS Foundation Trust, London, UK

Editorial Advisor
Craig Bailey MBBS FRCA
Consultant Anaesthetist, Guy's and
St Thomas' NHS Foundation Trust, London, UK

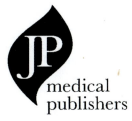

JP
medical
publishers

London • Philadelphia • Panama City • New Delhi

© 2014 JP Medical Ltd.
Published by JP Medical Ltd
83 Victoria Street, London, SW1H 0HW, UK
Tel: +44 (0)20 3170 8910   Fax: +44 (0)20 3008 6180
Email: info@jpmedpub.com   Web: www.jpmedpub.com

ISBN: 978-1-907816-59-8

British Library Cataloguing in Publication Data
A catalogue record for this book is available from the British Library

Library of Congress Cataloging in Publication Data
A catalog record for this book is available from the Library of Congress

JP Medical Ltd is a subsidiary of Jaypee Brothers Medical Publishers (P) Ltd, New Delhi, India

Commissioning Editor: Steffan Clements
Design: Designers Collective Ltd

Copy edited, typeset, indexed, printed and bound in India.

Foreword

If you are reading this then you must have some interest in the FRCA examination process, whether as a candidate, a college tutor or an educator. In my opinion it is the most rigorous but fairest test of knowledge of any medical specialty. The Royal College of Anaesthetists has invested an enormous amount of time, money and expertise in ensuring that both the Primary and Final FRCA examinations are robust, the results reproducible and the papers valid. It is a relevant examination; after 18 years as a consultant, I find that the principles tested remain as important to me today as they have ever been. However, the examination is in continuous flux, constantly being adapted in order that it remains fit-for-purpose, and I am extremely proud and honoured to be one of its examiners.

The Primary FRCA examination is, in effect, the gatekeeper to a career in anaesthesia: once success is achieved then the world of anaesthesia opens up to the trainee and anything is possible. However, acquiring that success necessitates serious preparation, and lots of it. The Primary multiple choice question (MCQ) paper tests knowledge of a wide curriculum and no candidate could ever 'wing it'. The candidate preparing for the Primary examination will have spent many a lonely night and weekend 'hitting the books', deprived of the company of friends and family. If it is any consolation the rewards for passing are tremendous. I clearly remember the day I passed the Primary examination – it felt like a huge weight had been lifted from my shoulders, I had more energy and was eager to get on with the rest of my life as an anaesthetist.

The Primary FRCA MCQ paper

Preparing for and sitting the Primary examination is expensive (currently £310) so it is foolhardy to attempt it without proper preparation. There are three sittings a year at various locations and a total of five attempts is allowed. Once the MCQ paper has been passed it is valid for three years.

The MCQ paper itself consists of 60 Multiple True/False (MTF) questions each worth 5 marks (20 in pharmacology, 20 in physiology and 20 in physics, clinical measurement and data interpretation), as well as 30 Single Best Answer (SBA) questions each worth 4 marks for a correct answer and consisting of any topics from the curriculum. This gives a maximum score of 420; there is no negative marking.

At the time of writing the pass rate for the previous four sittings was 55% (February 2012), 61% (June 2012), 49% (September 2012) and 51% (February 2013). There is a reason why there is such an apparently wide variation in the pass rate. If a fixed pass *mark* is set, then all candidates who obtain that mark or higher are passed. If the paper was easier than in previous years, then more candidates are likely to pass. Conversely, fewer are likely to pass if the examination is particularly difficult. On the other hand, if a certain pass *rate* is set, e.g. 60%, then a particularly good cohort may put at a disadvantage the borderline candidate who would have passed if the cohort were less competent. This is the reason the Angoff method of criterion referencing was introduced by the College.

Angoff referencing

This is a method of setting the pass mark based on the professional judgement of a group of experienced examiners. The Primary MCQ examination currently uses a modified Angoff referencing system whereby a number of examiners make independent judgements which are then used to set the standard.

The principle of standard setting is to set the pass mark for an examination by determining the minimum level of knowledge or skills required to pass that examination. In order to do this the examiners are asked to decide for each exam question the probability that a *minimally competent candidate* will *know* the correct answer. Minimally competent means a candidate who is of reasonable intelligence, with an average amount of clinical knowledge and who has done a reasonable amount of preparation. Such a candidate is often described as the borderline candidate, or one who has performed *just* well enough to pass the examination.

Due to the relatively large size of the Primary MCQ paper, examiners are given a version with alternate MTF questions and all the SBA questions. For each question the examiner gives a score from 0 to 10 for the probability of a borderline candidate knowing the correct answer.

Impossible					Probable					Certain
0	1	2	3	4	5	6	7	8	9	10

These numbers are summated to give a total for each examiner. Inevitably there will be a range of numbers across the 'Angoffing' group. Once all examiners' totals are returned, the examinations department calculates the average Angoff mark. Outliers are removed using a 1st and 3rd quartile calculation. It has been agreed that 12 or more examiners in any Angoffing group are required to give a reliable Angoff reference score.

Revision aids

There is a plethora of examination aids available, ranging from e-Learning to past papers published by the College itself, but they are not always as helpful as they could be. How often have you attempted practice questions, looked at the answers and not understood why 'B' was false and then had to look elsewhere for the reason behind the answer? This book does not suffer that fault because it provides comprehensive answers to all the questions, so you are left in no doubt as to why the answers are as they are. Preparation for the examination relies on this sort of analysis and on wider reading: there is no point in simply memorising answers.

The authors are young and their enthusiasm can be sensed throughout. Kariem El-Boghdadly and Imran Ahmad have spent a huge amount of time writing this book, and I truly believe that it is the best revision aid on the market. All the questions are closely based on the current curriculum and the answers have been painstakingly researched for accuracy. I feel sure that by the time you finish this book you will be in a fabulous position to take on the examination and pass.

You may want a career in our specialty but until you achieve success in the Primary FRCA examination you can never truly call yourself an anaesthetist.

Craig Bailey
July 2013

Preface

The FRCA has always been a challenging set of examinations. The recent addition of the Single Best Answer (SBA) format to the multiple choice question sections of both Primary and Final FRCA examinations has added to their difficulty. In order to succeed, candidates must use all the tools available to them to either increase their knowledge or improve their technique. We recognised that for the new examination format there were few good resources to support them in this, and our aim has been to provide the right resource to help candidates pass the rigorous Primary FRCA examination

This work has taken a huge amount of time and effort to put together. We have ensured that the full breadth of the syllabus is addressed and we have made every effort to write in the College's exam style. Detailed explanations reinforce understanding of the correct answers and are accompanied by references.

The SBAs are the most challenging aspect of the examination. We have included a wide range of science and clinical SBAs to assist the reader in improving exam technique. Again, references are provided to facilitate more in-depth reading around the topic in question.

We hope this book serves its intended purpose of helping the reader succeed in the Primary FRCA examination.

Good luck!

Kariem El-Boghdadly
Imran Ahmad
July 2013

C20449241

Contents

Bibliography

Al-Shaikh, Stacey S. Essentials of anaesthetic equipment. 4th edn. Edinburgh: Churchill Living-stone, 2013.

Brit.sh National Formulary, 63. London: British Medical Association and the Royal Pharmaceutical Society; March 2012.

Cross M, Plunkett E. Physics, Pharmacology and physiology for anaesthetists. Key Concepts for the FRCA. Cambridge: Cambridge University Press, 2008.

Davis PD, Kenny GNC. Basic physics and measurement in anaesthesia. Oxford: Butterworth-Heinemann; 5th edn. 2003.

Johnston I, Harrop-Griffiths W, Gemmell L (eds). AAGBI core topics in anaesthesia 2012. Chichester: Wiley-Blackwell, 2012.

Leslie RA, Johnson EK, Goodwin APL. Dr Podcast Scripts for the Primary FRCA. Cambridge: Cambridge University Press, 2011.

Magee P, Tooley M. The physics, clinical measurement and equipment of anaesthetic practice for the FRCA (Oxford Specialty Training: revision texts), 2nd edn. Oxford: Oxford University Press, 2011.

Peck TE, Hill, SA, Williams M (2008). Pharmacology for anaesthesia and intensive care, 3rd edn. Cambridge: Cambridge University Press.

Rang HP, Dale MM, Ritter JM, Moore PK. Pharmacology, 5th edn. Edinburgh: Churchill Livingstone; 2011.

Sasada M, Smith S. Drugs in anaesthesia and intensive care, 4th edn. Oxford: Oxford University Press, 2011.

Smith T, Pinnock C, Lin T. Fundamentals of anaesthesia (Cambridge Medicine), 3rd edn. Cambridge: Cambridge University Press, 2009.

West JB. Respiratory physiology: the essentials, 9th revised edn. Philadelphia: Lippincott Williams and Wilkins, 2011.

Yentis SM, Ip J, Hirsch N, Smith G. Anaesthesia and intensive care A–Z: an encyclopedia of principles and practice, 4th revised edn. Edinburgh: Churchill Livingstone, 2009.

Website of National Tracheostomy Safety Project. www.tracheostomy.org.uk (last accessed 01/10/2012).

Dedications

For N, S, R, S, Zs & D – Thank you for all of your patience, love and support.

Kariem

I would like to dedicate this book to my parents, wife, siblings and three children. You have always supported me. Thank you.

Imran

Chapter 1

Mock paper 1

60 MTFs and 30 SBAs to be answered in three hours

Questions: MTFs

Answer each stem 'True' or 'False'.

1. **Regarding the cardiac cycle, which of the following are true:**
    A   At the end of atrial systole, the mitral valve closes because the pressure in the left atrium exceeds that in the left ventricle
    B   At the end of isovolumetric contraction, the aortic valve opens at approximately 120 mmHg
    C   Isovolumetric relaxation signifies the beginning of diastole
    D   The pressure/volume trace of the right ventricle has the same morphology as the left ventricle
    E   The dicrotic notch appears on the left ventricle pressure trace

2. **Coronary blood flow:**
    A   Is approximately 500 mL/min
    B   In the left coronary artery is constant throughout the cardiac cycle
    C   In the right coronary artery is always greater than the left coronary artery
    D   In the right coronary artery occurs throughout the cardiac cycle
    E   In the left coronary artery peaks during systole

3. **The left ventricle:**
    A   Has a wall that is three times thicker than that of the right ventricle
    B   Takes about 2 seconds to fill during ventricular diastole at rest
    C   Is responsible for the 'apex beat'
    D   Ejects blood into the right coronary artery
    E   Contains papillary muscles connected to the aortic valves

4. **Regarding veins, which of the following are true:**
    A   They contain a third of the circulating blood volume
    B   Their pressure/volume curve is initially very steep
    C   Blood enters the venules at a lower pressure than larger veins
    D   Central venous pressure is the pressure at the point where the venae cavae enter the right atrium
    E   Standing results in a decrease in the venous pressure of veins above and below the level of the heart

5. **Regarding physiological dead space, which of the following are true:**
    A It decreases under general anaesthesia
    B It increases with hypovolaemia
    C It is the same as anatomical dead space
    D It requires knowledge of the P_{ECO_2} and P_{aO_2} to be calculated
    E Alveolar dead space is normally 150 mL

6. **Regarding pulmonary blood flow, which of the following is true:**
    A It is greatest in the uppermost lung when a subject is in the lateral position
    B Regional perfusion differences can be explained by the effects of hydrostatic pressure
    C Measurement of pulmonary blood flow requires knowledge of arterial carbon dioxide content
    D In West zone 1, alveolar pressure exceeds pulmonary arterial pressure
    E Hypoxic areas of lung have increased perfusion

7. **The respiratory centre receives afferents from:**
    A Pulmonary stretch receptors
    B Juxtaglomerular capillary receptors
    C Dorsal medullary neurones
    D Baroreceptors
    E Carotid sinus receptors

8. **The following substances undergo metabolism in the lungs:**
    A Angiotensin II
    B Acetylcholine
    C Noradrenaline
    D Leukotrienes
    E Prostaglandin A_2

9. **The following are true regarding the kidneys:**
    A They receive approximately 25% of the cardiac output
    B Each kidney has two renal arteries
    C Most of the renal blood flow is to the medulla
    D The vasa recta arise from the afferent arterioles
    E The renal arteries divide into interlobular and arcuate arteries

10. **Functions of the kidney include:**
    A Direct maintenance of intracellular fluid volume
    B Maintenance of extracellular potassium concentration
    C Gluconeogenesis
    D Production and secretion of angiotensinogen
    E Production of prostaglandins

11. **Glomerular filtration rate:**
    A Can be calculated using inulin and creatinine as indicators
    B Can be calculated using the formula urine concentration (U) × plasma concentration/urinary flow rate (V)

    C   Is about 125 L/min
    D   Is the same as the clearance of inulin
    E   Ceases when the mean systemic arterial pressure falls below 60 mmHg

12. **Regarding potassium balance, which of the following is true:**
    A   Approximately 60% is excreted in the urine and 40% in the faeces
    B   Approximately 99% is stored intracellularly
    C   Extracellular potassium is important for the regulation of potassium balance
    D   Acute regulation is controlled by aldosterone
    E   Most of the potassium filtered by the kidney is reabsorbed

13. **Regarding cerebral blood flow (CBF), which of the following is true:**
    A   The majority is in the white matter
    B   It is approximately 15% of cardiac output
    C   Two thirds are from the vertebral arteries
    D   Autoregulation maintains a constant CBF between a mean arterial pressure of 50 and 150 mmHg
    E   It is calculated using Fick's law

14. **Regarding cerebrospinal fluid (CSF), which of the following is true:**
    A   500 mL is produced every 24 hours
    B   At greater intracranial pressures, more CSF is produced
    C   Fluid passes from the 3rd ventricle via the foramen of Magendie
    D   Potassium concentrations are normally 2.5–3.5 mmol/L
    E   There is a lower concentration of protein in CSF than in the plasma

15. **Parasympathetic stimulation causes:**
    A   Lacrimation
    B   Increased insulin secretion
    C   Vasoconstriction
    D   Tachycardia
    E   Bronchodilation

16. **Regarding muscle spindles, which of the of following are true:**
    A   They are involved in maintenance of posture
    B   Efferent control is via γ-motor neurones
    C   Sensory supply involves only type II fibres
    D   They sense muscle tension
    E   The withdrawal reflex is polysynaptic

17. **Regarding daily nutrition, which of the following are true:**
    A   Energy requirements are mainly obtained from fats, minerals and vitamins
    B   The largest energy contribution as a percentage of intake is from dietary fats
    C   Per unit, proteins have the highest caloric value
    D   Essential amino acids are only synthesised in small quantities
    E   Fat-soluble vitamins include vitamins B, C, E and K

18. **Swallowing:**
    A   Is a voluntary process
    B   Involves the soft palate being pulled up
    C   Causes the larynx to be pulled up by the pharyngeal muscles
    D   Takes about 3 seconds from start to finish
    E   Is initiated at the tonsillar pillars

19. **Regarding hormone production, which of the following are true:**
    A   The kidneys produce calcitriol
    B   The thyroid gland produces calcitonin
    C   The stomach produces glucagon
    D   The liver produces cholecystokinin
    E   The anterior pituitary gland produces oxytocin

20. **Regarding haemoglobin, which of the following are true:**
    A   Adult haemoglobin is composed of two α- and two γ-subunits
    B   It contains iron in its ferrous state
    C   It contains four iron atoms
    D   It can bind eight molecules of oxygen to each haemoglobin chain
    E   Cooperative binding is due to the Bohr effect

21. **Bioavailability:**
    A   Is the fraction of administered substance that enters the systemic circulation
    B   Is higher for orally administered drugs than rectally administered drugs
    C   May be reduced by increasing first-pass metabolism
    D   Increases in the presence of hepatic enzyme inducers
    E   Is 100% for intravenous ketamine

22. **The following drugs can be administered transdermally:**
    A   Procaine
    B   Glyceryl trinitrate
    C   Clonidine
    D   Alfentanil
    E   Diclofenac

23. **The volume of distribution:**
    A   Is greater for fentanyl than morphine
    B   Of propofol is greater than total body water
    C   Is greater than 1 L/kg for most non-depolarising neuromuscular blocking drugs
    D   Is higher for highly protein-bound drugs
    E   Is the apparent volume that a drug disperses into to produce observed plasma concentrations

24. **The following drugs are excreted in the urine predominantly unchanged:**
    A   Diclofenac
    B   Epinephrine

   C   Lithium

   D   Ephedrine

   E   Digoxin

25. **The ideal intravenous anaesthetic agent would have the following properties:**

   A   High lipid solubility

   B   Lipid-soluble formulation

   C   Long half-life

   D   Analgesic at sub-anaesthetic concentrations

   E   Pre-prepared solution

26. **Thiopentone:**

   A   Is formulated as a sulphur salt

   B   Forms a neutral solution when dissolved in water

   C   Is stored in nitrogen

   D   Once administered, 80% is immediately available at pH 7.4

   E   Is safe to use in patients with porphyria

27. **Xenon:**

   A   Is a colourless gas with a pungent odour

   B   Is produced by fractional distillation of air

   C   Increases cardiac output by sympathetic stimulation

   D   Has a slower onset and offset time than desflurane

   E   Has a higher density and viscosity than nitrous oxide

28. **Tachyphylaxis:**

   A   Is synonymous with tolerance

   B   Occurs when larger doses are required to achieve a similar response

   C   Is seen with amphetamine

   D   May be due to a change in receptor structure

   E   Takes place over a short period of time

29. **The following local anaesthetics are esters:**

   A   Prilocaine

   B   Etidocaine

   C   Amethocaine

   D   Cocaine

   E   Ropivacaine

30. **Systemic vascular absorption of local anaesthetic is greater than epidural administration when given:**

   A   To the brachial plexus

   B   Caudally

   C   Subcutaneously

   D   To the femoral nerve

   E   Intercostally

31. **The following drugs have a vasodilator action:**
    - A   Prilocaine
    - B   Bendroflumethiazide
    - C   Diazoxide
    - D   Tramadol
    - E   Lidocaine

32. **Antiarrhythmic drugs:**
    - A   Are classified according to their site of action
    - B   Are classified according to their effects on the action potential
    - C   May belong to more than one class in the Vaughan Williams classification
    - D   Belong to class I as they slow phase 0 of the action potential
    - E   Such as adenosine belong to class III

33. **Regarding vasoactive drugs, which of the following is true:**
    - A   Dopamine is a synthetic analogue of dobutamine
    - B   Dopamine is a precursor of noradrenaline
    - C   Dobutamine can cause hypotension
    - D   Dobutamine acts on dopaminergic receptors
    - E   Dopamine causes peripheral dilatation at high doses

34. **The following are true regarding the mechanism of action of nitrates:**
    - A   They preferentially dilate large coronary arteries and arterioles
    - B   They redistribute blood from epicardial to endocardial regions
    - C   They have no effect on myocardial oxygen demand
    - D   The vascular endothelium should be intact for effective vasodilation
    - E   They are better arteriolar than venous dilators

35. **Suxamethonium:**
    - A   Is hydrolysed at the neuromuscular junction by cholinesterases
    - B   Has active metabolites
    - C   Is predominantly excreted in the urine
    - D   Produces a phase I block on repeated administration
    - E   Consists of two acetylcholine molecules joined by an ester link

36. **Bisquaternary aminosteroid drugs include:**
    - A   Pancuronium
    - B   Vecuronium
    - C   Mivacurium
    - D   Tubocurarine
    - E   Rocuronium

37. **The following are true of non-steroidal anti-inflammatory drugs:**
    - A   Paracetamol has anti-inflammatory properties
    - B   Aspirin has antipyretic properties
    - C   Diclofenac is 10% plasma protein bound
    - D   Paracetamol is 90% plasma protein bound
    - E   Ibuprofen has greater anti-inflammatory activity than analgesic activity

38. Morphine:

   A   Is a naturally occurring phenanthrene derivative
   B   Relaxes the gut sphincters and the sphincter of Oddi
   C   Causes nausea and vomiting via serotonergic (5HT) and muscarinic receptors
   D   Can precipitate chest wall rigidity
   E   Inhibits the release of adrenocorticotropic hormone and prolactin

39. Benzodiazepines:

   A   Bind to the α-subunit of gamma-aminobutyric acid $(GABA)_A$ receptors
   B   Act via second-messenger systems
   C   Are highly plasma protein bound
   D   Always have active metabolites
   E   Include zopiclone

40. These diuretics have the following unwanted effects:

   A   Furosemide and hypercalcaemia
   B   Bendroflumethiazide and hypocalcaemia
   C   Spironolactone and Conn's syndrome
   D   Mannitol and an increase in preload and cardiac output
   E   Bendroflumethiazide and leucopaenia and thrombocytopaenia

41. The following is true regarding electricity:

   A   Electrons can only pass from one atom to another under a potential difference
   B   Body fluids are generally bad conductors
   C   Insulators bind to their electrons more firmly then semiconductors
   D   Thermistors are insulators
   E   Diodes are semiconductors

42. Surgical diathermy:

   A   Typically uses frequencies of 1 kHz
   B   Is more likely to cause ventricular fibrillation than a direct current
   C   Relies on two connections to the patient, even with monopolar diathermy
   D   Contains a capacitor
   E   When bipolar, uses higher power than monopolar

43. Regarding the hazards of magnetic resonance imaging (MRI), which of the following is true:

   A   MRI involves the use of ionising radiation
   B   There is a risk of causing involuntary muscle contraction
   C   Patients may experience flashing lights and sensations of taste
   D   Patients with metal prosthetic joints should not undergo MRI
   E   Ferromagnetic objects are safe to use within the fringe field of the scanner

44. Regarding the gas laws, which of the following is true:

   A   Boyle's law states that at a constant temperature, the volume of a given mass of gas varies inversely to the absolute pressure
   B   Gay Lussac's law is the third perfect gas law

    C   The second gas law states that at a constant pressure, the volume of a gas is proportional to the absolute temperature

    D   They are corrected to a standard temperature of 273°F

    E   Dalton's law states that PV/T = constant

45. **The following statements about simple mechanics are true:**

    A   Power is defined as the work done when a force is applied in the direction of the force

    B   Power is measured in joules

    C   When the point of application of a force moves in the direction of the force energy is expended

    D   The power of breathing can be calculated by the area under the pressure/volume curve divided by time

    E   In respiratory muscles, most of the chemical energy is converted to mechanical energy

46. **Regarding humidity, which of the following is true:**

    A   Relative humidity is expressed in milligrams of water per liter of gas

    B   Humidity may be expressed as the pressure exerted by water vapour in a gas mixture

    C   As humidity increases, hair length shortens

    D   If a fully saturated gas is cooled, both the absolute and the relative humidity will fall

    E   A wet and dry bulb hygrometer measures ambient and relative humidity

47. **Regarding heat and temperature, which of the following is true:**

    A   Heat is a measure of the tendency of an object to gain or lose heat

    B   The SI unit for temperature is Celsius

    C   Temperature is the energy which can be transferred from a hotter object to a cooler one

    D   Zero Kelvin is absolute zero

    E   The triple point of water is at 273.16 K

48. **Regarding latent heat in anaesthesia:**

    A   Liquid ethyl chloride vapourises from the skin causing a cooling sensation

    B   Ethyl chloride is stored as a liquid in a glass ampoule under pressure

    C   Cooling of volatile anaesthetics makes them less volatile

    D   Carbon dioxide is stored in cylinders in gaseous form

    E   As nitrous oxide is emptied from a cylinder, the pressure remains constant until all the liquid has vapourised

49. **The following are true regarding fluids and flow:**

    A   Liquids are the only fluids

    B   During laminar flow, the fluid nearest to the wall has no flow

    C   In the middle of a pipe, the velocity is twice than that of the average velocity across the pipe, during laminar flow

    D   Turbulent flow requires less driving pressures than laminar flow

    E   Turbulent flow wastes more energy than laminar flow

50. **Regarding the principles of ultrasound, which of the following is true:**
   A   It is a form of mechanical energy
   B   It is produced from piezoelectric crystals which are compressed and decompressed
   C   The frequency is dependent on the compression pressures
   D   The wavelength is the reciprocal of the frequency
   E   The wave can pass through a vacuum

51. **The following are true regarding hazards of electrical equipment:**
   A   Under single fault conditions, type 1 CF equipment should have a leakage current of the order of 4 mA
   B   Type BF equipment is safe because the patient circuit is earthed
   C   Class II equipment has power cables only containing 'live' and 'neutral' conductors
   D   Class III equipment is defined as that which operates at 'safety extra low voltage' of less than 12 V
   E   A current-operated earth-leakage circuit breaker relies on an unacceptable current causing disintegration of a fuse that then breaks the circuit

52. **Nitrous oxide cylinders:**
   A   Have blue and white quartered shoulders
   B   Are pressurised to 4.4 bar
   C   Have a filling ratio of 0.75 in the UK
   D   Have pressure within them decreasing linearly
   E   Of size E have a capacity of 1800 L

53. **With regard to vacuum-insulated evaporators:**
   A   They store liquid oxygen at a pressure of 400 kPa
   B   They have an internal temperature of –118°C
   C   The mass of oxygen can be measured by weight
   D   If less oxygen is utilised, the internal temperature rises
   E   If pressure exceeds 17 bar, this causes opening of a safety valve

54. **Flowmeters such as rotameters:**
   A   Depend on gas density
   B   Rely on laminar flow at low flow rates
   C   Are accurate within 1%
   D   Reduce piped gas pressure
   E   Are inaccurate in the presence of static charge

55. **The emergency oxygen flush:**
   A   Delivers flow that bypasses the vapourisers
   B   Delivers at a pressure of 137 bar
   C   Has pressure-reducing valves to reduce barotrauma
   D   May lead to awareness
   E   Can deliver flow rates of 40–50 L/min

56. The following are maximum allowable environmental concentrations in the UK:

   A   Desflurane: 75 ppm
   B   Enflurane: 50 ppm
   C   Halothane: 25 ppm
   D   Isoflurane: 100 ppm
   E   Nitrous oxide: 25 ppm

57. The Lack breathing system:

   A   Is a Mapleson D arrangement
   B   Is most efficient for controlled ventilation
   C   Can be in coaxial or parallel arrangements
   D   Requires a fresh gas flow rate of two to three times the minute ventilation during spontaneous ventilation
   E   Vents exhaled gases through a 14 mm inner tube

58. The 12-lead electrocardiogram:

   A   Has a signal output of 1–2 mV
   B   Uses six bipolar leads
   C   Has a frequency response in monitoring mode of between 0 and 100 MHz
   D   Prints from an oscilloscope running at 25 mm/s
   E   CM5 arrangement optimally detects arrhythmias

59. Regarding statistical tests:

   A   A type I error involves rejecting a true null hypothesis
   B β-errors are the same as false negatives
   C   The power of a study must be calculated after data collection
   D   A power of 20% is acceptable
   E   The variance is the square root of the standard deviation

60. The following devices contain differential pressure transducers:

   A   Vacuum-insulated evaporators
   B   Paramagnetic analysers
   C   End-tidal carbon dioxide analysers
   D   Tec 6 vapourisers
   E   Pneumotachographs

Questions: SBAs

For each question, select the single best answer from the five options listed.

61. A 73-year-old man has had an asystolic cardiac arrest. You have successfully intubated him and cardiopulmonary resuscitation is underway.

Which is the most likely finding for this patient?

A   Blood pressure of 52/26 mmHg
B   End-tidal CO_2 of 0.4 kPa
C   A pH of 7.38
D   A standard bicarbonate of 38.1 mmol/L
E   A serum potassium of 7.8 mmol/L

62. A 68-year-old woman, who had a grade I intubation, is having an open reduction and internal fixation of an ankle fracture. She is being ventilated at a rate of 14 breaths per minute, with a peak inspiratory pressure of 36 cmH_2O, achieving a tidal volume of 210 mL.

Which of the following is the most appropriate statement regarding lung compliance?

A   The patient may have pulmonary oedema
B   Normally lung compliance is 500 mL/cmH_2O
C   During an asthma attack lung compliance decreases
D   The patient may have underlying emphysema
E   It may be plotted on a flow/volume loop

63. A 23-year-old man has sustained a traumatic intracranial haemorrhage with evidence of raised intracranial pressure (ICP). He is intubated and requires transfer to a specialist neurosurgical centre.

Which of the following is most likely to reduce his ICP?

A   Increasing his Pao_2 from 9.0 to 12 kPa
B   Sedation with ketamine
C   Reducing $Paco_2$ from 5.8 to 4.2 kPa
D   8 mg of dexamethasone
E   Fluid restriction

64. A 75-year-old man in the emergency department has a heart rate of 44 beats per minute and an unrecordable blood pressure. His pulses are not palpable.

What is the first drug this patient should receive?

A   Atropine
B   Adrenaline
C   Amiodarone
D   Ephedrine
E   Metaraminol

65. A 54-year-old woman is having a bunionectomy under general anaesthetic. You perform an ankle block using the landmark technique.

Which of the following nerves could a nerve stimulator be used to block?

    A Deep peroneal nerve
    B Saphenous nerve
    C Superficial peroneal nerve
    D Sural nerve
    E Tibial nerve

66. An 8-year-old girl (30 kg body weight) presents for tonsillectomy. You have prepared drugs and equipment.

Which calculation is correct?

    A Length of a nasal tube at the nares is 19 cm
    B Endotracheal tube size is 5.0 mm internal diameter
    C Laryngeal mask size is 2.0
    D Fentanyl dose is 15 µg
    E Intravenous paracetamol dose is 800 mg

67. A 34-year-old man has a rapid sequence induction for a perforated duodenal ulcer. Twenty minutes later his heart rate rises to 125 beats per minute, blood pressure decreases to 75/40 mmHg, airway pressures increase to 36 cmH$_2$O and cutaneous urticaria is rapidly spreading.

What is the most likely causative agent?

    A Atracurium
    B Succinylcholine
    C Latex
    D Morphine
    E Co-amoxiclav

68. A 68-year-old woman with chronic obstructive airways disease and rheumatoid arthritis presents for a total shoulder placement. You perform an interscalene nerve block using a nerve stimulator technique.

What is the most likely complication in this patient?

    A Recurrent laryngeal nerve palsy
    B Horner's syndrome
    C Pneumothorax
    D Vertebral artery puncture
    E Phrenic nerve palsy

69. A 44-year-old man (100 kg body weight) in the intensive care unit with acute respiratory distress syndrome is being ventilated with volume-controlled ventilation at tidal volumes of 620 mL, peak inspiratory pressures of 29 cmH$_2$O,

positive end-expiratory pressure (PEEP) of 6 cmH$_2$O and a FIO$_2$ of 0.9. His arterial blood gas demonstrates a Pao$_2$ of 6.9 kPa and a Paco$_2$ of 7.3 kPa.

What intervention is most likely to increase his Pao$_2$?

A   Increase the tidal volume
B   Increase the FIO$_2$
C   Increase the expiratory time
D   Increase the respiratory frequency
E   Increase the PEEP

70. A 22-year-old woman with a past medical history of asthma presents with difficulty in breathing, a respiratory rate of 28 breaths per minute, inability to complete sentences and wheeze. An arterial blood gas breathing room air reveals a Pao$_2$ of 8.5 kPa and a Paco$_2$ of 3.4 kPa. Five milligrams of nebulised salbutamol has been administered.

What is the next step in this patient's management?

A   Nebulised antimuscarinic agents
B   Check peak expiratory flow rates
C   Intubation and ventilation
D   Intravenous magnesium
E   Request a chest radiograph

71. While trying to attach a cylinder to the anaesthetic machine, you realise it does not fit appropriately. The pin index shows positions 3 and 5.

Which is the most likely cylinder?

A   Nitrous oxide
B   Oxygen
C   Air
D   Carbon dioxide
E   Entonox

72. A 36-year-old woman has oxygenation saturations of 96% on pulse oximetry but 88% on arterial blood gas oximetry analysis.

What is the most likely cause for this discrepancy?

A   Hyperbilirubinaemia
B   Indocyanine green dye
C   Methaemoglobinaemia
D   Carboxyhaemoglobin
E   Presence of nail varnish

73. While floating a pulmonary artery catheter, a pulmonary capillary wedge pressure of 15 mmHg is shown on the monitor.

This represents the pressure in which of the following?

 A Right atrium
 B Right ventricle
 C Left atrium
 D Left ventricle
 E Pulmonary artery

74. Using the flow of water through a pipe, driven by a mechanical pump as an analogy for electricity, the pressure difference between two points in the pipe would correspond to which of the following?

 A Current
 B Work
 C Voltage
 D Resistance
 E Power

75. A 20-year-old woman has arrived in the anaesthetic room for elective orthopaedic surgery. She is needle phobic and is insisting on a gaseous induction of anaesthesia.

 Which of the following would most efficiently and rapidly allow you to perform a gas induction?

 A Bain breathing system
 B Mapleson A breathing system
 C Mapleson B breathing system
 D Mapleson C breathing system
 E Mapleson D breathing system

76. A 75-year-old man has had emergency vascular surgery. He presented with a full stomach, therefore required a rapid sequence induction to secure his airway followed by prolonged surgery requiring significant blood transfusion.

 Which of the following extubation strategies is least appropriate?

 A Deep extubation
 B Laryngeal mask exchange
 C Airway exchange catheter
 D Remifentanil technique
 E Awake extubation

77. A 35-year-old man requires surgery to repair a lacerated biceps tendon. He had been assaulted and sustained a left-sided pneumothorax and a 5 cm stab wound to his right antecubital fossa.

 Which of the following ultrasound-guided upper limb blocks would be the most appropriate for surgery?

 A Interscalene
 B Supraclavicular
 C Infraclavicular

D Axillary

E Peripheral nerve block

78. The components of a circle breathing system attached to a standard anaesthetic machine include soda lime in a canister.

Which of the following is *incorrect* regarding soda lime?

A It contains a pink dye

B The dye changes to white when the soda lime is exhausted

C The size of the granules should be 4–8 mesh

D It consists of 95% sodium hydroxide

E Silica is added

79. A 35-year-old woman is having laparoscopic gynaecological surgery. She is anaesthetised and has a blood pressure of 110/60 mmHg and heart rate of 60 beats per minute as the surgeon is insufflating the peritoneum with gas. There is an immediate complication as a result of the pneumoperitoneum.

Which of the following emergency drugs would you first administer?

A Adrenaline

B Atropine

C Ephedrine

D Suxamethonium

E Metaraminol

80. You have chosen to use an infusion of remifentanil and propofol to induce and maintain anaesthesia for a patient undergoing elective surgery for a plastics procedure.

Which of the following is *least* likely to guarantee drug delivery using this technique?

A Use of non-return valves

B Keeping the cannulation site visible at all times

C Being aware of the uses and limitations of the infusions pumps

D Infusing intravenous fluids through the same cannula as the drugs

E Using a large proximal vein for infusion

81. A 46-year-old man is being anaesthetised for functional endoscopic sinus surgery to remove nasal polyps as a day case procedure.

Which of the following is most likely to reduce intraoperative bleeding?

A Hypotensive anaesthesia

B Normocarbia

C Reverse Trendelenburg tilt

D Use of Moffat's solution

E Normothermia

82. You are about to perform a fibreoptic intubation in a patient with a known difficult airway.

Which of the following would be the most appropriate method of preventing cross-contamination with a fibreoptic scope?

A   Cleaning
B   Sterilisation
C   Disinfection
D   Decontamination
E   Autoclaving

83. A 43-year-old woman having a laparoscopic cholecystectomy has an oxygen saturation which rapidly decreases to 80% on 100% inspired oxygen, peak airway pressures increase to 38 cmH$_2$O, and blood pressure reduces to 72/42 mmHg. Examination demonstrates absent breath sounds and a hyper-resonant percussion note on the left side of the chest.

What is the most appropriate immediate management?

A   Increase tidal volumes
B   50–100 µg of adrenaline
C   Needle decompression
D   Increase respiratory rate
E   Fluid bolus

84. A 68-year-old woman presents with shortness of breath and weakness. A 12-lead electrocardiogram shows a rate of 42 beats per minute with complete dissociation of P waves from QRS complexes.

What is the most likely jugular venous pressure (JVP) waveform that will be seen?

A   Absent JVP waveforms
B   Absent *a* waves
C   Raised JVP with normal waveforms
D   Large *v* waves
E   Cannon *a* waves

85. A 45-year-old man presents with a productive cough, shortness of breath and pyrexia. He has saturations of 91% on room air. An arterial blood gas sample (ABG) is performed but the plastic syringe is left for more than 60 minutes at room temperature prior to analysis.

What is the most likely erroneous result on the ABG analysis?

A   Reduced pH
B   Elevated Pao_2
C   Reduced $Paco_2$
D   Increased glucose
E   Reduced lactate

86. A 46-year-old woman is undergoing an open reduction and internal fixation of a tibial plateau fracture. She is breathing spontaneously through a laryngeal mask airway. Ten minutes following prosthesis insertion, her respiratory rate increases to 34 breaths per minute, oxygen saturations decrease to 88% with an F_{IO_2} of 0.5, end-tidal CO_2 reduces to 2.4 kPa and a petechial rash is noted on her chest.

What is the most likely diagnosis?

A   Haemorrhage
B   Anaphylaxis
C   Fat embolism syndrome
D   Venous thromboembolism
E   Myocardial ischaemia

87. A 28-year-old man with a traumatic brain injury is to be transferred to a neurosurgical centre 90 minutes away. He is intubated and being ventilated with an F_{IO_2} of 1.0 and a minute ventilation of 10 L per minute.

What is the minimum number of full size E oxygen cylinders that would be needed for transfer?

A   One size E oxygen cylinders
B   Two size E oxygen cylinders
C   Three size E oxygen cylinders
D   Four size E oxygen cylinders
E   Five size E oxygen cylinders

88. A 44-year-old woman is undergoing free flap surgery for breast reconstruction. The surgeons are concerned about microvascular perfusion in the donor tissue. The blood pressure decreases to 85/44 mmHg.

What is the most important variable to consider in order to optimise flap perfusion?

A   Blood pressure
B   Heart rate
C   Blood viscosity
D   Vessel calibre
E   Temperature

89. A 65-year-old man presents with a 12-hour history of fatigue, confusion and chest pain with a plasma normal troponin concentration. A 12-lead electrocardiogram shows a heart rate of 32 beats per minute with complete dissociation of P waves from QRS complexes.

Which drug is most likely to increase the heart rate in this patient?

A   Isoprenaline
B   Atropine
C   Phenylephrine
D   Salbutamol
E   Noradrenaline

90. A 66-year-old man with severe chronic obstructive airways disease presents for a laparoscopic hernia repair as a day case.

Which is the most appropriate anaesthetic agent to use in this patient?

A   Bupivacaine
B   Desflurane
C   Sevoflurane
D   Remifentanil
E   Lidocaine

Answers: MTFs

1. **A** False
   B False
   C True
   D True
   E False

   The atria and ventricles contract in sequence, which results in a cycle of pressure and volume changes (see **Figure 1.1a** and **b**). During atrial systole, blood flows from the atria through the atrioventricular valves and into the ventricles. The volume of blood in a ventricle at the end of the filling phase is the end-diastolic volume (about 120 mL in adults). As soon as the left ventricular pressure rises above the left atrial pressure, the mitral valve closes (A). This is the beginning of isovolumetric contraction.

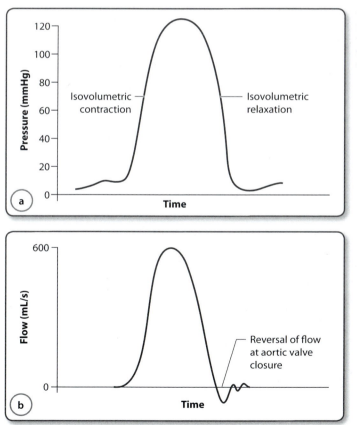

Figure 1.1 (a) The pressure/time curve for the left ventricle. (b) The flow/time curve for the left ventricle.

During isovolumetric contraction the ventricle is a closed chamber, allowing a steep pressure rise, generated as a result of increasing ventricular wall tension. When the ventricular pressure exceeds aortic pressure, usually approximately 80 mmHg, then the aortic valve opens, isovolumetric contraction ends and ejection into the aorta begins (B).

At the end of the ejection phase, the aortic and pulmonary valves close and once again the ventricles become closed chambers; this is isovolumetric relaxation. As the pressure in the ventricles falls below atrial pressure, the atrioventricular valves open and blood then flows from the atria into the ventricles. Both mitral and aortic valves are closed during isovolumetric relaxation, and there is a rapid fall in pressure; this is the first stage of diastole (C).

Both the left and right ventricles have the same pressure/volume traces or morphology, but the pressures are lower in the right ventricle (D).

The dicrotic notch is seen on the aortic pressure trace and is as a result of the elastic recoil of the aortic walls after the aortic valve closes. It is not seen in the left ventricular pressure trace (E).

2. A False

    B False

    C False

    D True

    E False

Coronary blood flow is approximately 200–250 mL/min in an average adult and comprises about 5% of the total cardiac output (A).

Flow in the right coronary artery is greater than that in the left during systole, but less during diastole. The blood flow within the left coronary artery varies throughout the cardiac cycle (B).

Flow through the right coronary artery occurs throughout the cycle as the transmitted intracavity pressures are low compared with the left ventricle, where the higher pressures lead to compression of the coronary vessels and left coronary blood flow almost ceases during systole (see **Figure 1.2**) (C, D, E).

Coronary blood flow is least during systole and mostly occurs during diastole.

The coronary perfusion pressure (CPP) determines the maximum pressure perfusing the coronary arteries and can be quantified by:

CPP = aortic-diastolic pressure − left ventricular end-diastolic pressure.

The above equation demonstrates that the greatest perfusion occurs during diastole.

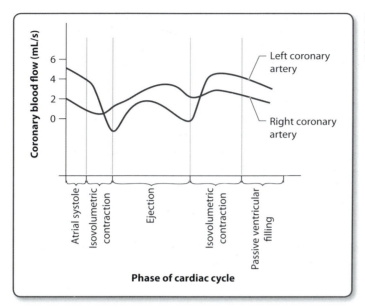

Figure 1.2 Left and right coronary arterial blood flow in different phases of the cardiac cycle.

3. A True
    B False
    C True
    D True
    E False

The left ventricular wall is about three times thicker than the right, as it has to generate much higher pressures to provide blood flow in the systemic circulation (A). Ejection of blood is produced by a reduction in both diameter and length of the chamber.

At rest, ventricular diastole typically lasts for approximately 0.5 second, which is about two-thirds of the cardiac cycle (B).

When the chamber of the left ventricle contracts, it twists forward and the apex taps against the chest wall; this can be palpated in the left fifth intercostal space as the 'apex beat' (C).

Both the right and left coronary arteries arise from the aorta immediately above the cusps of the aortic valve to receive blood from the left ventricle (D).

The papillary muscles of the left ventricle are connected to the cusps of the mitral valve by chordae tendineae, not to the aortic valves (E).

4. A False
    B True

C False

D True

E False

Peripheral veins and venules are thin-walled, voluminous vessels that hold roughly two-thirds of the circulating volume (A). Venules have a diameter of 0.01–0.2 mm with veins having a diameter of 0.2–5.0 mm, together collectively being known as capacitance vessels. In contrast, arterioles and small arteries are known as resistance vessels as they are responsive to autonomic supply and can constrict and dilate to control blood flow.

The effect of pressure on venous volume is very steep between 0 and 10 mmHg, due to the easily distensible walls (B). This allows the volume to increase relatively easily per unit rise in pressure.

Blood enters the venules at a pressure of about 12–20 mmHg, but by the time it reaches larger veins, such as the axillary or femoral vein, the pressure falls to about 10 mmHg (C).

Central venous pressure is usually measured directly by a catheter placed in the superior vena cava, via the internal jugular or subclavian veins (D).

On standing the pressure increases in any blood vessel below the level of the heart and decreases above the heart; this is due to gravity acting on the column of fluid between the heart and the vessel (E).

5. A False

    B True

    C False

    D False

    E False

Physiological dead space increases under general anaesthesia and in hypovolaemic patients as shown in **Table 1.1** (A, B).

Table 1.1 The causes of increased and decreased dead space		
Anatomical dead space		**Alveolar dead space**
Increased	**Decreased**	**Increased**
Neck extension	Neck flexion	Pulmonary embolism
Jaw protrusion	Low tidal volumes	Pulmonary disease
Increased tidal volumes	General anaesthesia	Hypovolaemia
Neonates and the elderly	Intubation	Hypotension
Bronchodilation	Tracheostomy	General anaesthesia
Anticholinergics	5-hydroxytryptamine	Intermittent positive pressure ventilation
Catecholamines	Histamine	Positive end-expiratory pressure

Physiological dead space is the sum of anatomical dead space (normally 150 mL) and alveolar dead space (normally 0 mL); thus, it is not the same as the anatomical dead space (C, E). It is normally approximately 30% of tidal volume (i.e. $V_D/V_T = 0.3$) and is calculated by the Bohr equation (see Answer 3.61). The Bohr equation requires the knowledge of the arterial partial pressure of CO_2 (Pa_{CO_2}) and the expired partial pressure of CO_2 (PE_{CO_2}) (D):

$$\frac{V_D}{V_T} = Pa_{CO_2} - \frac{PE_{CO_2}}{Pa_{CO_2}}$$

There are a number of factors that affect the anatomical dead space and alveolar dead space as classified in **Table 1.1**.

6. A False

    B True

    C False

    D True

    E False

Pulmonary blood flow is greatest in the dependent areas of the lung. Thus, when standing, perfusion is greatest at the bases, and in the lateral position perfusion is greatest in the lower lung (A). This is due to the effect of hydrostatic pressure whereby gravity increases perfusion pressure in the lungs by 1 cmH$_2$O for every centimetre in height below the level of the heart (B).

The Fick principle may be utilised in the measurement of pulmonary blood flow. This states that O_2 consumption per unit time ($\dot{V}_{O_2}$) is equal to the amount of O_2 taken up by the blood in the lungs per unit time (i.e. the blood flow times the arterial oxygen content (Ca_{O_2}) – venous oxygen content ($C\bar{v}_{O_2}$) difference) (C).

$$\dot{V}_{O_2} = \dot{Q}\,(Ca_{O_2} - C\bar{v}_{O_2})$$

Therefore:

$$\dot{Q} = \frac{\dot{V}_{O_2}}{(Ca_{O_2} - C\bar{v}_{O_2})}$$

The lung is divided into three zones defined by the relationship between pulmonary arterial (Pa), pulmonary venous (Pv) and alveolar pressures (PA). In zone 1, $PA>Pa>Pv$, thus capillaries are closed and no flow occurs (D). This does not occur normally but in areas where it does occur it is defined as an area of alveolar dead space. Zone 2 may be a region in the middle of the lung, where $Pa>PA>Pv$ and blood flow is determined by the arterial-alveolar pressure difference. Finally, zone 3 is often at the bottom of the lung, where $Pa>Pv>PA$ and blood flow is determined by the arterial–venous pressure difference.

Hypoxic areas of the lung undergo vasoconstriction (hypoxic pulmonary vasoconstriction, HPV) to prevent blood flow to poorly ventilated alveoli, thus reducing shunt (E).

7. **A** True

    B False

    C False

    D True

    E False

The control of breathing involves sensors with afferent fibres to central controllers that then feed effector targets. The location and function of each of these areas can be summarised as follows:

- Central controllers
    - The respiratory centre is responsible for the rhythmic inspiratory and expiratory patterns and includes:
        - The medullary respiratory centre
        - The apneustic centre in the lower pons
        - The pneumotaxic centre in the upper pons
- Sensors
    - Central chemoreceptors
        - On the ventral medullary surface (C)
        - Stimulated by a reduction in CSF pH (i.e. an increase in H^+ ion concentration) caused by metabolic acidosis or an increased $P\text{co}_2$
        - Not affected by $P\text{o}_2$
    - Peripheral chemoreceptors
        - Aortic bodies giving vagal afferents and carotid bodies giving glossopharyngeal nerve afferents (E)
        - Stimulated by elevated $P\text{co}_2$ in a linear fashion, increase in H^+ ions and a reduction in $P\text{o}_2$ below 8–10 kPa
    - Lung receptors
        - Pulmonary stretch receptors (A)
        - Juxtapulmonary capillary (J) receptors (B)
        - Irritant receptors
        - Bronchial C fibres
    - Other receptors
        - Nose and upper airway receptors
        - Arterial baroreceptors (D)
        - Joint and muscle receptors
        - Higher centres: pain, temperature, anxiety
- Effectors
    - Respiratory muscles

8. **A** False

    B False

    C True

    D True

    E False

Other than the heart, the lungs are the only other organ that receives the whole circulating blood volume. Therefore, the lungs are involved in a number of metabolic processes (see **Table 1.2**) including noradrenaline and leukotriene metabolism (C, D).

Table 1.2 Metabolic functions of the lungs		
Removal/inactivation	**No effect**	**Conversion**
Bradykinin – 80%	Angiotensin II	Angiotensin I to II by angiotensin-converting enzyme (ACE)
5-hydroxytryptamine (5-HT; serotonin)	Vasopressin (antidiuretic hormone, ADH)	
Noradrenaline	Dopamine	
Prostaglandins E_2 and $F_{2\alpha}$	Histamine	
Leukotrienes	Prostaglandin A_2 (E)	

Although angiotensin II is formed in the lungs by the action of angiotensin-converting enzyme (ACE) on angiotensin I, it is metabolised to angiotensin III in red blood cells and vascular endothelium (A). It is therefore not metabolised in the lungs.

Acetylcholine is hydrolysed in the plasma and post-synaptic membranes, but not directly in the lungs (B).

Other functions of the lung include phospholipid synthesis (e.g. surfactant), involvement in immune and coagulant function, and acting as a reservoir of blood (between 500 and 900 mL at any given moment). This latter feature explains the decreased blood pressure on release of an elevated intrathoracic pressure, as seen during the Valsalva manoeuvre (see Question 2.89).

9. **A** True

   B False

   C False

   D False

   E True

Despite the kidneys being small (weighing approximately 130 g each), together they receive nearly a quarter of cardiac output, or 500 mL/min/100 g (about 1.2 L/min) (A).

Blood is supplied to the kidneys via the renal artery, which is a branch of the aorta. There are typically two renal veins and one renal artery per kidney (B).

The distribution of blood flow to different regions varies, with 90% of renal blood flow to the cortex and only 10% to the medulla (C). Despite this the inner medulla still receives a higher blood flow per gram of tissue than most other organs.

The vasa recta arise from the inner cortical efferent arterioles, which also supply the peritubular capillaries (D). The vasa recta provide the only blood supply to the renal medulla.

The high-pressure renal arteries first divide into several interlobar arteries and these in turn divide into arcuate arteries, which give off the interlobular arteries at right angles (see **Figure 1.3**) (E).

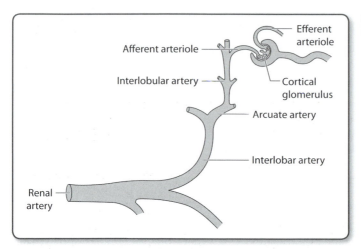

Figure 1.3 Divisions of renal arterial supply.

10. **A** False

B True

C True

D False

E True

The kidneys maintain the constancy of the extracellular fluid volume (ECFV) and the extracellular osmolality by balancing the intake and excretion of sodium and water (A). The osmolality of the ECFV is strictly controlled to avoid large fluctuations in volume and osmolality within the intracellular compartment, as this is in osmotic equilibrium with the ECFV. They do not directly maintain intracellular fluid volume.

The kidneys maintain the concentration of extracellular potassium constant as well as the pH of the blood, by adjusting the excretion of hydrogen ions and bicarbonate (B).

Gluconeogenesis is the process of formation of glucose from substrate, including lactate and pyruvate, occurring predominantly in the liver with a smaller contribution from the kidneys (C). Other metabolic functions of the kidneys include arginine formation and peptide hydrolysis.

The kidneys produce the proteolytic enzyme renin from the juxtaglomerular apparatus, which it releases into the bloodstream. Renin acts on angiotensinogen, which is produced in the liver, to form angiotensin I (D). This is then converted to the highly active angiotensin II by cleaving two amino acids. Angiotensin II causes thirst and stimulates the release of aldosterone.

In addition to the regulation of the ECFV and ion concentration, the kidneys are a source of hormones, such as prostaglandins, angiotensin II and erythropoietin (E).

11. A True

   B False

   C False

   D True

   E False

Both inulin and creatinine have the suitable properties required to measure glomerular filtration rate (GFR) (A). Inulin is a carbohydrate which is infused into the bloodstream, whereas creatinine is already present in the blood as a breakdown product of muscle metabolism.

The formula for calculating GFR is UV/P, where U is the urine concentration of the indicator, V is the urine flow rate and P is the plasma concentration of the indicator (B). The GFR is normally approximately 125 mL/min for a normal adult (C).

Inulin, once injected, is completely filtered to enter the tubule and all of it enters the urine; therefore, the rate of filtration of inulin will equal the rate of excretion (D).

GFR is constant at mean systemic arterial pressures above 80 mmHg, so the filtration pressure is kept constant in this range by altering the pre-arteriolar and arteriolar resistance. Filtration significantly reduces but does not cease below a mean pressure of 60 mmHg (E).

12. A False

   B True

   C True

   D False

   E True

About 50–150 mmol of potassium (K^+) is resorbed daily in which about 90% of the K^+ is excreted in the urine and about 10% in the faeces (A).

About 98–99% of the total body K^+ stores are intracellular, mostly in muscle cells, but also in the liver and the erythrocytes (B).

Extracellular K^+ only accounts for about 1% of the total body store; one of the main functions of this extracellular store is to mediate the regulation of the whole K^+ balance of the body (C).

The acute regulation of extracellular K^+ is achieved largely by the release of insulin, which promotes the uptake of K^+ from the extracellular compartment in to the intracellular compartment. Aldosterone, adrenaline and alkalosis all promote the cellular uptake of K^+, but are not as rapid in their management as insulin (D).

About 70% of K^+ is reabsorbed by the end of the proximal convoluted tubule, about 20% at the loop of Henle and the rest is reabsorbed in the distal convoluted tubule (E).

13. **A** False

B True

C False

D True

E False

Cerebral blood flow (CBF) is approximately 15% of cardiac output, 700 mL/min (50 mL/100 g/min) of which the grey matter receives the majority (A, B). The blood supply is two thirds from the internal carotid arteries and one third from the two vertebral arteries (C). The two systems merge at the anterior and posterior communicating arteries to form the circle of Willis. CBF remains constant between mean arterial pressures (MAPs) of 50–150 mmHg – above this range there is a sharp increase in CBF, with a decrease in CBF below this range (D).

CBF can be measured using the Fick principle. This states that the uptake/release of a substance, e.g. O_2 ($\dot{V}o_2$), by an organ is the product of the blood flow ($\dot{Q}$) through that organ and the arteriovenous difference in content ($Cao_2–C\bar{v}o_2$) (see Question 1.6). This is applied using the Kety–Schmidt technique where 10% N_2O is inhaled for 10–15 minutes, and the jugular venous concentration is measured and assumed to be the same as the brain concentration. Fick's law, however, describes the rate of diffusion across a membrane being proportional to the concentration gradient (E).

14. **A** True

B False

C False

D True

E True

Cerebral spinal fluid (CSF) is a clear, colourless fluid surrounding the brain that protects it from traumatic damage and helps regulate intracranial pressure (ICP). It has characteristics and properties as follows:

- Production
  - Total volume is 100–150 mL (10% of intracranial volume), produced at a rate of 0.3 mL/min by choroid plexuses in lateral, third and fourth ventricles
  - 500 mL is produced a day (A)
  - Formed by plasma filtration and secretion
  - Production of CSF is independent of ICP (B)
- Circulation
  - Lateral ventricles to the third ventricle via foramen of Monro
  - Third to fourth ventricle via aqueduct of Sylvius
  - Fourth ventricle down the spinal cord or over cerebral hemispheres via midline foramen of Magendie or lateral foramen of Luschka (C)
  - Absorbed from dural venous sinuses via arachnoid villi
- Composition
  - Normal CSF reference values in **Table 1.3** (D)

- CSF proteins are only 1% of plasma levels, while calcium and glucose levels are 50–60% of plasma levels (E)
- Chloride and magnesium levels, however, are greater in the CSF than the plasma

Table 1.3 Reference values for cerebrospinal fluid

Constituent	Concentration
Sodium	135–145 mmol/L
Potassium	2.5–3.5 mmol/L
Chloride	115–125 mmol/L
Calcium	1–1.5 mmol/L
Magnesium	1.2–1.5 mmol/L
Glucose	2.7–4.2 mmol/L
Urea	1.5–6.0 mmol/L
Lymphocytes	$0–5 \times 10^6$/L
Protein	0.2–0.4 g/L

15. A True

B True

C False

D False

E False

Parasympathetic stimulation is responsible for the 'rest and digest' actions in the autonomic nervous system, of which the Vagus nerve carries approximately three quarters of the fibres. Vasoconstriction, tachycardia and bronchodilation are all sympathetically mediated effects, while lacrimation and insulin production are parasympathetic effects.

The following are effects of parasympathetic stimulation:

- Ophthalmic: pupillary and ciliary constriction; lacrimation (A)
- Cardiovascular: bradycardia, reduced contractility; vasodilation in skeletal muscle, coronary, pulmonary, renal and viscera (C, D)
- Pulmonary: bronchoconstriction; increased secretions (E)
- Gastrointestinal: increased motility and secretions; sphincteric relaxation
- Metabolic: increased secretion of insulin and glucagon (B)
- Genitourinary: detrusor muscle contraction, sphincteric relaxation; penile erection

16. A True

B True

C False

D False

E True

Muscle spindles are formed from intrafusal muscle fibres that respond to changes in length, rather than muscle tension, whereby contraction of muscles causes shortening of muscle spindles, an important mechanism in maintaining posture (A, D).

When muscle spindles are passively stretched, they transmit impulses directly to efferent γ-motor neurones via either type Ia or type II fibres (B, C). This is the monosynaptic stretch reflex. However, γ-motor neurone activity can be modulated by descending spinal cord pathways, which may alter the resting tone and sensitivity of muscles. These features make muscle spindles suitable for sensing and modifying posture. Golgi tendon organs are responsible for sensing muscle tension.

The withdrawal reflex is a polysynaptic reflex, as there are interneurones between sensory signals and motor elements of the reflex (E).

17. **A** False

    B False

    C False

    D True

    E False

Energy requirements are primarily provided by proteins, fats and carbohydrates (A). Vitamins and minerals are required in small quantities but do not provide significant energy supplies.

The energy contribution of carbohydrates is about 60% of the total, while fats provide about 25–30% of the energy (B). The remaining energy is provided by proteins.

One gram of fat provides about 40 kJ of energy, while 1 g of protein provides about 17 kJ as does 1 g of carbohydrates (C).

Essential amino acids are those that cannot be synthesised by humans or only in very small amounts; therefore, they need to be part of a healthy diet (D). The essential amino acids include valine, leucine, isoleucine, threonine, methionine, phenylalanine, tryptophan and lysine.

Fats are largely superfluous in the diet, provided that there is a supply of the essential fatty acids, such as linoleic acid, and the fat-soluble vitamins, such as A, D, E and K (E).

18. **A** False

    B True

    C False

    D False

    E True

Swallowing is an involuntary reflex (A). It is preceded by the voluntary act of collecting food on the tongue and propelling the bolus into the pharynx by raising the tongue.

As the bolus of food enters the pharynx, it stimulates the swallowing receptors. This triggers the swallowing reflex, which is a series of autonomic pharyngeal muscular contractions.

First, the soft palate is pulled upwards to close the posterior nares, thus preventing food from entering the nasal cavities (B).

The palatopharyngeal folds are pulled medially so that well-masticated food passes posteriorly into the pharynx, and larger objects are impeded.

The vocal cords are strongly approximated, the larynx is pulled upwards and anteriorly by the neck muscles, not the pharyngeal muscles, and the epiglottis swings backwards over the opening of the larynx (C). This all prevents food from entering the larynx, while enlarging the opening of the oesophagus.

At the same time the upper oesophageal sphincter relaxes, allowing food to easily pass into the upper oesophagus.

The whole process, which includes the trachea closing, the oesophagus opening and propelling of the food bolus from the pharynx to the oesophagus, takes about 1–2 seconds (D).

The most sensitive tactile areas of the pharynx for the initiation of swallowing lie around the pharyngeal opening, with the tonsillar pillars having the greatest sensitivity (E).

19. **A** True

   B True

   C False

   D False

   E False

A hormone is a regulatory substance released by a single or group of cells or organ that has an effect at a distant site. Common hormones can be seen in **Table 1.4**.

Calcitriol is the active form of vitamin D that acts to increase plasma calcium levels and is produced in cells of the proximal tubule of the renal nephron (A).

Calcitonin is generated by the thyroid parafollicular (C) cells to reduce serum calcium concentrations (B).

Glucagon is a peptide hormone synthesised in the α-cells of the pancreatic islets of Langerhans that increase blood glucose concentrations (C).

Cholecystokinin is a peptide hormone that is produced in the small intestinal and duodenal mucosa in response to fat and protein in chime (D). It increases gastric transit time to allow further digestion of fats.

Both oxytocin and vasopressin (antidiuretic hormone, ADH) are released from the posterior pituitary but are produced in the hypothalamus (E).

Table 1.4 Sites of hormone production

Organ	Hormone
Adrenal cortex	Aldosterone, cortisol, androgens
Kidneys	Calcitriol
Testes	Testosterone
Ovaries	Oestrogen, progesterone
Thyroid	T3 (triiodothyronine), T4 (thyroxine), calcitonin
Adrenal medulla	Adrenaline, noradrenaline
Mast cells	Histamine
Pancreas	Insulin, glucagon
Parathyroids	Parathyroid hormone
Stomach and small intestine	Gastrin, secretin, cholecystokinin, gastric inhibitory peptide
Anterior pituitary	Human growth hormone, prolactin, adrenocorticotropic hormone, melanocyte stimulating hormone, thryoid stimulating hormone, follicle stimulating hormone, luteinising hormone
Hypothalamus	Oxytocin, antidiuretic hormone

20. **A** False

   B True

   C True

   D False

   E False

Haemoglobin is a molecule that is designed to increase the oxygen carrying capacity of blood >50 times, and is made of four polypeptide globin chains. The adult circulation contains HbA (two α-chains and two β-chains) as well as 2–3% HbA2 (two α-chains and two δ-chains) (A). Fetal haemoglobin contains two α-chains and two γ chains.

Each globin chain has a porphyrin-derived haem group with a central iron atom in its ferrous state (Fe^{2+}) able to carry one O_2 molecule; therefore, up to four molecules of O_2 can be carried per haemoglobin (B, C, D). It is methaemoglobin that carries iron atoms in the ferric state (Fe^{3+}). Haemoglobin has a number of characteristic effects that it demonstrates:

- Cooperativity: binding of one O_2 molecule breaks non-covalent salt links between globin chains that increase affinity for further O_2 molecules to bind. This effect is more pronounced with the second and third molecule of O_2 that bind and is the underlying cause of the sigmoid-shaped oxyhaemoglobin dissociation curve
- Bohr effect: higher $P\text{co}_2$ reduces the affinity of haemoglobin for O_2 (E)
- Haldane effect: increases affinity of deoxygenated haemoglobin for CO_2

21. A True

B False

C True

D False

E True

Bioavailability is the fraction of a drug dose that reaches the systemic circulation compared with a standard, usually intravenous, route of administration (A). Thus, any drug administered via the intravenous route has a bioavailability of 100% (E). By plotting a plasma concentration over time curve for the same dose of oral and intravenous drug administration (see **Figure 1.4**), the bioavailability can be calculated by:

$$\text{Bioavailability} = \frac{\text{AUC oral}}{\text{AUC IV}}$$

where AUC is area under the curve and IV is intravenous.

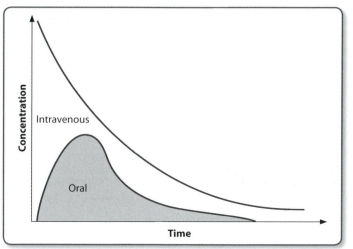

Figure 1.4 Bioavailability of a drug from oral and intravenous administration.

Bioavailability can be affected by a number of factors, including:

- **First-pass metabolism:** drugs absorbed from the gastrointestinal tract enter the portal vein and thence to the liver, where they undergo metabolism prior to reaching the systemic circulation. This is minimised with sublingual and rectal routes of administration which have a higher bioavailability than the oral route (B, C)
- **Hepatic enzymes:** induction of hepatic enzymes increases first-pass metabolism thereby reducing bioavailability, while hepatic enzyme inhibition reduces metabolism, thus increasing bioavailability (D)
- **Physicochemical properties:** small or liquid drugs are more readily absorbed when compared with large drug preparations. Interaction with other orally delivered substances may reduce absorption, thus reducing oral bioavailability

- **Gastrointestinal properties:** any cause for delayed gastric emptying or malabsorption may reduce oral bioavailability

22. A False

   B True

   C True

   D False

   E True

Transdermal drug delivery depends on drug factors and patient factors as shown in **Table 1.5**.

Table 1.5 Factors affecting transdermal drug delivery	
Drug factors	**Patient factors**
Lipophilic and hydrophilic	Good regional blood flow
Short half-life	Intact skin
Low melting point	
Low molecular weight (<500 Da)	
High potency	
Unionised	

Prilocaine, not procaine, is a component of the topical local anaesthetic cream EMLA (eutectic mixture of local anaesthetic) and can be delivered transdermally (A).

Glyceryl trinitrate is a vasodilator that can be administered as transdermal patches (B).

Clonidine is a versatile α_2-adrenoceptor agonist that can be administered orally, transdermally, intramuscularly, intravenously or intrathecally (C).

Alfentanil is a synthetic piperidine opioid receptor agonist that is only delivered via the intravenous route (D).

Diclofenac is a non-steroidal anti-inflammatory drug that can be administered orally, intravenously, rectally or transdermally (E).

Commonly used transdermally applied drugs include:

- Fentanyl
- Buprenorphine
- Diclofenac
- EMLA (2.5% lidocaine, 2.5% prilocaine)
- Amethocaine

23. A True

   B True

   C False

D True

E True

The volume of distribution (*V*d) is the theoretical volume in which a drug would have to disperse in order to achieve observed plasma concentrations (E). Because it is only a theoretical volume, it may potentially be larger than total body water. Highly protein bound drugs also have a high volume of distribution, while highly polar or charged drugs do not cross membranes easily and stay within the central compartment, leading to small volumes of distribution (D).

The *V*d of fentanyl is 4.0 L/kg, while that of morphine is 3.5 L/kg, reflecting its lipid solubility that is 600 times greater than that of morphine (A).

As propofol is highly lipid soluble, it has a volume of distribution of 4 L/kg, which is greater than total body water (B).

Non-depolarising neuromuscular blocking drugs all have volumes of distribution of <0.30 L/kg because they are highly polar drugs (C).

24. **A** False

    B False

    C True

    D True

    E True

Diclofenac is significantly metabolised in the liver by phase I and II metabolism, while exogenous epinephrine (adrenaline) is metabolised in the liver by catechol-*O*-methyl transferase to metadrenaline and metnoradrenaline (A, B).

Lithium, ephedrine and digoxin are all renally excreted without undergoing a significant degree of metabolism (C, D, E).

The following drugs are excreted predominantly unchanged in the urine and can be remembered by the mnemonic **ACED LMNOP G**:

Aminoglycosides

Cephalosporins

Ephedrine

Digoxin

Lithium

Milrinone/Mannitol

Neostigmine

Oxytetracycline

Penicillins

Drugs that are excreted unchanged in the urine are likely to need dose adjustment in renal failure.

25. A True

    B False

    C False

    D True

    E True

The ideal intravenous anaesthetic agent would have the following properties:

- High lipid solubility (A)
- Water-soluble formulation (B)
- Short half-life (C)
- Analgesic properties at low doses (D)
- Pre-prepared solution (E)
- Rapid recovery, with no accumulation after infusion
- Minimal cardiovascular and respiratory depression
- Antiemetic properties
- Painless on injection
- No interaction with other drugs
- No histamine release
- Long shelf life at room temperature
- No histamine release
- No hypersensitivity reactions

26. A False

    B False

    C True

    D False

    E True

Thiopentone is the sulphur analogue of the oxybarbiturate pentobarbitone. It is formulated as a sodium salt, sodium thiopentone and appears as a yellow powder in a glass vial (A).

Sodium thiopentone is a weak acid with a pKa value of 7.6. When dissolved in water, it forms an alkaline solution (B).

The free acid that is formed in solution is highly insoluble and would precipitate out of solution. To prevent the formation of the free acid, sodium thiopentone is stored in glass vials containing nitrogen, while sodium carbonate is added to react with water to produce hydroxide ions (C). This forms an alkaline solution, thus preventing the accumulation of hydrogen ions and therefore the undissociated acid.

At physiological pH, only 12% of the administered sodium thiopentone is actually available in the active form, which is non-protein bound and unionised (D). The rapid onset is due to the high lipid solubility of the drug and the fact that the brain receives a relatively large blood flow. Emergence after a single bolus dose is due to rapid redistribution into well-perfused tissues such as the liver followed by the skin and muscle.

Sodium thiopentone may precipitate an acute porphyric crisis and is absolutely contraindicated in patients suffering from porphyria (E).

27. A False

B True

C False

D False

E True

Xenon is a non-toxic inert odourless gas, making up only 0.0000087% of the atmosphere and is produced by the fractional distillation of air (A, B).

It does not alter myocardial contractility and may cause a small reduction in heart rate and hence cardiac output (C). Xenon does not sensitise the myocardium to catecholamines.

Xenon has a minimum alveolar concentration of 71% and has a very low blood:gas partition coefficient of 0.14, as a result its onset and offset of action are faster than desflurane, sevoflurane and nitrous oxide (D).

Xenon is three times denser and nearly twice as viscous as nitrous oxide, although the Fink effect of diffusion hypoxia is not a feature of xenon (E).

Xenon has a molecular weight of 131.2, a boiling point of –108°C, is non-flammable and does not support combustion. It undergoes virtually no metabolism in the body.

28. A False

B False

C True

D True

E True

Tolerance occurs when larger doses of a drug are required to achieve a given response, often due to altered receptor sensitivity such as in chronic opioid use (A).

Tachyphylaxis, however, is the reversible, acute decrease in response to a given dose of drug after repeated administration and is synonymous with desensitisation, which takes place over a longer period of time (B, E). The underlying mechanisms include:

- Change in receptor structure (D)
- Loss of receptors
- Reduction in mediators
- Increased breakdown of drug
- Physiological adaptation

Examples include ephedrine and amphetamine depleting amine stores (C).

29. A False

    B False

    C True

    D True

    E False

Local anaesthetics can be classified as esters or amides depending on the intermediate chains (see **Figure 1.5**). Esters contain the —CO.O— linkage and undergo hydrolysis in the plasma. They include amethocaine, cocaine and procaine (C, D). Amides contain the amide (—NH.CO—) linkage chain and undergo hepatic metabolism. All amides contain an 'i' followed by the suffix 'caine', including bupivacaine, etidocaine, lignocaine, prilocaine and ropivacaine (A, B, E).

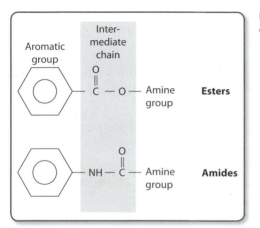

Figure 1.5 Chemical structure of ester and amide classes of local anaesthetic.

30. A False

    B True

    C False

    D False

    E True

Systemic absorption of local anaesthetics is greater than epidural administration when given via the caudal injection or intercostal injection (B, E). Systemic concentrations are lowest when administered subcutaneously, to plexuses or to large distal nerves (see **Figure 1.6**).

Systemic vascular absorption is dependent on:

- Local anaesthetic characteristics
- Use of vasoconstrictor
- Location of injection

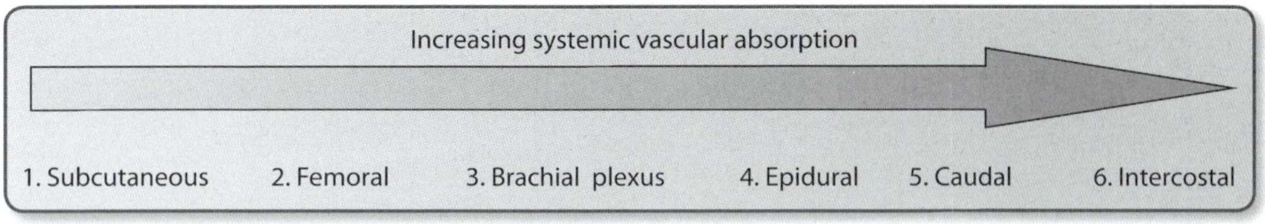

Increasing systemic vascular absorption

1. Subcutaneous   2. Femoral   3. Brachial plexus   4. Epidural   5. Caudal   6. Intercostal

Figure 1.6 Systemic absorption of local anaesthetics.

31. A True

 B True

 C True

 D False

 E True

Most local anaesthetic agents, including prilocaine and lidocaine, cause vasodilatation at low concentrations with vasoconstriction at higher concentrations (A, E). Cocaine however is a pure vasoconstrictor. Bendroflumethiazide has an antihypertensive effect by inhibiting Na^+/Cl^- co-transport in the distal convoluted tubule, leading to a diuresis, but also exerts a direct vasodilator effect (B).

Diazoxide is structurally similar to bendroflumethiazide and acts as a vasodilator by modulating cyclic adenosine monophosphate levels in arteriolar smooth muscle cells (C).

Tramadol has no significant vascular effects when administered via the intravenous route (D).

32. A True

 B True

 C True

 D True

 E False

Antiarrhythmic drugs can be categorised according to the cardiac tissue that they affect (see **Table 1.6**) (A). This may be useful when specific arrhythmias need to be treated.

The Vaughan Williams classification is based on the electrophysiological action on isolated cardiac fibres (B). There are four classes in this classification, more recently a 5th class has been added, as shown in **Table 1.7**.

Some drugs have more than one action and can belong to more than one class, but they all have a dominant effect that allows them to be classed accordingly (C).

Class I antiarrhthymic drugs have local anaesthetic properties that exhibit membrane stabilising activity and affect conduction, refractoriness and the action potential (D). They are further subdivided into Ia, Ib and Ic, but they all slow phase 0 of the action potential to different degrees. Class Ic has the most potent

Table 1.6 Site of action of antiarrhythmic agents

Site of action	Drugs
Sinuatrial node	Beta-blockers
	Class IV drugs
	Digoxin
Atrioventricular node	Class Ic and IV drugs
	Beta-blockers
	Digoxin
	Adenosine
Ventricles	Class I and III drugs
Atria	Class Ia and Ic drugs
	Beta-blockers
	Class III drugs
Accessory pathways	Class Ia and III drugs

Table 1.7 The modified Vaughan Williams classification

Class	Mechanism of action	Drugs
I a	Block Na^+ channels, prolong refractory period	Disopyramide, procainamide, quinidine
I b	Block Na^+ channels, shorten refractory period	Lidocaine, mexiletine, phenytoin
I c	Block Na^+ channels, no effect on refractory period	Flecainide, propafenone
II	β-adrenoceptor blockade	Atenolol, propranolol
III	K^+ channel blockade	Amiodarone, bretylium, sotalol
IV	Ca^{2+} channel blockade	Diltiazem, verapamil
V*	Miscellaneous	Adenosine (E), digoxin, magnesium sulphate

*Antiarrhythmic agents that do not fit into any of the original classes described by Vaughan Williams in 1970 were later classified into class V.

sodium channel blocking action; therefore, it leads to reduction in phase 0 rapid depolarisation. The weakest sodium channel effects, thus the least effect on phase 0, are from class Ib drugs such as lidocaine.

33. **A** False

   B True

   C True

   D False

   E False

Dobutamine is a synthetic analogue of dopamine and is a β-adrenoceptor-stimulating agent (A). Dopamine is a catecholamine-like agent used for the treatment of severe heart failure and cardiogenic shock.

Dopamine is the precursor of noradrenaline and releases noradrenaline from stores in the nerve endings in the heart (B). The conversion of dopamine to noradrenaline occurs in granulated vesicles and is dependent on the enzyme dopamine β-hydroxylase.

Dobutamine is a derivative of isoprenaline with predominantly β_1-adrenoceptor activity, thus making it a potent inotrope. It does, however, also have β_2-stimulating effect, which causes peripheral vasodilatation. This may result in hypotension and a fall in the diastolic pressure with a reflex tachycardia (C).

Dobutamine acts on adrenergic receptors in the following order: $\beta_1 > \beta_2 > \alpha$. It has no action on dopaminergic receptors (D).

Dopamine stimulates the heart by both β- and α-adrenergic responses and causes vasodilatation through its action on dopaminergic receptors. At high doses (>10 μg/kg/min), dopamine causes predominant α-adrenoceptor stimulation with peripheral vasoconstriction, increased peripheral vascular resistance and reduced renal blood flow (E).

34. **A** True

    B True

    C False

    D False

    E False

In preference to small coronary arteries, nitrates dilate the large coronary arteries and arterioles with diameters >100 μm (A).

Nitrates redistribute blood flow along collateral channels and from epicardial to endocardial regions (B). They also relieve coronary spasm and dynamic stenosis, especially at epicardial sites, including the coronary arterial constriction induced by exercise.

Nitrates increase the venous capacitance, causing pooling of blood in the peripheral veins and thereby reducing venous return and ventricular volume. There is less mechanical stress on the myocardial wall and the myocardial oxygen demand is reduced. In addition to this, there is a fall in aortic systolic pressure, which further reduces myocardial oxygen demand (C).

The basic mechanism of nitrates (NO_3^-) is conversion to nitrites (NO_2^-) followed by enzyme-mediated release of unstable nitric oxide (NO). For some vasoactive agents an intact vascular endothelium is required, but nitrates vasodilate whether or not the endothelium is physically intact or functional (D). The NO produced then stimulates the enzyme guanylate cyclase to produce cyclic guanosine monophosphate (cyclic GMP). This reduces the levels of calcium in the vascular monocyte and therefore vasodilatation occurs. Nitrates are better venous than arteriolar dilators (E).

35. A False

 B True

 C False

 D False

 E False

Suxamethonium is a depolarising muscle relaxant. It is hydrolysed by plasma cholinesterase to choline and succinylmonocholine, leaving only 20% to reach the neuromuscular junction (A). Succinylmonocholine is a weakly active ester of succinic acid with choline (B). Because of the rapid metabolism of suxamethonium, only 10% is excreted via the kidneys in the urine (C).

It produces a 'phase I' block in which there is a train-of-four ratio of >0.7, no fade to a 1 Hz stimulus with no post-tetanic facilitation. Repeated administration may produce a 'phase II' block similar to that of non-depolarising muscle relaxants, demonstrating a reduced train-of-four ratio of <0.7, fade on 1 Hz stimulation and post-tetanic facilitation present (D).

Suxamethonium has a structure of two acetylcholine molecules joined through acetyl groups (E). By binding to nicotinic acetylcholine receptors, suxamethonium depolarises the membrane; however, due to the lack of plasma cholinesterase at the neuromuscular junction, it remains attached to the acetylcholine receptors thereby preventing any further activation, and thus causing neuromuscular blockade.

36. A True

 B False

 C False

 D False

 E False

The aminosteroid neuromuscular blocking drugs are large, bulky, polar molecules containing a steroid ring. They can be monoquaternary (containing a single N^+—CH_3 group) such as vecuronium and rocuronium, or bisquaternary (containing two N^+—CH_3 groups) such as pancuronium. Of note, pancuronium is the bisquaternary analogue of vecuronium thereby making it more potent (A, B). Mivacurium is a benzylisoquinolinium, along with atracurium and *cis*-atracurium, while tubocurarine is a monoquaternary alkaloid (C, D, E).

37. A True

 B True

 C False

 D False

 E False

Non-steroidal anti-inflammatory drugs (NSAIDs) are a group of diverse drugs with variable analgesic, antipyretic and anti-inflammatory properties. The extent and effect of common NSAIDs can be seen in **Table 1.8**.

Table 1.8 Features of non-steroidal anti-inflammatory drugs

Drugs	Plasma protein binding (%)	Analgesic and antipyretic action	Anti-inflammatory action
Aspirin	85	+++	++
Diclofenac	99	+	+++
Ibuprofen	99	+	+
Ketorolac	99	++	+
Paracetamol	10	+++	++

Thus, paracetamol has moderate anti-inflammatory properties, while aspirin has significant antipyretic action (A, B). Most NSAIDs are highly protein bound except paracetamol that is only 10% protein bound (C, D). Ibuprofen is an equipotent analgesic and anti-inflammatory agent (E).

38. A True

B False

C False

D True

E True

Morphine is a naturally occurring opiate with a phenanthrene structure comprising three fused benzene rings (A). It causes constriction of the gut sphincters and spastic immobility of the bowel, resulting in constipation. It also causes contraction of the sphincter of Oddi, causing an increase in the intraluminal pressure within the biliary tree (B).

Morphine stimulates the chemoreceptor trigger zone via 5-HT$_3$ and dopaminergic receptors. This explains the nausea-inducing effect of morphine (C). Muscarinic receptors are not activated by morphine to cause nausea and vomiting.

Morphine and other opioids can cause chest wall rigidity (D). This is thought to be as a result of dopaminergic and GABA pathways in the substantia nigra interacting with the opioid receptors.

Morphine inhibits the release of adrenocorticotropic hormone, prolactin and gonadotrophic hormones (E). It may also increase the secretion of vasopressin (antidiuretic hormone, ADH) that can cause water retention and hyponatraemia.

39. A True

B False

C True

D False

E False

Benzodiazepines are hypnotic drugs that act on the α-subunit of GABA$_A$ receptors to open the ligand-gated chloride (Cl$^-$) channel causing hyperpolarisation of post-synaptic neuronal membranes predominantly (A). They therefore do not act via second messenger systems (B). Baclofen, however, acts via metabotropic GABA$_B$ receptors, activating second messenger systems.

Benzodiazepines are generally highly protein bound and usually have active metabolites; however, lorazepam is glucuronated to inactive metabolites (C, D).

Zopiclone, along with zolpidem and zaleplon, is non-benzodiazepine 'Z-drug' that lacks the benzodiazepine chemical structure but binds to GABA$_A$ receptors in a similar fashion (E).

40. A False

B False

C False

D True

E True

The biochemical effects of furosemide include hyponatraemia, hypokalaemia, hypochloraemic alkalosis, hypomagnesaemia and hyperuricaemia. These effects are also caused by the thiazide diuretics, but furosemide can also cause hypocalcaemia by increasing Ca^{2+} excretion (A).

Bendroflumethiazide causes hypercalcaemia as a result of reduced renal excretion (B).

Spironolactone is a competitive aldosterone antagonist; therefore, it not only reduces the excretion of K$^+$ but also increases the excretion of Na$^+$ and water. As a result of its action, it is used to treat ascites, Conn's syndrome (primary hyperaldosteronism) and nephrotic syndrome (C).

Mannitol is administered as an intravenous infusion and is usually given as a loading dose followed by an infusion. The loading dose for the treatment of raised intracranial pressure is about 1 g/kg, followed by an infusion of between 0.1 and 0.2 g/kg. As a result of these large infusion volumes, the initial circulating volume is increased which increases the preload and cardiac output (D).

The haematological effects of bendroflumethiazide include haemolytic anaemia, aplastic anaemia, leucopaenia, thrombocytopaenia and agranulocytosis (see **Table 4.8**) (E).

41. A False

B False

C True

D False

E True

Electricity is the flow of electrons from one atom to another under the influence of a potential difference or under the influence of a changing magnetic field (A).

The electrons in a conductor are loosely bound; therefore, they can readily move when influenced by a potential difference. Bodily fluids are good conductors as they contain positive and negative ions, and these can move when a potential difference is applied to them, thereby conducting electricity (B).

The electrons in insulators are firmly bound to their atoms; therefore, they do not conduct electricity; thermistors are semiconductors (C, D).

The outer electrons in semiconductors are more firmly bound to their atoms than in conductors, but less firmly bound than in insulators. Diodes and transistors are semiconductors (E).

42. **A** False

    B False

    C True

    D True

    E False

Surgical diathermy typically uses high-frequency currents in the region of 1 MHz (A).

The passage of lower frequency currents through the body can cause muscular contractions and ventricular fibrillation. The lower frequency of alternating current or the use of direct current is more likely to cause ventricular fibrillation than using high-frequency diathermy currents (B).

When using monopolar diathermy two connections are made to the patient: one is the patient plate (or neutral plate) and the other is the active (or cutting) electrode. When using bipolar diathermy, two connections are also made, but this is through the two ends of the forceps; a diathermy plate is not required (C).

Isolating capacitors are placed within the diathermy apparatus to increase safety of the equipment and reduce the risk of accidental burns to the patient in the event of the diathermy pad becoming detached (D).

Bipolar diathermy uses lower power than monopolar diathermy (E).

43. **A** False

    B True

    C True

    D False

    E False

MRI does not involve the use of ionising radiation (A). There is little evidence of serious adverse effects as a result of the magnetic field. Various recommendations exist, but generally continuous exposure should be limited to a magnetic flux density of 0.2 T and short exposures to 5 T.

If the magnetic field gradient is switched, then eddy currents can be induced and this has the potential of inducing small currents in any biological conductors, especially nerve fibres, which can cause involuntary muscle contraction (B). There is also a small risk of causing breathing difficulties and inducing ventricular fibrillation as a result of these eddy currents.

In the presence of very strong fields, patients may experience flashing lights and various taste sensations (C).

Joint and dental prostheses are safe as they are usually non-ferromagnetic and are firmly fixed in the patient, thus cannot be dislodged by the magnetic field of the scanner (D). They may however distort MRI images.

Ferromagnetic objects are attracted to the scanner even in the fringe field, which can extend for a few metres (E).

44. A True

   B False

   C True

   D False

   E False

Boyle's law is the first perfect gas law. If, at a constant temperature, the volume (V) of a gas is decreased, then the pressure (P) will increase by the same proportion (A). This principle can be used to calculate the volume of gas remaining in a cylinder when the pressure on the pressure gauge is known.

The second perfect gas law is Charles's law or Gay Lussac's law (B). This states that at a constant pressure the volume of a given mass of gas varies directly with the absolute temperature (T) (C). The third perfect gas law states that at a constant volume the absolute pressure of a given mass of gas varies directly with the absolute temperature. Combining the three perfect gas laws gives us the formula:

$$\frac{P \times V}{T} = \text{constant}$$

The perfect gas laws are usually corrected to a standard temperature of 273.15 K (0°C) and a standard pressure of 101 kPa (760 mmHg) (D). This is because gases are affected by temperature and pressure.

Dalton's law of partial pressures is not one of the perfect gas laws but refers to a mixture of gasses within a container (E). It states that in a mixture of gases the pressure exerted by each gas is the same as that which it would exert if it alone were occupying the container.

45. A False

   B False

   C True

   D True

   E False

Power is the rate of work, or the amount of work performed over time (A). It is measured in watts (W) with one watt equalling one joule (J) per second(s): $1 W = 1 J/s$ (B).

Energy is always expended and work is done when the point of application of a force moves in the direction of the force (C). It is measured in joules, the energy expended when applying a force of one newton (N) through a distance of one metre (m).

The area under a pressure/volume curve for ventilation is the work done. If power is the rate of work done, then the power of breathing can be calculated by dividing the work done (the area under the curve) by the time (D).

There are various energy changes that take place during the respiratory cycle. It must be remembered that energy cannot be created or lost, but it is converted from one form to another. So, most of the chemical energy generated by the respiratory muscles is converted to heat energy, with only a small proportion converted to mechanical energy (E).

46. A False

   B True

   C False

   D False

   E False

Humidity is the amount of water vapour present in gas, and it may be expressed in many ways. Absolute humidity is the mass of water vapour present in a volume of gas and is expressed in milligrams of water per litre of gas. Relative humidity is the amount of water vapour at a particular temperature, and this is expressed as a percentage of the amount that would be held if the gas were fully saturated (A).

Humidity may also be expressed as the pressure exerted by water vapour in a gas mixture (B).

If gas saturated with water vapour is cooled, then it will condense out water vapour. The amount of condensed water vapour will be the amount held at the original temperature minus the amount it can hold at the new lower temperature. The absolute humidity will therefore fall, but the relative humidity remains at 100% (D).

The hair hygrometer is one method used to measure relative humidity, and it operates on the principle that hair length increases if the humidity increases (C).

The wet and dry bulb hygrometer allows the measurement of the ambient humidity, while relative humidity is obtained from a set of tables and is not directly measured (E).

47. A False

B False

C False

D True

E True

Heat is the energy that can be transferred from a hotter object to a cooler object down this temperature gradient (A).

The SI unit for temperature is the Kelvin (K) and not Celsius (B).

Temperature is a measure of the tendency of an object to gain or lose heat (C).

Absolute zero is the zero reference point on this scale and 0 K is equivalent to −273°C (D).

The triple point of water is the temperature at which it exists as a solid, liquid and gas simultaneously. This is at 273.16 K or 0.01°C (E).

48. A True

B True

C True

D False

E False

Latent heat is the heat absorbed or released when a substance changes its state at a constant temperature. As liquid ethyl chloride vapourises from the skin surface, it requires the latent heat of vapourisation to do so, which is gained from the skin. This results in cooling of the skin as heat is taken away from its surface (A).

Within glass ampoules ethyl chloride is stored under pressure as a liquid to ensure it does not vapourise until it has left the ampoule and contacts skin (B).

When volatile anaesthetics are vapourised, they lose latent heat and the vapourised liquid takes heat from the remaining fluid as well as the vapouriser. This can cause a fall in temperature of the remaining volatile anaesthetic, which makes them less volatile (C).

Nitrous oxide, carbon dioxide and oxygen may all be stored in liquid form when in cylinders, oxygen being a liquid in the vacuum-insulated evaporator (D).

As nitrous oxide is emptied from a cylinder, the liquid form is converted to gas which requires latent heat of vapourisation. This is taken from the remaining liquid and cylinder walls, which cools and may cause the water vapour in the air to condense outside the cylinder. Because of this cooling, there is a rapid fall in vapour pressure inside the cylinder, which is indicated on the pressure gauge (E).

49. A False

  B True

  C True

  D False

  E True

Fluids are any form of matter that change shape under shear forces and can either be liquids or gases (A).

The flow of fluids can be described either as laminar or turbulent. Laminar flow is flow in layers, or laminae, of fluid running parallel to each other. In a pipe, the layers nearest to the wall will have the lowest velocity, and the layer closest to the wall will probably have no flow (B). The velocity profile across the pipe during laminar flow is parabolic, with the highest flow in the centre. The peak velocity in the centre is twice the average across the pipe at equilibrium (C). There is minimum energy loss during laminar flow.

During turbulent flow, eddies, vortices and currents are developed which result in energy loss in the form of heat, friction and noise (E). The driving pressure required for turbulent flow is greater than that required for an equivalent laminar flow rate (D).

50. A True

  B True

  C False

  D True

  E False

Ultrasound is mechanical energy in the form of high-frequency vibrations (A).

It is generated by electrically deforming a piezoelectric crystal, which causes it to compress and decompress the medium to which the crystal is coupled (B). The wavelength is the distance occupied by one oscillation when seen graphically.

The changes in pressure created by the crystal travel through the medium; the distance between the points of maximum pressure is also the wavelength. The frequency is not dependent on the compression pressures; in fact it is the wavelength that is dependent on the compression pressures (C). The wavelength of ultrasound is generally the reciprocal of the frequency (D). The wave is propagated by the movement of particles; therefore, it is unable to travel through a vacuum (E).

51. A False

  B False

  C True

  D False

  E False

Under single-fault conditions, type 1 CF equipment should have leakage currents under 50 µA (A).

Type BF equipment is floating, and may be either class I, II or III, thus is not, by definition, earthed (B).

Safety classification of equipment can be based on either:

- The means of protection it provides
  - Class I – any accessible conducting part of the equipment is connected to an earth wire. Live, neutral and earth wires never come in contact with each other
  - Class II – also called 'double-insulated' as all accessible parts have two layers of insulation. Power cables only contain 'live' and 'neutral' conductors with a single fuse (C)
  - Class III – the equipment does not need electrical supply >50 V DC or 24 V AC; called 'safety extra-low voltage' (SELV) and still provides a theoretical risk of microshock (D)
- The maximum leakage currents permissible
  - Type B – safe for external patient connection. Under single-fault conditions, equipment has leakage currents of 500 mA if class I or 100 mA if class II
  - Type BF – like type B, but the part connected to the patient is isolated (floating)
  - Type CF – safe for direct connection to the heart with isolated circuits. Leakage currents must be under 50 mA if class I or 10 mA if class II. Includes electrocardiogram leads and pressure transducers

Current-operated earth leakage circuit breakers (COELCB) consist of a live wire and a neutral wire attached to a relay circuit breaker. Faulty currents (e.g. high leakage current) lead to a magnetic field between the live and neutral wires that induce the relay to break the circuit. There is no fuse in COELCBs (E).

52. **A** False

   B False

   C True

   D False

   E True

Nitrous oxide is stored in cylinders with French blue bodies and shoulders; Entonox is stored in cylinders with white and blue quartered shoulders (A). With a boiling point of −88°C and a critical temperature of 36.5°C, nitrous oxide exists as a liquid in cylinders with a vapour layer above.

It is stored at a pressure of 4400 kPa (44 bar), which decreases slowly until all the liquid is utilised with only vapour remaining at which point the pressure decreases rapidly (B). The slow decrease in cylinder pressures is due to the latent heat of vapourisation cooling the cylinder, thereby reducing the vapour pressure. Thus, cylinder pressures do not decrease in a linear fashion (D).

If nitrous oxide cylinders were full of liquid, then increasing temperature would risk the expansion of liquid, thus creating the risk of potential explosion. Therefore, the mass of gas in a cylinder divided by the mass of water required to fill that cylinder is termed the 'filling ratio', and in the UK the filling ratio is 0.75 (C).

Size E cylinders are attached directly to the anaesthetic machine and have a capacity of 1800 L, while size J cylinders are used in cylinder manifold and hold 18,000 L of nitrous oxide (E).

53. A False

   B False

   C True

   D True

   E True

A vacuum-insulated evaporator supplies oxygen to piped gas supplies in hospitals. It is composed of a double-insulated steel tank with a vacuum to maintain internal temperatures. Oxygen is stored as a liquid at −160°C which is below its critical temperature of −118°C, with an internal pressure of approximately 7 bar (700 kPa), not 400 kPa (A, B).

Up to 1500 L of liquid oxygen may be stored and the mass of the liquid can be measured either by weighing the vessel or by differential pressure gauges comparing pressures at the liquid bottom and vapour top of the cylinder (C).

When oxygen evaporates, the temperature of the vessel reduces due to the latent heat of vapourisation, further contributing to the maintenance of a low temperature. However, with reduced use of oxygen, the contribution of latent heat of vapourisation is reduced, therefore temperatures rise (D). With a rise in temperature, the internal pressure rises, and when this exceeds 17 bar, a safety valve opens allowing escape of vapourised oxygen (E). This leads to a further vapourisation, and thus a desired reduction in the temperature once again.

54. A True

   B True

   C False

   D False

   E True

Rotameter is the trade name of flowmeters that are constant-pressure, variable orifice devices composed of a conical tube that is wider at the top and a bobbin that varies in height depending on the flow rates. Opening of a needle valve at the bottom of the flowmeter allows gas into the tube, with higher flow rates allowing the bobbin to float higher within the tube. As the bobbin is of fixed dimensions, the distance between the bobbin and the wall of the tube increases as flow increases (see **Figure 1.7**). Thus, at low flow rates, the orifice is narrow and long allowing laminar flow depending on gas *viscosity*, while at higher flow rates the orifice is wider and flow is turbulent depending on gas *density* (A, B).

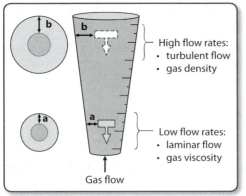

Figure 1.7 Rotameter.

High flow rates:
• turbulent flow
• gas density

Low flow rates:
• laminar flow
• gas viscosity

Gas flow

Flowmeters are 2.5% accurate but are only calibrated for the individual gases they are to be used for (C). Accuracy can be reduced by dirt within the flowmeter tubes, static electricity build-up (up to 35% inaccurate) and back pressure from the common gas outlet of up to 10% (E). Flowmeters have no effect on piped gas pressures (D).

55. A True

   B False

   C False

   D True

   E True

The emergency oxygen flush is designed to provide 100% oxygen flow that bypasses flowmeters and vapourisers at piped gas pressures of 4 bar (400 kPa) and flow rates of 35–75 L/min to the common gas outlet (A, B, E). Because it bypasses both flowmeters and vapourisers, it may therefore dilute anaesthetic gases potentially leading to awareness (D). It is a non-locking device that does not have any pressure reducing or regulating valves; therefore, the delivered pressure of 4 bar may potentially lead to barotrauma (C).

56. A False

   B True

   C False

   D False

   E False

In 1996, the Health and Safety Commission issued maximally accepted 8-hour time-weighted average concentrations for the UK:

• Enflurane: 50 particles per million (ppm) (B)
• Halothane: 10 ppm (C)
• Isoflurane: 50 ppm (D)
• Nitrous oxide: 100 ppm (E)

These levels vary in different countries. No definite acceptable level was set for desflurane at the time of publication (A).

57. **A** False

B False

C True

D False

E True

The Lack system is a coaxial version of the Mapleson A (Magill) breathing system that can also be in a parallel arrangement (A, C). It consists of a 14 mm inner tube attached to an adjustable pressure-limiting valve for exhaled gases and a 30 mm outer tube supplying the fresh gas flow (E).

It is efficient for spontaneously ventilating patients, requiring 70 mL/kg/min fresh gas flow, but is inefficient for controlled ventilation requiring a fresh gas flow rate of two to three times the minute ventilation (B, D). The most efficient Mapleson breathing system for controlled ventilation is the Mapleson D system, or Bain circuit.

58. **A** True

B True

C False

D True

E False

The electrocardiogram is a device monitoring cardiac electrical activity using silver/silver chloride gel covered electrodes at specific sites on the skin. At the cardiac level, electrical potentials in the range of 90 mV are generated, but this signal is reduced as it passes through tissues, leaving a signal output of 1–2 mV (A). The initial signal is increased by a differential amplifier that may be set at a monitoring mode (frequency of 0.5–40 Hz) or diagnostic mode (frequency of 0.05–100 Hz) (C). The differential amplifier minimises noise and signal interference using the principles of common mode rejection, whereby interference that is the same between two leads is eliminated. The signal output is displayed via an oscilloscope or on paper running at 25 mm/s with a signal of 1 mV/cm (D).

There are six bipolar leads: I, II, III, aVR, aVL and aVF (note that 'aV' stands for 'augmented voltage') and there are six unipolar leads: V1–V6 (B). In anaesthetic practice, the configurations of three skin electrodes used include:

- Lead II: right arm, left arm and indifferent electrodes; arrhythmia detection
- CM5: right arm electrode on manubrium, left arm electrode on the 5th intercostal space, anterior axillary line and the indifferent electrode is on the left shoulder; sensitive for detecting ischaemia (E)
- CB5: right arm electrode on right scapula, left arm electrode on the 5th intercostal space, anterior axillary line and the indifferent electrode is on the left shoulder; used in thoracic anaesthesia

59. A True

B True

C False

D False

E False

The null hypothesis (H_0) states that no difference exists between two sample groups. The null hypothesis must be set prior to conducting any clinical trial, and if a difference between the two samples is detected, the null hypothesis must be rejected. It is liable to sources of error and two outcomes of error are possible: Type I or type II errors.

A type I error is also known as an α-error or a false positive. A difference is found when one does not truly exist causing incorrect rejection of the null hypothesis (A). It is most commonly due to a high p-value or a small sample size.

A type II error is also known as a β-error or a false negative (B). No difference is found when one does indeed exist causing incorrect acceptance of the null hypothesis. It is most commonly due to small sample sizes.

The power of a study should be calculated prior to conducting the study as it indicates what sample size is required (C). The power measures the probability of a difference being detected when one exists and is calculated as $1 - \beta$. A power of 80% or above (i.e. $\beta < 20\%$) is sufficient for a study to be adequately powered (D).

Standard deviation (SD) is a measure of spread around central tendency of data:

$$SD = \sqrt{\frac{\Sigma(\bar{x} - x)^2}{n-1}}$$

where Σ is the sum of the difference of each value (x) from the mean ($\bar{x}$) divided by the number of values (n). The mean ± 1 SD should include 68% of data points, ± 2 SD include 96% of all data points and ± 3 SD include 99% of all data points.

Variance (SD^2) is thus calculated by (E):

$$\text{Variance} = \frac{\Sigma(\bar{x} - x)^2}{n-1}$$

60. A True

B True

C False

D True

E True

Differential pressure transducers work by detecting a difference in pressure between two sides of a given sensor. Although many devices utilise this principle, it may be argued that all devices measuring pressure are differential pressure transducers, giving the difference between atmospheric pressure and device pressure. The overall design is one that compares a measurement sample with a reference sample to give a pressure difference, which can be analysed and interpreted (see **Figure 1.8**).

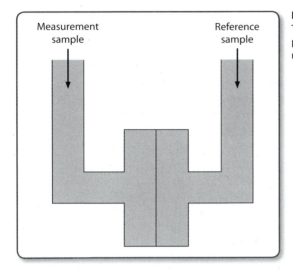

Figure 1.8 Differential pressure transducer. The transducer detects the difference in pressures between measurement and reference samples.

The vacuum-insulated evaporator uses a differential pressure transducer between the top and bottom of the cylinder to calculate the mass of liquid oxygen remaining within the vessel (A).

Paramagnetic analysers are rendered particularly accurate using the principles of differential pressure (B). A reference gas of 21% oxygen is compared with a measured gas with a set concentration of oxygen. When exposed to a magnetic field, the paramagnetic properties of oxygen cause it to be attracted to the field, leading to a difference in pressure between both chambers that is proportional to the partial pressure of oxygen.

End-tidal carbon dioxide analysers do not incorporate differential pressure transducers in their design (C).

Tec 6 desflurane vapourisers contain a differential pressure transducer between the fresh gas flow channel and the vapourising channel, which is then interpreted and electronically alters the gas flow accordingly (D).

Pneumotachographs can be designed in a number of ways, one which uses the Pitot tube design. One tube faces the direction of gas flow, while the other faces the opposite direction, being the reference tube. The pressure difference between the two tubes is proportional to the flow rate squared (E).

Answers: SBAs

61. B End-tidal CO_2 of 0.4 kPa

In a cardiac arrest, there is no cardiac output, therefore no perfusion of the lungs. This is an extreme form of dead space involving both lungs. Although arterial CO_2 might be elevated, the end-tidal CO_2 will be low if there is effective cardiopulmonary resuscitation (CPR) or zero if there is ineffective CPR. Asystolic patients will have no blood pressure and are more than likely going to have a metabolic and/or respiratory acidosis; therefore, the bicarbonate is likely to be low. Elevated serum potassium may cause cardiac arrest, but this is not necessarily true.

Weil MH, Bisera J, Trevino RP, Racklow EC. Cardiac output and end-tidal carbon dioxide. Crit Care Med 1985; 13:907–909.

62. A The patient may have pulmonary oedema

Compliance (C) is defined as the change in volume (ΔV) per unit change in pressure (ΔP) and it reflects the elastic recoil of an organ:

$$C = \Delta V/\Delta P.$$

In the lung, ΔP is the difference in pressure between alveolar pressure measured at the mouth when there is no gas flow and intrapleural pressure measured by a balloon in the lower third of the oesophagus. Normal lung compliance (C_{lung}) is 150–200 mL/cmH$_2$O (1.5–2.0 L/kPa). Chest wall compliance (C_{chest}) is normally 200 mL/cmH$_2$O (2.0 L/kPa), where ΔP is the difference between alveolar pressure and intrapleural pressure. Total thoracic compliance (C_{total}) is 85–100 mL/cmH$_2$O (0.85–1 L/kPa) and is related to both C_{lung} and C_{chest}:

$$1/C_{total} = 1/C_{chest} + 1/C_{lung}.$$

Repeated pressure and volume readings can be plotted on a pressure/volume loop that is approximately linear during normal tidal volume breathing. However, the curves demonstrate *hysteresis*, meaning that the inflation and deflation curves are different (see **Figure 1.9**). This is because of the need to initially overcome surface tension upon inflation or inspiration.

Lung compliance can be either static or dynamic. Static compliance refers to the stiffness of the lung and chest wall, i.e. alveolar stretchability and is measured when there is no gas flow. Dynamic compliance is related to airway resistance during equilibration of gases at end-inspiration or end-expiration. Dynamic compliance is usually less than static compliance.

Because compliance is relative to body size, specific compliance is calculated as:

$$\text{Specific compliance} = C_{total}/\text{FRC}.$$

Pulmonary oedema increases lung compliance due to the interstitial oedema. However, asthma has been shown to reduce lung compliance, a pathology related

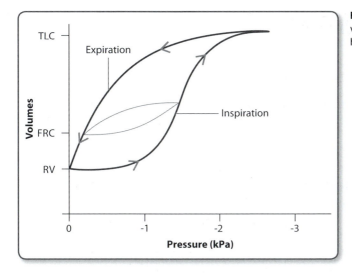

Figure 1.9 Lung pressure/volume loops demonstrating hysteresis.

to a loss of elastic recoil at total lung capacity and increased compliance of airways in spite of airway oedema. Emphysema also increases lung compliance, again due to loss of elastic recoil.

Compliance can be affected by the following factors (see Table 2.1):

- Increased compliance: surfactant, emphysema, old age, acute asthma (reason unclear)
- Reduced compliance: pulmonary fibrosis, pulmonary venous engorgement, pulmonary oedema, ARDS, pneumonia, neonates, extremes of lung volumes, chronic bronchitis (dynamic)

Wenzel S. Severe asthma in adults. Am J Respir Crit Care Med 2005; 172:149–160.
West JB. Respiratory physiology: the essentials, 9th edn. Baltimore: Lippincott Williams & Wilkins; 2012.

63. C Reducing $Paco_2$ from 5.8 to 4.2 kPa

There are a number of factors affecting intracranial pressure (ICP), and management of traumatic brain injury is aimed at reducing secondary injury. Target $Paco_2$ should be 4.5–5.0 kPa, with a reduction in cerebral blood flow of approximately 2–4% for each 0.13 kPa reduction in $Paco_2$. Avoidance of hypoxia is vital, but the ICP does not significantly increase above a Pao_2 of 6.7 kPa. Another management target is avoidance of hypotension and fluid restriction in the immediate phase that reduces mean arterial pressure (MAP), thereby reducing cerebral perfusion pressure (CPP): CPP = MAP – (ICP + CVP). Dexamethasone may reduce cerebral oedema secondary to tumours, but there is no evidence that it affects traumatic brain injury. There are a number of anaesthetic drugs that affect ICP (see **Table 1.9**).

Curry P, Viernes D, Sharma D. Perioperative management of traumatic brain injury. Int J Crit Illn Inj Sci 2011; 1:27–35.

Table 1.9 Anaesthetic drugs affecting intracranial pressure (ICP)	
Increased ICP	**Decreased ICP**
Ketamine	Barbiturates, etomidate, propofol
Volatile agents	Opioids
Suxamethonium (transient)	

64. B Adrenaline

This patient is in pulseless electrical activity (PEA) cardiac arrest. The Resuscitation Council (UK) published their latest guidelines in 2010 that modified the application of atropine in cardiac arrest situations. It is no longer recommended for use in PEA or asystolic cardiac arrests due to a poor evidence base. The first-line pharmacological therapy should be administration of 1 mg adrenaline via the intravenous or intraosseous routes.

Nolan J, Soar J, Lockey A. Advanced life support, 6th edn. London: Resuscitation Council; 2011.

65. E Tibial nerve

An ankle block may be performed to provide analgesia or anaesthesia for forefoot operations. It requires blockade of the deep and superficial peroneal nerves, sural nerve, saphenous nerve and tibial nerve. As the tibial nerve is the only one that has a motor component beyond the site of block, it is the only nerve that a nerve stimulator may identify. Stimulation of the tibial nerve leads to plantar flexing of the toes via contraction of the flexor digitorum longus and flexor hallucis longus. The tibial nerve also provides sensory supply to the medial aspect of the ankle and foot.

Kopka A, Serpell MG. Distal nerve blocks of the lower limb. Cont Educ Anaesth Crit Care Pain 2005; 5 (5): 166–170.

66. A Length of a nasal tube at the nares is 19 cm

Drug dosing and equipment calculation is an important aspect of preparation for paediatric anaesthesia. The important calculations for equipment and drug dosing are as follows:

Equipment

- Endotracheal tube internal diameter size = (Age/4) + 4
- Length of oral endotracheal tube at lips = (Age/2) + 12
- Length of nasal endotracheal tube at nares = (Age/2) + 15
- Laryngeal mask sizes as defined by **Table 1.10.**

Drug dosing: for details of drug dosing for paediatric anaesthesis see **Table 1.11.**

Therefore, this patient should have a size 6.0 mm endotracheal tube at 16 cm at the lips for an oral tube and 19 cm at the nares for a nasal endotracheal tube. The patient should have a size 2.5 or 3 laryngeal mask airway.

Table 1.10 Paediatric laryngeal mask airway (LMA) sizes

LMA size	Patient weight (kg)
1	<5
1.5	5–10
2	10–20
2.5	20–30
3	30–50

Table 1.11 Drug dosing for paediatric anaesthesia

Drug	Dose
Analgesics	
Paracetamol	15 mg/kg intravenous (7.5 mg/kg if weight is < 10 kg)
	40 mg/kg loading dose per rectum
	15 mg/kg every 4–6 hours
Ibuprofen	10 mg/kg
Diclofenac	1 mg/kg
Codeine	0.5 mg/kg
Fentanyl	1 µg/kg
Morphine	0.1–0.2 mg/kg
Antiemetics	
Dexamethasone	0.1–0.2 mg/kg
Ondansetron	0.1–0.2 mg/kg

Girgis, Sanders. The BADS Paediatric Dose Table. Journal of One-day Surgery 2004; 14:65–8.
South Thames Retrieval Service. Clinical Guidelines. http://www.strs.nhs.uk/educationandguidelines/
guidelines.aspx (Last accessed 01/10/2012).

67. B Succinylcholine

The clinical features described are in keeping with a diagnosis of anaphylaxis.
Anaphylaxis is an IgE-mediated type 1 hypersensitivity reaction caused under
anaesthesia by the substances shown in **Table 1.12**.

Thus, in this patient, it is most likely to be due to the use of succinylcholine during
rapid sequence induction. However, formal allergy testing would be mandatory.

Association of Anaesthetists of Great Britain and Ireland. Suspected anaphylactic reactions associated
with anaesthesia. Anaesthesia 2009; 64:199–211.

Table 1.12 Anaesthetic causes of anaphylaxis

Agent	Frequency (%)	Notes
Neuromuscular blocking drugs	60	Most commonly succinylcholine and rocuronium, rarely atracurium or mivacurium
Latex	20	Most commonly in atopic patients, healthcare workers, fruit allergy
Antibiotics	15	Penicillins and cephalosporins account for 70% of antibiotic-related anaphylaxis
Colloids	4	Most commonly to gelatins, rare with starches
Opioids	Uncommon	Usually due to histamine release
Local anaesthetics	Rare	May be related to preservatives
Anaesthetic agents	Very rare	Rare with propofol, very rare with thiopental, never reported with volatile agents

68. E Phrenic nerve palsy

An interscalene brachial plexus block is indicated for shoulder, humeral or elbow surgery. It may be performed using the landmark technique in the interscalene groove at the level of C6, ultrasound guidance or a nerve stimulator eliciting deltoid and biceps contraction.

Nearly 100% of patients have a phrenic nerve block; therefore, the block should only be performed unilaterally. Other complications include a stellate ganglion block causing Horner's syndrome in up to 25% of patients, recurrent laryngeal nerve palsy in up to 10% of patients and vagal nerve damage. Vertebral artery and other vessel puncture may occur, and intrathecal or epidural injunction may also take place. Pneumothorax is rare but more common in patients with chronic obstructive airways disease, thus care must be taken in this patient.

Nicholls B, Conn D, Roberts A. The Abbott pocket guide to practical peripheral nerve blockade. Maidenhead: Abbott Anaesthesia; 2010.
Urmey WF, Talts KH, Sharrock NE. One hundred percent incidence of hemidiaphragmatic paresis associated with interscalene brachial plexus anesthesia as diagnosed by ultrasonography. Anesthesia and Analgesia 1991; 72: 498–503.

69. E Increase the positive end-expiratory pressure (PEEP)

Acute respiratory distress syndrome (ARDS) is traditionally defined by the American-European Consensus Conference (1994) as:

- Acute onset
- Bilateral infiltrates on chest X-ray
- Absence of left atrial hypertension
- A $Pa_{O_2}:Fi_{O_2}$ ratio of <200 mmHg (26.7 kPa)

A more recent consensus definition of ARDS has now replaced this definition. The Berlin definition (2012) involves:

- Onset of ARDS within 7 days of a defined event (e.g. sepsis)
- Bilateral opacities consistent with pulmonary oedema on either chest X-ray or CT scan
- Respiratory failure not fully explained by cardiac failure or fluid overload; objective assessment with echocardiography should be performed.

ARDS is caused by either pulmonary or extrapulmonary pathology, both producing hypoxia due to an increase in both shunt and dead space

Treating hypoxia is best achieved with alveolar recruitment. This can be done by increasing the mean airway pressures, either by increasing the positive end-expiratory pressure (PEEP) or prolonging the inspiratory time. The ARDSnet trial have recommended a lung-protective strategy for ventilating patients with ARDS, and the recommendations include:

- Use of pressure-controlled ventilation
- Aim for tidal volumes of 6 mL/kg of ideal body weight
- Plateau pressures of <30 cmH_2O
- PEEP of 10–12 cmH_2O
- Titrate FIO_2 to a PaO_2 of 8 kPa
- Permissive hypercapnia of 8 kPa, increasing the respiratory rate to reduce the $PaCO_2$

In this patient, increasing the tidal volumes will increase peak airway pressures and have minimal effect on mean airway pressures. The patient already has an FIO_2 of 0.9; thus, increasing the FIO_2 will have minimal effect on hypoxia and will not aid alveolar recruitment. Increasing the expiratory time will only shorten the inspiratory time, lead to higher peak airway pressures and reduce alveolar recruitment. Increasing the respiratory rate will have a greater effect on offloading CO_2 than oxygenation and will be of limited benefit in this scenario.

The Acute Respiratory Distress Syndrome Network. Ventilation with lower tidal volumes as compared with traditional tidal volumes for acute lung injury and the acute respiratory distress syndrome. N Engl J Med 2000; 342:1301–1308.
The ARDS Definition Task Force. Ranieri VM, Rubenfeld GD, et al. Acute respiratory distress syndrome: the Berlin definition. JAMA 2012; 307:2526–2533.

70. A Nebulised antimuscarinic agents

This patient has evidence of acute severe asthma, which is defined by the British Thoracic Society (BTS) as any one of:

- Peak expiratory flow rate (PEFR) of 33–50% of best or predicted
- Respiratory rate of 25 breaths per minute or more
- Heart rate or 110 beats per minute or more
- Inability to complete sentences in one breath

Life-threatening asthma as defined by BTS (2012) guidelines includes:

- PEFR of <33% best or predicted
- SpO_2 <92%
- Quiet chest, cyanosis or reduced respiratory effort
- Arrhythmia or hypotension
- Altered consciousness
- 'Normal' $PaCO_2$ of 4.6–6.0 kPa

- Severe hypoxia with Pao_2 of <8.0 kPa
- Acidosis

The immediate treatment of acute severe asthma in adults is:

- Oxygen to maintain Spo_2 94–98%
- Nebulised salbutamol 5 mg or terbutaline 10 mg (β_2-agonists)
- Nebulised ipratropium bromide 0.5 mg (antimuscarinic)
- Oral prednisolone 40–50 mg or intravenous hydrocortisone 100 mg
- Chest radiograph only if pneumothorax or consolidation is suspected or patient requires intubation
- If life-threatening asthma, then also:
  - Consider ventilation
  - Consider intravenous magnesium sulphate 1.2–2 g via intravenous infusion
  - More frequent salbutamol nebulisers

This patient does not yet require intubation and ventilation, and there is no evidence of requirement for chest radiography at this current stage. PEFR assessment should be performed after immediate treatment as the diagnosis of acute severe asthma is already made. Intravenous magnesium should only be used once conventional therapy has been used and not been successful.

British Thoracic Society/Scottish Intercollegiate Guidelines Network. British Guideline on the Management of Asthma. January 2012 (http://www.brit-thoracic.org.uk/Portals/0/Guidelines/AsthmaGuidelines/sign101%20Jan%202012.pdf) (Last accessed 01/10/2012).

71. A Nitrous oxide

The pin index system is a safety mechanism designed to avoid attachment of the incorrect cylinder to the wrong yoke on the anaesthetic machine. Each gas has a specific pin index to ensure the valve block holes correspond to the machine yoke (see **Figure 1.10**). The pin index system positions for the common gases are shown in **Table 1.13**.

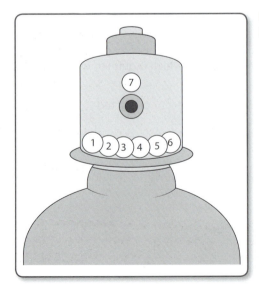

Figure 1.10 The pin index system showing pin positions.

Table 1.13 Pin index system positions for the common gases

Gas	Pin index system positions
Nitrous oxide	3 and 5
Oxygen	2 and 5
Air	1 and 5
Carbon dioxide	1 and 6
Entonox	7

Al-Shaikh B, Stacey S. Essentials of anaesthetic equipment, 3rd edn. Edinburgh: Churchill Livingstone; 2007.

72. D Carboxyhaemoglobin

Pulse oximetry uses the principle of light absorption based on Beer's and Lambert's laws. They are accurate above 70% to ±2%, below which the saturation is extrapolated from studies. Pulse oximeters under read in presence of:

- Indocyanine green dye
- Methaemoglobinaemia
- Methylene blue dye
- Nail varnish

It over-reads, as in this patient, in the presence of carboxyhaemoglobin because the absorption coefficient is similar to that of oxyhaemoglobin, causing the readings to be 96%.

Pedersen T, Moller AM, Pedersen BD. Pulse oximetry for perioperative monitoring: Systematic review of randomized, controlled trials. Anesth Analg 2003; 96:426–431.
Al-Shaikh B, Stacey S. Essentials of anaesthetic equipment, 3rd edn. Edinburgh: Churchill Livingstone; 2007.

73. C Left atrium

The tip of the catheter is placed in the pulmonary artery tree where it is wedged. Once wedged the pulsatile waveform is lost to continuous low pressure reading; this is the pulmonary artery occlusion pressure or the pulmonary capillary wedge pressure; and it is an accurate representation of the left atrial pressure. However, the presence of the mitral valve means that the pressure analysed is more directly related to the left atrium, although the left ventricular pressure can be inferred from this. Because the pressure being measured is beyond the right atrium, ventricle and pulmonary artery, it is not related to these three pressures.

Levick JR. An introduction to cardiovascular physiology, 5th edn. London: Hodder Arnold; 2010.

74. C Voltage

The water pressure difference between two points would correspond to the voltage difference in an electrical circuit. If there is a water pressure difference between two points, then water will flow from one point to the other and this would allow the water to do work, such as rotate the blades in a turbine. Similarly, work is done by the flow of an electric current in a circuit driven by a voltage difference; the current which is generated could then provide power to an electrical device such as a light bulb. If the water pump is not working, then there will be no pressure difference generated so the turbine blades will not rotate, similarly if there is no flow of current then the bulb will not light up.

Davis PD, Kenny GNC. Basic physics and measurement in anaesthesia, 5th edn. Boston: Butterworth-Heinemann; 2003.

75. B Mapleson A breathing system

Mapleson A breathing systems are the most efficient for spontaneous ventilation, and the fresh gas flows required are equal to alveolar minute ventilation. This system is not efficient for controlled ventilation, as it would require fresh gas flows three times the minute ventilation. Mapleson B and C systems are not efficient for spontaneous or controlled ventilation; however, the B system is more efficient than the A and C systems for controlled ventilation.

The Bain system is a coaxial version of the Mapleson D breathing system. This system is not efficient for spontaneous ventilation, requiring a fresh gas flow of about twice the alveolar minute ventilation, but is efficient during controlled ventilation.

Mapleson WW. Editorial I: Fifty years after – reflections on 'The elimination of rebreathing in various semi-closed anaesthetic systems'. Br J Anaesth 2004; 93:319–321.

76. A Deep extubation

This patient would be classed as an 'at risk' extubation; he has a full stomach, has undergone emergency surgery taking several hours and lost significant amount of blood requiring blood transfusion. The patient may not be able to maintain his own airway after the tracheal tube has been removed. An 'at-risk' extubation is characterised by the concern that once extubated, airway management may be difficult. A deep extubation should not be performed in such a patient. Deep extubation should only be performed in 'low-risk' extubation cases; these are routine extubations where reintubation could be managed without difficulty if required.

All the other options are appropriate techniques for 'at-risk' extubations, but must be performed by clinicians who are experienced in the technique.

Difficult Airway Society Extubation Guidelines Group. Popat M, Mitchell V, et al. Difficult Airway Society Guidelines for the management of tracheal extubation. Anaesthesia 2012; 67:318–340.

77. D Axillary

This patient has a pneumothorax on the contralateral side to where the block will be performed. Either a supraclavicular, infraclavicular or axillary nerve block will provide appropriate analgesic coverage for the area where surgery will be performed. The dermatomal distribution for this is region is C5, C6 and T1 where the sensory innervation will be from the median and ulnar nerves.

For a supraclavicular block, the brachial plexus is blocked at the level of the divisions and when performed under ultrasound guidance, the risk of pneumothorax is reduced, but not completely eliminated, even by experienced practitioners. Therefore, there is still a risk of pneumothorax, which must be avoided as the patient already has a pneumothorax on the contralateral side.

An interscalene block would not provide adequate cover for an incision over the antecubital fossa. There is also a high chance of phrenic nerve palsy on the ipsilateral side, thus the patient would be at risk of respiratory distress as he already has a pneumothorax on the left and a phrenic nerve palsy on the right could further compromise ventilation. This is a further reason for not choosing this block.

Axillary and infraclavicular blocks both cover a similar area, which will be adequate for surgery in the antecubital fossa. But there is still some associated risk of pneumothorax when performing an infraclavicular block, even if guided by ultrasound.

Therefore, the most appropriate block would be an axillary nerve block, this will provide adequate coverage to the antecubital fossa and has no risk of pneumothorax. A peripheral nerve block is less likely to be as effective as an axillary block in this circumstance.

Perlas A, Lobo G, Lo N, et al. Ultrasound-guided supraclavicular block: outcome of 510 consecutive cases. Reg Anesth Pain Med 2009; 34:171–176.

78. D It consists of 95% sodium hydroxide

In the circle breathing system soda lime is added to absorb exhaled carbon dioxide. As a result fresh gas flows may be low and, compared with all the Mapleson breathing systems, this makes the circle breathing system a very efficient and economical one. It also causes minimal pollution.

The soda lime is placed in a canister which has two ports: one to deliver fresh gases to the patient and another to receive exhaled gases via unidirectional valves. Soda lime is made of 94% calcium hydroxide, 5% sodium hydroxide and a small amount of potassium hydroxide.

A dye is added which indicates when the soda lime is exhausted; this can either be from pink to white or white to violet. Silica is added to stop the granules from disintegrating into dust particles, which could be inhaled by the patient. The soda lime granules are 4–8 mesh in size, but they can also be made into spherical shapes of 3–4 mm in size.

Al-Shaikh B, Stacey S. Essentials of anaesthetic equipment, 3rd edn. Edinburgh: Churchill Livingstone; 2007.

79. B Atropine

The patient has a low heart rate at this point, and one of the commonest complications of pneumoperitoneum is bradycardia as a result of stimulation of the Vagus nerve due to rapid peritoneal stretching. The combination of a pre-existing low heart rate and vagal stimulation will most likely cause a bradycardia requiring immediate atropine administration and temporary cessation of air insufflation.

Metaraminol would make the bradycardia worse, so should not be administered in this scenario.

Ephedrine and adrenaline could be administered, but there is nothing to suggest that the blood pressure has been compromised, and therefore the first line of treatment should be atropine, followed by ephedrine if the blood pressure is compromised.

There are many complications associated with gas insufflation for laparoscopic surgery including:

- Trauma to intra-abdominal viscera and great vessels
- Gas embolus if gas is insufflated into a blood vessel
- Pneumothorax
- Pneumomediastinum
- Subcutaneous emphysema
- Caval compression

Perrin M, Fletcher A. Laparoscopic abdominal surgery. Contin Educ Anaesth Crit Care Pain 2004; 4:107–110.

80. E Using a large proximal vein for infusion

The Safe Anaesthesia Liaison Group has published guidelines in 2009 to help guarantee the administration of drugs during total intravenous anaesthesia. This was after a number of incidences of awareness as a result of inadequate drug delivery.

Non-return or one-way valves prevent the backflow of the anaesthetic drugs into the intravenous fluid lines, therefore guaranteeing the delivery of these drugs to the patient.

Monitoring the cannulation site at regular intervals is a simple way to reduce the risk of inadequate drug delivery by ensuring that accidental disconnection, backtracking of anaesthetic drugs or displacement of the cannula are noted early.

Infusing fluids through the same cannula as the anaesthetic drugs will help ensure their delivery because if the fluid infusion abruptly stops or suddenly flows at a very fast rate, occlusion or disconnection of the cannula could be the cause and this can then be investigated and resolved.

The use of a large vein as opposed to a smaller vein does not further guarantee drug delivery.

Safe Anaesthesia Liaison Group. Guaranteeing drug delivery in total intravenous anaesthesia. London: National Patient Safety Agency; October 2009.

81. A Hypotensive anaesthesia

Intraoperative bleeding is one of the major problems of this type of surgery and can lead to complications such as impairing the surgeon's vision, increasing the duration of surgery and increasing the risk of intracranial and orbital complications. Blood loss is primarily dependent on cut vessels, but can be reduced considerably by a reduction in the mean arterial pressure. Controlled hypotension deliberately and predictably decreases mean arterial pressure to limit intraoperative blood loss and is the method most likely to reduce intraoperative bleeding.

Normocarbia will prevent increased blood flow to the head and neck region as a result of vasodilation which would otherwise occur with hypercarbia. The reverse Trendelenburg position helps reduce local blood flow to the capillary bed by having the patient in a slightly head-up position. However, neither of these techniques is as effective as hypotensive anaesthesia.

Moffat's solution is a sprayed onto the nasal mucosa to induce vasoconstriction, reduce intraoperative bleeding, reduce congestion of the nose and act as a local anaesthetic. It consists of a combination of cocaine, adrenaline and sodium bicarbonate. This is often required within a multimodal approach for generating a bloodless field but is usually insufficient in isolation. Surgeons often supplement Moffat's solution with lignocaine and adrenaline injections intraoperatively because it rarely guarantees a bloodless field.

Hypothermia has been shown to increase intraoperative blood loss and the need for blood transfusion due to hypothermia-induced impairment of platelet function; this is more likely to occur with a core temperature of 35–35.7°C, therefore will have less influence on this short duration surgery.

Allman KG, Wilson IH. Oxford handbook of anaesthesia, 3rd edn. Oxford: Oxford University Press; 2011.

82. D Decontamination

Decontamination is the process of removing contaminants such that they are unable to reach a site in sufficient quantities to initiate an infection or other harmful reaction. The process of decontamination always starts with cleaning and is followed by disinfection or sterilisation. Fibrescopes are classed as intermediate risk equipment (do not penetrate the skin or enter sterile cavities) so decontamination by cleaning followed by disinfection is an acceptable method of cleaning this type of equipment.

Cleaning is the process of physically removing foreign material from an object without necessarily destroying any infective material. An example of manual cleaning is washing, and automated cleaning is performed using an ultrasonic bath or low-temperature steam.

Disinfection is the process of rendering an object free from all pathological organisms except bacterial spores. Chemicals used for disinfection are glutaraldehyde 2%, alcohol 60–80%, chlorhexidine 0.5–5% and hydrogen peroxide. Pasteurisation is the process of using heat to destroy pathogenic organisms without destroying bacterial spores. It is an alternative to chemical disinfection.

Sterilisation is the process of rendering an object completely free of all visible infectious agents including bacterial spores. This can be done using chemicals such as ethylene oxide and glutaraldehyde 2%, using radiation like gamma irradiation, or using heat such as the autoclave.

Sabir N, Ramachandra V. Decontamination of anaesthetic equipment. Contin Educ Anaesth Crit Care Pain 2004; 4:134–135.

83. C Needle decompression

This patient is demonstrating clinical features of a tension pneumothorax with hypoxia, elevated airway pressures and hypotension. This is a recognised risk of laparoscopic surgery and requires immediate recognition and treatment with insertion of a cannula in the second intercostal space, midclavicular line on the affected side. An intercostal chest drain should then be inserted for this life-threatening emergency.

Adrenaline may be used but would not treat the underlying cause. Optimising ventilatory parameters would not treat the cause and may worsen any tension by increasing the size of the pneumothorax. Administration of intravenous fluid boluses would be of benefit but would not be addressing the underlying cause.

Hayden P, Cowman S. Anaesthesia for laparoscopic surgery. Contin Educ Anaesth Crit Care Pain 2011; 11:177–180.

84. E Cannon *a* waves

The jugular venous pressure (JVP) is assessed by viewing the height and pulsations of the jugular veins with the patient sitting at 45° and the head turned slightly away. It has a characteristic double-pulsatile waveform pattern, distinguishing it from arterial pulsations (see **Figure 1.11**):

- *a* wave: atrial contraction
- *c* wave: bulging of the closed tricuspid valve at the start of isovolumetric right ventricular contraction
- *x* descent: atrial relaxation
- *v* wave: venous return against a closed tricuspid valve
- *y* descent: atrial relaxation while emptying into the right ventricle

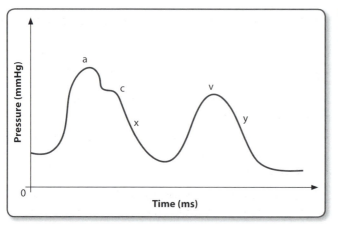

Figure 1.11 The jugular venous pressure (JVP) waveform.

Abnormalities of the JVP waveform may reflect underlying pathology:

- Absent JVP may be present in patients who are intravascularly deplete
- Elevated JVP (>4 cm above the sternal angle) with normal waveforms may reflect right heart failure and fluid overload
- Elevated JVP with absent waveforms may be caused by superior vena cava obstruction
- Cannon *a* waves are caused by atrial contraction against a closed tricuspid valve such as in complete heart block
- Absent *a* waves may be seen in atrial fibrillation
- Large *v* waves is a feature of tricuspid regurgitation
- Elevated JVP with deep *x* and *y* descents may be seen with constrictive pericarditis

The electrocardiographic findings in this patient are consistent with complete atrioventricular dissociation, as is seen in complete heart block. Thus, the most likely JVP waveforms will be cannon *a* waves.

Levick JR. An introduction to cardiovascular physiology, 5th edn. London: Hodder Arnold; 2010.

85. A Reduced pH

Once an arterial blood gas (ABG) sample is collected, it should be analysed as soon as possible. Within the ABG syringe cellular metabolism continues. Dissolved oxygen is utilised; however, this is only of a limited quantity and anaerobic metabolism ensues and carbon dioxide is produced, thereby increasing the $Paco_2$. Anaerobic metabolism persists utilising glucose stores and producing lactate. The overall effect of delayed analysis of an ABG sample can be summarised as follows:

- Reduced pH
- Reduced Pao_2
- Increased $Paco_2$
- Reduced glucose
- Increased lactate

Other errors in analysis of an ABG sample include:

- Air bubbles in syringe: may incorrectly increase Pao_2, saturation and pH of the sample
- Clotting of the sample: may incorrectly increase the potassium concentration of the sample
- Dilution of the sample with arterial line saline flush or liquid heparin: may incorrectly increase Pao_2 while decreasing $Paco_2$, glucose, lactate, haemoglobin and potassium
- Accidental venepuncture during ABG sample collection: may incorrectly decrease Po_2 and saturations, while increasing Pco_2

Wennecke G, Juel G. Avoiding pre-analytical errors in blood gas testing. Radiometer Medical ApS; 2008.

86. C Fat embolism syndrome

This patient has clinical features of fat embolism syndrome. This condition occurs when fat from the bone marrow enters the circulation and restricts right ventricular outflow by increasing pulmonary artery pressures. It most frequently occurs after major trauma, but bone fixation may also cause it. The classical triad of clinical features includes:

- Respiratory symptoms: tachypnoea, dyspnoea, pulmonary oedema, hypoxia
- Neurological features: confusion, drowsiness
- Petechial rash: usually on chest wall, axilla or conjunctiva

Other clinical features include tachycardia, pyrexia, retinal emboli on fundoscopy, renal dysfunction, thrombocytopaenia, anaemia, increased erythrocyte sedimentation rate and fat macroglobulinaemia. Treatment is predominantly supportive.

Haemorrhage would present with cardiovascular as well as respiratory changes, and a rash is not a common presentation for acute haemorrhage. Although anaphylaxis may have a similar presentation, the rash is not typically petechial but urticarial. In addition, cardiovascular changes usually predominate in anaphylaxis. Venous thromboembolism is possible, yet in the time frame described it is less likely. Finally myocardial ischaemia does not usually present with a rash.

Gupta A, Reilly CS. Fat embolism. Contin Educ Anaesth Crit Care Pain 2007; 7:148–151.

87. B Two size E oxygen cylinders

Calculation of the volume of oxygen cylinders required for a transfer depends on two factors: the oxygen delivered and the duration of the transfer.

Oxygen delivered = $F_{IO_2} \times$ minute volume

Oxygen delivered = 1.0×10 L/min

Oxygen delivered = 10 L/min

A size E oxygen cylinder contains a volume of 680 L of oxygen, thus would last for 68 minutes in total. A journey of 90 minutes would therefore require a minimum of 2 size E oxygen cylinders, as this would provide enough oxygen to last 136 minutes.

Shouman YM. More information from the pressure gauge of oxygen cylinders. Anesth Analg 2004; 99;307–308.

88. D Vessel calibre

Blood flow to the flap is determined predominantly by the Hagen–Poiseuille equation:

$$\text{Flow} = \frac{\Delta P \pi r^4}{8 \eta l}$$

where η is fluid viscosity, l is length of the tube, r is the radius of the tube and ΔP is pressure gradient along the tube.

Although the blood pressure and viscosity play an important role in microvascular perfusion, a change in the calibre or radius of vessels leads to a change in blood flow to the power of 4. Therefore, it is the vessel radius that is the most important variable.

Temperature may affect a combination of variables including viscosity and vessel radius; however, it is ultimately the radius that is vital.

Although heart rate may affect the cardiac output, it may not necessarily increase flap perfusion to the extent of vessel diameter.

Adams J, Charlton P. Anaesthesia for microvascular free tissue transfer. BJA CEPD Reviews 2003; 3:33–37.

89. A Isoprenaline

This patient has symptomatic complete heart block that is due to complete atrioventricular (AV) dissociation. The ideal pharmacological agent for this patient would be one with positive chronotropic effects, mediated via β_1-adrenoceptors. Anticholinergic drugs such as atropine would be ineffective because they would act to increase the atrial rate but have no effect on ventricular rate because of the AV dissociation.

Isoprenaline is a potent synthetic β_1- and β_2-adrenoceptor agonist with no α-adrenoceptor effects. Thus, it has positive inotropic and chronotropic effects, increasing the cardiac output. It was thought to be the ideal drug for patients with complete heart block.

Phenylephrine is a pure α_1-adrenoceptor agonist with no β-effects, therefore would not have any effect on heart rate or contractility in this patient.

Salbutamol is predominantly a β_2-adrenoceptor agonist; thus, it induces smooth muscle relaxation and vasodilatation. It will have no direct effects to increase myocardial contractility or heart rate.

Noradrenaline predominantly acts via α_1-adrenoceptors to causes peripheral vasoconstriction, hypertension and, potentially, a reflex bradycardia, although this reflex may be absent in a patient with complete AV dissociation. Noradrenaline has minimal influence on increasing heart rate in patients with complete heart block, and therefore would not be indicated in this patient.

Sasada M, Smith S. Drugs in anaesthesia and intensive care, 4th edn. Oxford: Oxford University Press; 2011.

90. C Sevoflurane

Laparoscopic hernia repairs are most frequently done under general anaesthetic, although there a few reports of regional anaesthetic techniques being used but this is not common practice. General anaesthesia is required to ensure optimal ventilation, avoidance of excessive build-up of CO_2 and abdominal discomfort despite adequate regional blockade. Therefore, lidocaine and bupivacaine would not be ideal agents in this patient.

Under general anaesthesia, the ideal agent in this patient would be sevoflurane because it provides bronchodilator properties that would be of benefit to patients with chronic obstructive airways disease (COAD). Desflurane is irritative to airways and can precipitate bronchospasm, particularly in patients with COAD.

Although a remifentanil infusion would provide intraoperative analgesia and blood pressure control, it is not an anaesthetic agent in itself, and therefore cannot be used in isolation.

Molinelli BM, Tagliavia A, Bernstein D. Total extraperitoneal preperitoneal laparoscopic hernia repair using spinal anesthesia. JSLS 2006; 10:341–344.

Chapter 2

Mock paper 2

60 MTFs and 30 SBAs to be answered in three hours

Questions: MTFs

Answer each stem 'True' or 'False'.

1. **Regarding lung compliance, which of the following are true:**
   A   Specific compliance is related to total lung capacity
   B   It is less in a child than in an adult
   C   Lung compliance is less than total thoracic compliance
   D   It is normally 150–200 mL/cmH$_2$O
   E   It is reduced in the supine position

2. **Regarding closing capacity, which of the following are true:**
   A   Closing volume is approximately 10% of vital capacity in normal subjects
   B   It is the same as functional residual capacity in a standing adult
   C   It is reduced when intrathoracic pressures are high
   D   It increases with age
   E   It may be measured using helium

3. **In a lung unit with a high ventilation/perfusion ($\dot{V}/\dot{Q}$) ratio:**
   A   Alveolar PCO$_2$ reduces
   B   End-capillary PCO$_2$ approaches 0 kPa
   C   The ratio could represent the lung bases
   D   An increase in FIO$_2$ will normalise the $\dot{V}/\dot{Q}$ mismatch
   E   Alveolar gas equilibrates with inspired gas

4. **Regarding the oxyhaemoglobin dissociation curve, which of the following are true:**
   A   It is shifted to the left with alkalosis
   B   It demonstrates a reduced affinity of haemoglobin for oxygen with increased 2,3 diphosphoglycerate levels
   C   The P_{75} determines the position of the curve
   D   The Haldane effect suggests that haemoglobin has a higher affinity for oxygen in more alkaline environments
   E   The normal P_{50} is 3.5 kPa

5. **During the cardiac cycle:**
    A   Atrial contraction results in approximately 60% of its volume delivered to the left ventricle
    B   The *c* wave seen on the atrial pressure curve occurs during isovolumetric contraction
    C   The *x* descent on the atrial pressure curve occurs after the *c* wave and is as a result of the aortic valve opening
    D   The *y* descent on the atrial pressure wave occurs after the mitral valve opens
    E   There is a prominent *c* wave seen on the atrial pressure curve in tricuspid regurgitation

6. **Regarding cardiac conduction, which of the following are true:**
    A   The resting cell membrane is 100 times more permeable to sodium than potassium
    B   The Donnan effect describes how negatively charged molecules are held inside the cell
    C   The Nernst equation determines the contribution of multiple ions across a membrane
    D   Cardiac pacemaker cells maintain a stable resting membrane potential
    E   The cell membrane is impermeable to organic phosphates

7. **During exercise:**
    A   All phases of the cardiac cycle shorten equally
    B   Systole is the main factor limiting the maximum heart rate
    C   Passive filling still has an important role
    D   The cardiovascular changes are mainly caused by circulating catecholamines
    E   There is a relatively greater increase in stroke volume than heart rate

8. **Regarding capillary permeability, which of the following are true:**
    A   It is calculated by measuring solute diffusion rate and the concentration difference across the wall
    B   Solute diffusion rate can be calculated directly and indirectly
    C   Radiolabeled albumin cannot be used as it is a macromolecule in measurement of capillary permeability
    D   The 'osmotic transient method' and the 'multiple indicator diffusion method' are both ways of measuring the concentration difference across the capillary wall
    E   The passage of water and solutes across the capillary wall is purely a passive process

9. **Autoregulation of blood flow to the kidney:**
    A   Occurs between a mean systemic blood pressure of 80 and 200 mmHg
    B   Does not occur in the denervated kidney
    C   Is mediated by changes in resistance within the interlobar arteries
    D   Is not influenced by the arterioles of the cortical nephrons
    E   Results in a directly proportional increase in the glomerular filtration rate

10. **Which of the following statements are true:**

   A In the proximal tubule, the primary drive for water reabsorption is isotonic osmolar reabsorption

   B The thick ascending limb of the loop of Henle is relatively impermeable to water

   C The distal convoluted tubule receives hypertonic fluid from the loop of Henle

   D Antidiuretic hormone acts at the distal convoluted tubules

   E Urea plays an important role in the concentration of urine

11. **Aldosterone:**

   A Is produced in the zona fasciculata of the adrenal cortex

   B Is synthesised from cholesterol

   C Secretion is lowest in the morning and highest in the evening

   D Secretion is stimulated by reduced blood volume and hyperkalaemia

   E Causes sodium retention and potassium excretion

12. **Which of the following are true regarding disturbances of acid/base balance:**

   A A high protein intake in the diet can result in a metabolic alkalosis

   B Starvation results in a metabolic acidosis

   C Acidosis occurs with incomplete oxidation of carbohydrate

   D The increased metabolism of organic anions can cause an acidosis

   E A diet high in vegetable matter produces alkaline urine

13. **Regarding the stomach, which of the following are true:**

   A It is usually the distal portion which expands on filling

   B Its mucosa consists of chief cells and parietal cells only

   C Emptying is dependent on signals from the stomach and duodenum

   D The duodenum depresses the pyloric pump of the stomach

   E Gastrin has an inhibitory effect on stomach emptying

14. **Regarding jaundice, which of the following are true:**

   A It develops when plasma bilirubin levels are >6 μmol/L

   B In the pre-hepatic form results from elevated levels of unconjugated bilirubin

   C A deficiency of glucuronyl transferase results in hepatic jaundice

   D All causes of hepatic jaundice result in dark urine

   E In the post-hepatic form there are high levels of stercobilinogen

15. **The following factors decrease liver blood flow:**

   A Supine posture

   B Hypoxia

   C Positive pressure ventilation

   D Food

   E Volatile anaesthetics

16. **Regarding abnormalities in body temperature, which of the following are true:**

   A During fever the hypothalamic thermostat is set at a lower temperature

   B In heat exhaustion the body temperature is usually high

    C   A high external temperature and relative humidity may lead to reduced heat loss by radiation, conduction and evaporation

    D   The elderly have a reduced perception of cold

    E   Fever occurs following release of immunoglobulins

17. **Hormone secretion by endocrine glands:**

    A   Is not influenced by the nervous system

    B   Can be inhibited by chemical changes in the blood

    C   Is usually continuous

    D   Is stimulated and inhibited by other hormones

    E   Exhibits positive and negative feedback mechanisms

18. **Insulin:**

    A   Accelerates the transport of glucose into the cells

    B   Increases glycogenesis

    C   Decreases lipogenesis

    D   Secretion is stimulated by adrenocorticotrophic hormone

    E   Release is inhibited by the parasympathetic nervous system

19. **The following will reduce cerebral blood flow:**

    A Pa_{CO_2} of 9.0 kPa

    B   Core body temperature of 34.6°C

    C   Isoflurane

    D   Fentanyl

    E   Thiopentone

20. **The following will result in a transfusion reaction:**

    A   Group A patient receiving group AB blood

    B   Group O patient receiving group AB blood

    C   Group AB patient receiving group B blood

    D   Group O patient receiving group A blood

    E   Group AB patient receiving group O blood

21. **The hepatic extraction ratio for a drug is affected by:**

    A   Protein binding

    B   Hepatic blood flow

    C   pKa

    D   Hepatic enzyme capacity

    E   Lipid solubility

22. **Regarding the time constant, which of the following are true:**

    A   It is directly proportional to the rate constant

    B   It is the time taken for the plasma concentration to reduce by half

    C   87% of the process is complete after 2 time constants

    D   An increase in volume of distribution will increase the time constant

    E   The time constant for alfentanil is less than its half-life

23. **The following drugs demonstrate zero-order kinetics:**

   A   Clonidine
   B   Paracetamol
   C   Aspirin
   D   Methanol
   E   Theophylline

24. **The following drugs preferentially bind to α_1-glycoprotein rather than albumin:**

   A   Morphine
   B   Propofol
   C   Phenytoin
   D   Paracetamol
   E   Thiopentone

25. **Regarding barbiturates, which of the following are true:**

   A   Thiobarbiturates are as lipid soluble as the oxybarbiturates
   B   Thiopentone has the lowest protein binding of all the barbiturates
   C   Their mechanism of action is unknown
   D   Thiopentone is the sulphur analogue of pentobarbitone
   E   Barbiturates are all derived from urea and malonic acid

26. **Ketamine has the following effects:**

   A   Stimulation of the sympathetic nervous system
   B   Decreased myocardial oxygen requirements
   C   Bronchodilatation
   D   Dissociation between the thalamocortical and limbic systems
   E   Less emetogenic than other induction agents

27. **The following increases the rise in alveolar concentration of inhaled anaesthetics:**

   A   Using a 50:50 mixture of oxygen and air
   B   A high heart rate and blood pressure
   C   An increase in alveolar ventilation
   D   A high inspired concentration of volatile anaesthetic
   E   A small functional residual capacity (FRC)

28. **Paracetamol:**

   A   Is classified as a non-steroidal anti-inflammatory drug
   B   Inhibits cyclo-oxygenase
   C   Exhibits antipyretic actions by inhibition of leukotrienes
   D   Is metabolised in the liver to glucuronide conjugates only
   E   Has an oral bioavailability of about 80%

29. **Regarding opioid receptors:**

   A σ is classified as an opioid receptor
   B μ_2 receptors produce the analgesic effects of opioids

    C   κ has three receptor subtypes
    D   They are generally located postsynaptically
    E   They are all reversed by naloxone

30. **Regarding the use of antiarrhythmic drugs:**
    A   Quinidine is active against both atrial and ventricular arrhythmias
    B   Flecainide is the first-line drug used for ventricular arrhythmias
    C   Disopyramide is active against both atrial and ventricular ectopics
    D   β-blockers should not be used to treat Wolff–Parkinson–White syndrome
    E   Sotalol demonstrates class I properties

31. **Amiodarone:**
    A   Is chiefly a class I antiarrhythmic with powerful class III activity
    B   Is effective in atrial fibrillation because of its effects on the superior pulmonary veins
    C   Requires a small oral loading dose
    D   Is used for treating recurring ventricular fibrillation
    E   Can cause side effects affecting the eyes, skin and liver

32. **The following drugs are inodilators:**
    A   High-dose dopamine
    B   Milrinone
    C   High-dose adrenaline
    D   Dobutamine
    E   Sodium nitroprusside

33. **Regarding local anaesthetics, which of the following are true:**
    A   Potency is related to lipid solubility
    B   Protein binding is inversely proportional to duration of action
    C   They are weak acids
    D   They are less ionised below their pKa
    E   Speed of onset is increased in the unionised state

34. **Eutectic mixture of local anaesthetic (EMLA):**
    A   Contains 2.5% procaine
    B   Has a higher melting point than the individual components
    C   Has a breakdown product of para-aminobenzoic acid
    D   Lasts for >120 minutes
    E   Can cause methaemoglobinaemia

35. **The following are recognised complications of suxamethonium:**
    A   Bradycardia
    B   Liver failure
    C   Myotonia
    D   Gastric reflux
    E   Anaphylaxis

36. **The following anticholinesterases have a quaternary amine structure:**

    A   Edrophonium
    B   Neostigmine
    C   Pyridostigmine
    D   Physostigmine
    E   Pralidoxime

37. **The following antimicrobials are correctly classified:**

    A   Ciprofloxacin is a penicillin
    B   Clarithromycin is a 4-quinolone
    C   Gentamicin is an aminoglycoside
    D   Cefuroxime is a third-generation cephalosporin
    E   Meropenem is a β-lactam

38. **Midazolam:**

    A   Has an oral bioavailability of 80%
    B   Has the active metabolite 1α-hydroxymidazolam
    C   Is unionised at pH 3.5
    D   Is lipid soluble in solution
    E   Is >90% plasma protein bound

39. **Tricyclic antidepressants:**

    A   Block uptake 1
    B   Are agonists at α_1-adrenoceptors
    C   Include phenelzine
    D   Take weeks to act
    E   Cause urinary retention

40. **The main sites of action of the following diuretics are correct:**

    A   Carbonic anhydrase inhibitors: distal convoluted tubule
    B   Thiazide diuretics: distal convoluted tubule
    C   Potassium sparing diuretics: proximal convoluted tubule
    D   Aldosterone antagonists: distal convoluted tubule
    E   Osmotic diuretics: thick ascending limb of the loop of Henle

41. **Regarding magnetism, which of the following are true:**

    A   A magnetic field is the region where a current-carrying conductor exerts its effects
    B   A changing magnetic field can produce an electric current
    C   The magnetic field strength is the power of the magnetic field in air
    D   Diamagnetic materials increase magnetic flux
    E   The unit of magnetic flux is the tesla

42. **Which of the following statements are true:**

    A   Alternating current (AC) and direct current (DC) cannot be combined
    B   An ampere is the flow of 6.24×10^{18} electrons per minute past a point

    C   A galvanometer works by the interaction of electricity and magnetism

    D   Potential difference is based on current flow and energy production

    E   The strongest point of a magnetic field in a coiled wire with a current flowing through it is at the end of the coil

43. **Concerning electrical safety, which of the following are true:**

    A   The high voltage supplied from a power station is reduced by a capacitor

    B   The live wire from the substation to the hospital is connected to earth

    C   The effect of an electric shock depends on current flow

    D   Skin and tissue have high impedance

    E   Antistatic shoes allow the safe dissipation of electrostatic charges

44. **In a gas cylinder at 100 kPa pressure:**

    A   If it contained air, the pressure exerted by oxygen would be approximately 21 kPa

    B   If it contained Entonox, the pressure exerted by nitrous oxide would be 50 kPa

    C   Oxygen would have twice the number of molecules as nitrogen in an identical cylinder and conditions

    D   The pressure is equivalent to 750 mmHg

    E   If it contained oxygen, then it would be a liquid at room temperature

45. **Regarding exponential functions, which of the following are true:**

    A   A 'wash-in' curve is an example of an exponential process

    B   A constant flow generator will produce an exponential curve when volume is plotted against time for inspiration

    C   The multiplication of cancer cells plotted against time would produce a 'wash-in' curve

    D   The expiration of gas from the lungs plotted against time would produce a 'wash-out' curve

    E   The 'wash-out' curves for dye dilution techniques are the same as for thermodilution when calculating cardiac output

46. **The following are derived SI units:**

    A   Newton

    B   Fahrenheit

    C   Watt

    D   Coulomb

    E   Joule

47. **The following physical laws are correct:**

    A   The critical temperature is the temperature at which a substance cannot be liquefied

    B   The critical pressure is the vapour pressure of a substance at its critical temperature

    C   Dalton's law states that in a mixture of gases the pressure exerted by each gas is the same

D Avogadro's hypothesis states that equal volumes of gases at the same temperature and pressure contain equal numbers of molecules
E The pseudocritical temperature is the temperature below which a mixture of substances cannot be separated

48. **Regarding humidification, which of the following are true:**
    A Inspired gas has 100% relative humidity by the time it reaches the alveoli in normal breathing
    B Heat and moisture exchangers can have hydrophobic or hygroscopic membranes
    C Heat and moisture exchangers have high thermal conductivity
    D Heated breathing tubes increases the inspired gas humidity
    E Pneumatic, but not ultrasonic, nebulised humidifiers can be heated

49. **Regarding core temperature, which of the following are true:**
    A The core compartments are composed of well-perfused tissues of uniform temperature
    B Core temperature reflects the amount of heat generated in the heart, brain and liver
    C The posterior hypothalamus contains the centre for temperature regulation
    D The deep tissues of the limbs contribute to the central core temperature
    E The core tissues contribute 90% of the thermal input to the thermoregulatory system

50. **Regarding Reynold's number, which of the following are true:**
    A It is used to calculate whether flow will be laminar or turbulent
    B A low number means there will be turbulent flow
    C Between 2000 and 4000, flow may be laminar and turbulent
    D Flow is required to calculate Reynold's number
    E Fluid density and viscosity are not required to calculate Reynold's number

51. **Regarding electrical hazards, which of the following are true:**
    A A current of 50 mA may cause ventricular fibrillation if applied directly to the myocardium
    B The current required to cause ventricular fibrillation is higher with AC than it is with DC
    C An increase in frequency increases the stimulation effect
    D Impedance is directly proportional to current flow
    E Wet skin increases resistance

52. **Oxygen cylinders:**
    A Have a pin index of 1 and 5
    B Contain oxygen in the liquid state
    C Have white and black quartered shoulders
    D Are usually size J in cylinder banks
    E Have a pressure which decreases exponentially as the cylinder empties

53. **Entonox:**

    A   Has a pseudocritical temperature of 36.5°C
    B   Is stored in cylinders at 4400 kPa
    C   May allow hypoxic mixtures to be delivered initially when used in cold environments
    D   Cylinders should be stored horizontally
    E   Cylinders require a two-stage demand pressure regulator for use

54. **The following can be used to measure flow:**

    A   Thermistor
    B   Ultrasound
    C   Wright respirometer
    D   Pitot tube
    E   Infrared

55. **The Tec Mark 6 vapouriser:**

    A   Is heated at 39°C
    B   Has wicks and baffles to ensure full vapour saturation
    C   May contain a bimetallic strip
    D   Has all the fresh gas flow entering the vapourising chamber
    E   Requires an electric supply

56. **Passive scavenging systems:**

    A   Contain valves opening at 1 kPa
    B   Have 22 mm connectors which are attached to adjustable pressure-limiting valves
    C   Are driven by patient expiration
    D   Do not require a power supply
    E   May have flow within them reversed

57. **The Bain breathing system:**

    A   Is less efficient as its length increases
    B   Is a Mapleson D system
    C   Can be bulky at the patient end
    D   Can be tested using the Venturi principle
    E   Has an internal volume of <500 mL

58. **The following are true regarding measurement of oxygen saturations using a saturations probe:**

    A   Measurement related to distance traveled by a path of light
    B   It utilises at least two light-emitting diode electrodes
    C   It relies on spectrophotometry
    D   Red wavelength of 940 nm absorbs oxyhaemoglobin
    E   It only interprets non-constant components of absorption

59. **Severinghaus electrodes:**
    A   Have hydrogen ion sensitive glass electrodes
    B   Are slow response devices
    C   Contain platinum reference electrodes
    D   Are affected by temperature
    E   Are in a bicarbonate bath

60. **Non-invasive blood pressure devices over-read in the following situations:**
    A   Obese patients
    B   Hypotensive patients
    C   Atrial fibrillation
    D   Shivering
    E   Small cuffs

Questions: SBAs

For each question, select the single best answer from the five options listed.

61. The pressure waveform while floating a pulmonary artery catheter reads 24/14 mmHg.

What is the most likely location of the catheter tip?

A   Superior vena cava
B   Right atrium
C   Right ventricle
D   Pulmonary artery
E   Pulmonary capillary

62. A healthy 26-year-old man develops laryngospasm after extubation following a laparoscopic appendicectomy. Despite application of $10\,cmH_2O$ continuous positive airway pressure and administration of 50 mg propofol, the laryngospasm continues and you elect to reintubate the patient. Following intubation, pink frothy secretions are noted in the endotracheal tube, basal crackles are auscultated and the oxygen saturations are 91% with an F_{IO_2} of 0.7.

What is the most likely mechanism of this complication?

A   Reduced interstitial hydrostatic pressure
B   Increased capillary hydrostatic pressure
C   Excessive fluid administration
D   Reduced capillary oncotic pressure
E   Increased interstitial hydrostatic pressure

63. A 5-year-old, 20-kg boy presents for a circumcision under general anaesthetic for a paraphimosis. A caudal block with local anaesthetic is performed following induction of anaesthesia.

Which local anaesthetic regimen would be most suitable?

A   16 mL of 0.25% bupivacaine
B   8 mL of 0.5% bupivacaine
C   6 mL of 1% lidocaine
D   10 mL of 0.25% bupivacaine
E   5 mL of 0.75% ropivacaine

64. A 74-year-old man presents with a ruptured abdominal aortic aneurysm requiring an urgent laparotomy. He is normally on warfarin for rate controlled atrial fibrillation. His international normalised ratio preoperatively is 9.4.

What is the most appropriate method for reversal of warfarin in this patient?

A   Oral vitamin K
B   NovoSeven (recombinant factor VIIa)
C   Beriplex (prothrombin complex concentrate)
D   Cross-matched fresh frozen plasma
E   Cryoprecipitate

65. A 48-year-old man with a history of type II diabetes mellitus and gout presents after a contrast CT scan with anuria and confusion. His blood results are:

Na$^+$	142 mmol/L	pH	7.31
K$^+$	5.3 mmol/L	HCO$_3^-$	19.3 mmol/L
Urea	18.0 mmol/L	BE	−6.8
Creatinine	216 mmol/L	Lactate	3.4
Glucose	8.0 mmol/L	Cl$^-$	106 mmol/L

Which is most likely to be true?

A Confusion is due to low chloride
B The anion gap is <20 mmol/L
C Treatment should involve *N*-acetylcysteine
D Plasma osmolality is 310 mOsm/kg
E The patient requires haemodialysis

66. A 28-year-old man has climbed to an altitude of 6 km. He remains conscious and communicative.

What is the most important physiological mechanism for acclimatisation?

A Increased minute ventilation
B Increased sensitivity of central chemoreceptors
C Increased 2,3-diphosphoglycerate
D Increased erythropoietin
E Increased renal excretion of bicarbonate

67. A 30-year-old woman had an epidural inserted for labour analgesia 16 hours previously. Multiple attempts at insertion were performed and she now complains of an occipital headache that is worse on standing.

What is the most appropriate treatment option?

A Co-codamol
B Hydration
C Epidural blood patch
D Sumatriptan
E Oral caffeine

68. A 56-year-old woman undergoing a laparoscopic hysterectomy that has lasted 2 hours and now has a tympanic temperature of 35.2°C.

What is the most appropriate method for preventing heat loss?

A Intravenous fluid warmer
B Heated mattress
C Forced air warmer
D Warmed blankets
E Heat and moisture exchange filters

69. A 24-year-old man presents following a stab wound to his abdomen. His blood pressure is 68/42 mmHg, heart rate is 142 beats per minute, capillary refill time is 7 seconds and his peripheries feel cool to touch.

    What is the most appropriate method of administering fluids to this patient?

    A   Quadruple lumen central venous catheter
    B   Intraosseous cannula
    C   20 gauge external jugular cannula
    D   14 gauge peripheral cannula
    E   Peripherally inserted central catheter

70. If the flow of blood through the circulation is used as an analogy to electricity, which of the following pairs is *not* correct?

    A   Blood flow is analogous to electrical current
    B   Pulsatile blood pressure is analogous to voltage
    C   Vascular resistance is analogous to electrical impedance
    D   Elasticity of the arterial wall is analogous to resistors
    E   Storage vessels are analogous to capacitors

71. Which of the following methods used to reduce pollution in the operating theatre is least useful?

    A   Low-flow anaesthesia
    B   Regular air exchanges in theatre
    C   Scavenging
    D   Use of a heat and moisture exchanger filter (HME filter)
    E   Use of total intravenous anaesthesia

72. A 22-year-old man has a traumatic laceration to dorsal aspect of his index finger, requiring tendon repair. You perform an ultrasound-guided axillary brachial plexus block.

    Which of the following nerves does not need to be anaesthetised when performing this block for surgery?

    A   Radial nerve
    B   Median nerve
    C   Ulnar nerve
    D   Musculocutaneous nerve
    E   Intercostobrachial nerve

73. A 28-year-old patient with respiratory papillomatosis requires excision of numerous intra-tracheal papillomas.

    Which of the following techniques would be the most appropriate to oxygenate and ventilate the patient during the procedure?

    A   Endotracheal intubation
    B   Laryngeal mask airway
    C   Tracheostomy

D   High-frequency jet ventilation
E   Spontaneous ventilation

74. A 59-year-old man in intensive care unit has a tracheostomy in situ for long-term ventilatory support. You have noticed that there is an air leak around the cuff so decide to change the tracheostomy tube.

Which of the following is *not* a component of a standard tracheostomy tube?

A   Introducer
B   Flanges for attachment
C   Inner cannula
D   15 mm connector
E   Beveled tip

75. A 6-year-old boy breathing air has oxygen saturations of 85% via pulse oximetry, but the arterial blood gas reading shows an oxygen saturation of 99%.

Which of the following is the most likely explanation for this discrepancy?

A   Methaemoglobinaemia
B   Hypoperfusion
C   Hyperbilirubinaemia
D   Methylene blue
E   Severe vasoconstriction

76. In preparing a 45-year-old man for extubation, you attach a peripheral nerve stimulator to assess the extent of neuromuscular blockade.

Which of the following is the *least* precise method of assessing depth of neuromuscular blockade?

A   Tetanic stimulation
B   Single burst twitch response
C   Train-of-four stimulation
D   Double burst stimulation
E   Post-tetanic potentiation

77. The hospital policy where you work states that all re-usable clinical instruments must be sterilised before use in any clinical setting.

Which of the following is a method used for sterilisation of these instruments?

A   Glutaraldehyde 2% for 20 minutes
B   Hydrogen peroxide 6–7.5% for 30 minutes
C   Boiling at 100°C for 1 minute
D   Pasteurisation
E   Ethylene oxide gas

78. A 43-year-old man is in the recovery room having had surgery for an inguinal hernia repair. Despite receiving dexamethasone and ondansetron he is still nauseated, so you decide to prescribe metoclopramide.

Which one of the following is *not* an action of metoclopramide?

A   Prokinesis
B   Increased gastric emptying
C   Dryness of mouth
D   Increased lower oesophageal sphincter tone
E   Extra-pyramidal effects

79. An 83-year-old woman on long-term steroids is receiving a blood transfusion due to a haemoglobin level of 7 g/dL following an episode of haematemesis. Soon after starting the transfusion, she develops dyspneoa, tachycardia and flushing.

Which of the following complications of blood transfusion is *least* likely to be the cause of her symptoms?

A   Transfusion-related graft-vs-host disease
B   Transfusion-related acute lung injury
C   Allergic reaction to protein
D   Reaction due to bacterial contamination
E   Air embolism

80. A 45-year-old man had a heart transplant 5 years ago.

Which one of the following drugs is most likely to increase the heart rate in this patient?

A   Atropine
B   Glycopyrrolate
C   Cyclizine
D   Noradrenaline
E   Glyceryl trinitrate

81. A 22-year-old woman presents with a Glasgow Coma Score (GCS) of 3/15 following an intracranial haemorrhage. She is intubated, not making any ventilatory efforts and is thought to be brainstem dead.

Which cranial nerve is *not* tested during brainstem death testing?

A   Optic nerve
B   Hypoglossal nerve
C   Facial nerve
D   Abducens nerve
E   Glossopharyngeal nerve

82. A 43-year-old woman has had a total thyroidectomy. Post-operatively she has an altered voice. A nasendoscopy is performed and her right vocal cord is in the midline while the left is lateral at rest.

What is the most likely pattern of nerve damage this patient has received?

A   Complete right superior laryngeal nerve palsy
B   Partial right recurrent laryngeal nerve palsy

C   Complete right recurrent laryngeal nerve palsy
D   Partial left recurrent laryngeal nerve palsy
E   Complete left superior laryngeal nerve palsy

83. A 33-year-old woman presents with palpitations due to supraventricular tachycardia with a heart rate of 165 beats per minute. She has a blood pressure of 132/84 mmHg, a Glasgow Coma Score of 15/15 and no chest pain. Vagal manoeuvres have been attempted but her rhythm remains unchanged.

What would be the next most appropriate management?

A   6 mg adenosine
B   1.25 mg bisoprolol
C   62.5 μg digoxin
D   300 mg amiodarone
E   5 mg verapamil

84. A 56-year-old man presents with pneumonia. He is referred to the intensive care unit for management of sepsis.

Which of the following does not contribute to the diagnosis of sepsis?

A   White blood cell count $<4.0 \times 10^9$
B   Temperature <36°C
C   Systolic blood pressure <90 mmHg
D   Heart rate >90 beats per minute
E   Respiratory rate >20 breaths per minute

85. A 31-year-old woman has a rapid sequence induction for an emergency Caesarean section. Following delivery of the baby, the obstetricians are concerned that the uterus is not contracting well and the woman continues to bleed.

What is the most likely anaesthetic cause of uterine atony in this patient?

A   Nitrous oxide
B   Atracurium
C   Sevoflurane
D   Thiopentone
E   Morphine

86. A 37-year-old woman has recently been started on an anti-arrhythmic agent for a Wolff–Parkinson–White syndrome. It is thought to block sodium channels and have no effect on the refractory period of cardiac muscle.

What is the most likely drug that the patient has been started on?

A   Disopyramide
B   Flecainide
C   Lidocaine
D   Quinidine
E   Bretylium

87. The oxygen saturation of fetal blood in the descending aorta is approximately 55%, while that in the umbilical vein is 80%.

   How does the fetal circulation ensure delivery of the most saturated blood to the brain?

   A   The umbilical venous blood bypasses the liver via the ductus venosus
   B   The ductus arteriosus shunts blood to the arch of the aorta
   C   Blood from the inferior vena cava mainly passes through the foramen ovale
   D   The oxyhaemoglobin dissociation curve shifts to the right
   E   High pulmonary vascular resistance reduces cardiac output through the lungs

88. A 29-year-old parturient at 38 weeks gestation presents with loin pain, dysuria, tachycardia and fever. She is diagnosed with sepsis due to pyelonephritis.

   What physiological change in pregnancy is most likely to give septic women a high risk of haemodynamic collapse?

   A   Hypoalbuminaemia
   B   Physiological anaemia
   C   Increased stroke volume
   D   Increased left ventricular mass
   E   Reduced systemic vascular resistance

89. A 67-year-old man has a laryngectomy and neck dissection for laryngeal cancer. At the end of the operation, the surgeon asks you to perform a Valsalva manoeuvre in order to look for bleeding points.

   Which of the following changes does *not* occur with a Valsalva manoeuvre in a healthy patient?

   A   Increased venous return in phase 1
   B   Tachycardia in phase 1
   C   Baroreceptor activation in phase 2
   D   Pulmonary blood pooling in phase 3
   E   Reflex bradycardia in phase 4

90. A 59-year-old patient in the intensive care unit has an arterial Po_2 of 13.3 kPa and a venous Po_2 of 5.3 kPa with an Fio_2 of 0.3.

   What is the most likely pathogenesis for his admission?

   A   Cardiogenic shock
   B   Anaemia
   C   Cyanide poisoning
   D   Pulmonary oedema
   E   Asthma

Answers: MTFs

1. A False

    B True

    C False

    D True

    E True

Compliance (C) is defined as the change in volume (ΔV) per unit change in pressure (ΔP) and reflects the elastic recoil of an organ:

$$C = \Delta V/\Delta P$$

Specific compliance is related to the functional residual capacity, not total lung capacity (A), and lung compliance is usually 200 mL/cmH$_2$O; therefore, it is more than total thoracic compliance (85–100 mL/cmH$_2$O) (C, D). The compliance in a child is lower than an adult (B). For example, a 70 kg adult with a tidal volume of 7 mL/kg has a compliance of approximately 100 mL/cmH$_2$O (500 ml/5 cmH$_2$O). However, in a 20 kg child the tidal volume will be 140 mL with the same inflation pressure as an adult of approximately 5 cmH$_2$O, therefore the compliance will be 28 mL/cmH$_2$O (140 mL/5 cmH$_2$O). There are a number of factors that reduce compliance including the supine position (see **Table 2.1**) (E) (see Answer 1.62.).

Table 2.1 Factors affecting lung compliance

Reduced compliance	Increased compliance
Pulmonary fibrosis	Surfactant
Pulmonary venous engorgement	Emphysema
Pulmonary oedema	Old age
Acute respiratory distress syndrome	Acute asthma
Neonates	
Extremes of lung volumes	
Pneumonia	
Chronic bronchitis (dynamic)	

2. A True

    B False

    C False

    D True

    E True

Closing capacity (CC) is the lung volume at which airway closure occurs, which is closing volume plus residual volume. Closing volume is about 10% of the vital capacity (VC) in young normal subjects, but it increases gradually with age and is about 40% of VC aged 65 (A, D). When CC equals or exceeds the functional residual capacity (FRC) airway closure takes place. CC equals FRC in neonates and infants, in 40-year-old subjects when supine and in 65-year-old subjects when upright (B). Other factors increasing CC include asthma, raised intrathoracic pressures and smoking (C). CC may encroach on FRC when the FRC is reduced such as in pregnancy, obesity or general anaesthesia.

Measurement of CC involves either nitrogen or helium concentration analysis as marker gases (E). In Fowler's method, similar to dead space measurement, a maximum inspiration of 100% O_2 or helium is taken and rapid gas analysers continuously plot the concentrations on slow expiration following this **(Figure 2.1)**.

- Phase I: dead space gas with no nitrogen or helium is present
- Phase II: mixture of dead space and alveolar gas with some marker gas
- Phase III: plateau of alveolar gas
- Phase IV: closure of upper airways causing a rise in the marker gas: closing volume

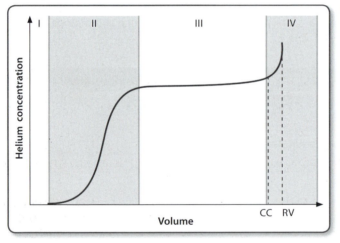

Figure 2.1 Helium dilution curve demonstrating CC.

3. **A** True

    B True

    C False

    D False

    E True

A lung unit with a high $\dot{V}/\dot{Q}$ ratio is better ventilated than perfused, which could represent dead space. Alveolar gases equilibrate with inspired air; therefore, alveolar P_{CO_2} reduces, alveolar P_{O_2} increases and end-capillary gas pressures mirror this with a reduced end-capillary P_{CO_2} (A, B, E). The top of the lungs has a high $\dot{V}/\dot{Q}$ ratio, while the bottom has a lower $\dot{V}/\dot{Q}$ ratio (C). Because areas with a high $\dot{V}/\dot{Q}$ are poorly perfused, increasing the F_{IO_2} will not sufficiently improve the mismatch (D).

4. **A** True

   B True

   C False

   D False

   E True

The position of the oxyhaemoglobin dissociation curve is determined by the P_{50} which is the partial pressure of O_2 at which haemoglobin is 50% saturated (C). This is normally 3.5 kPa (E), but is affected by a number of factors as shown in **Table 2.2**.

Table 2.2 Factors affecting position of the oxyhaemoglobin dissociation curve

Left shift (increased O_2 affinity, P_{50} <3.5 kPa)	Right shift (reduced O_2 affinity, P_{50} >3.5 kPa)
Reduced P_{aCO_2}	Elevated P_{aCO_2}
Alkalosis (A)	Acidosis
Hypothermia	Hyperthermia
Reduced 2,3-diphosphoglycerate	Elevated 2,3-diphosphoglycerate (B)
Carbon monoxide	Pregnancy
Methaemoglobinaemia	Haemoglobin S
Fetal haemoglobin	Altitude

The P_{75} is the partial pressure of O_2 at which haemoglobin is 75% saturated and usually corresponds to venous blood at 5.3 kPa. It does not determine the position of the curve.

The Bohr effect is the shift of the oxyhaemoglobin dissociation curve to the right in response to a rise in either P_{aCO_2} or a fall in pH. The Haldane effect however is the phenomenon where deoxygenated haemoglobin has a higher affinity for CO_2 than oxygenated haemoglobin (D).

5. **A** False

   B True

   C False

   D True

   E False

In resting subjects, the atrial contraction enhances ventricular filling by about 15–30% (A). In exercising patients, where the heart rate is high and there is less time for passive ventricular filling, the atrial contraction becomes more important.

During isovolumetric contraction, there is a small rise in atrial pressure, which is seen in the left atrial pressure trace as the c wave (B). It occurs as a result of the bulging back of the mitral valve into the left atrium.

The x descent is a fall in atrial pressure that occurs as a result of ventricular contraction, thereby lengthening the atria and causing a pressure drop (C).

Once the mitral valve opens blood flows into the ventricle from the left atrium causing a pressure drop in the atrium, described as the y descent (D).

As the atria fill, atrial pressure begins to rise, producing the v wave. The v refers to the simultaneously occurring ventricular systole. Tricuspid regurgitation results in a prominent v wave and the loss of the c wave and x descent (E).

6. A False

    B True

    C False

    D False

    E True

The resting membrane potential is due to the high concentration of potassium ions in intracellular fluid and the high permeability of the cell membrane to potassium ions compared with other ions. The cell membrane is about 100 times more permeable to potassium than sodium (A). Additionally, the intracellular potassium concentration is about 35 times higher than the extracellular concentration. Therefore, there is always a tendency for potassium to diffuse out of the cell down a concentration gradient.

The Donnan effect (or Gibbs–Donnan effect) describes the phenomenon where charged particles that cannot diffuse across a membrane have an effect on the distribution of other charged particles (B). Proteins and phosphates hold negatively charged molecules inside the cell; thus, the inside of the cell is negative with respect to the outside and these negatively charged molecules cannot cross the cell membrane (E).

The Nernst equation calculates the membrane potential for an individual ion at equilibrium (C). The equilibrium potential is equal in magnitude to the outward-driving effect of the concentration gradient or chemical potential.

$$E_x = \frac{RT}{zF} \cdot \ln \frac{[C_o]}{[C_i]}$$

where E_x is the relationship between equilibrium potential of ionic substance X and the ionic concentration ratio, R is the gas constant, T is absolute temperature, z is ionic valency, F is Faraday's constant, C_o is ion concentration outside the cell, and C_i is ion concentration inside the cell.

It is the Goldman equation that examines the contribution of multiple ions across the membrane.

Cardiac pacemaker cells exhibit automaticity, lacking a stable membrane potential and instead spontaneously decaying towards threshold (pre-potential) (D).

7. A False

    B False

    C True

    D False

    E False

During exercise, the heart has the ability to increase cardiac output in direct proportion to total oxygen consumption.

Exercise requires the heart to adapt in order to optimise three key parameters. Firstly, pulmonary blood flow must be increased by increasing right ventricular output, thus enhancing gas exchange. Secondly, blood flow through the working muscle must be increased by local metabolic vasodilatation thereby reducing the resistance to blood flow through the muscle. Finally, a stable blood pressure must be maintained by a variable degree of vasoconstriction in non-active tissues.

Although exercise shortens the duration of the cardiac cycle, the various phases do not shorten in equal amounts. Diastole is curtailed more than systole as heart rate increases (A).

Diastole is the chief factor limiting the maximum heart rate, as refilling of the ventricles during this phase is crucial (B).

Passive filling does have an important role during exercise, although atrial systole has a relatively greater contribution (C).

The cardiovascular changes during exercise are mainly brought about by a change in autonomic nerve activity (D). There is an increase in sympathetic drive and a reduction in parasympathetic activity. There is a rise in plasma catecholamine levels, but this contributes less to the overall cardiovascular changes.

The increase in stroke volume is relatively smaller than the increase in heart rate (E). This is because the stroke volume is limited by the size of the heart chambers and the time available for filling and ejection.

8. A False

    B True

    C False

    D True

    E True

Permeability of a membrane is defined as the rate of diffusion of solute across a unit area of membrane per unit of concentration difference. To determine capillary membrane permeability, three sets of measurements are required (A):

- The rate of solute transfer
- The membrane area
- The concentration difference across the wall

Solute diffusion rate can be measured directly by optical methods in cannulated capillaries perfused with dyes or fluorescent markers. Indirectly, the Fick principle can be used to calculate the whole organ transfer of rapidly diffusing solutes across the whole microvascular bed (B).

Recording the extravascular accumulation of radiolabeled albumin after intravascular injection can assess capillary permeability to plasma macromolecules (C).

In the 'osmotic transient' method, a solute such as glucose is injected intra-arterially and the average concentration difference across the capillary walls is calculated from the osmotic pressure that is generated. This can only be done in isolated, artificially perfused tissues.

The 'multiple indicator diffusion' technique can be applied to organs *in situ* and relies on the analysis of solute exchange along a capillary, usually using radiolabeled albumin (D).

There is no energy expenditure by the endothelium of the capillary walls in the transport of water or solute across the walls. Fluid movement is as a result of hydraulic flow down the pressure gradient. Solute exchange is due to passive diffusion down concentration gradients (E).

9. **A** True

    B False

    C False

    D False

    E False

Between mean systemic blood pressures of 80 and 200 mmHg, the renal blood flow remains almost constant as a result of autoregulation (A). Only minor changes in the glomerular filtration rate are seen within this range as a result.

Even the denervated kidney exhibits autoregulation, as it is the intrinsic ability of the organ to regulate its blood flow over a range of systemic mean arterial pressures (B).

Autoregulation is largely influenced by changes in resistance of the interlobular arteries as well as resistance in afferent and efferent arterioles of the cortical nephrons (D). It is not affected by changes in resistance of the larger interlobar arteries (C).

The glomerular filtration rate is constant above a mean pressure of about 80 mmHg; below this level there is no autoregulation and the glomerular filtration rate falls sharply, nearly ceasing below 60 mmHg (**Figure 2.2**) (E).

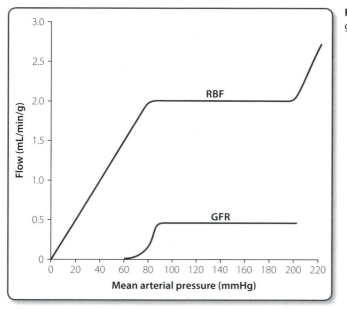

Figure 2.2 Autoregulation of glomerular filtration rate.

10. **A** False

   B True

   C False

   D True

   E True

About two-thirds of tubular fluid is reabsorbed in the proximal tubule, and the main driving force for water reabsorption is Na^+ reabsorption, which is followed by Cl^- and HCO_3^- reabsorption (A). This creates a small osmotic gradient along which water passively diffuses out (isotonic reabsorption). Therefore, the main drive for water reabsorption in the proximal tubule is Na^+ reabsorption.

In the thick ascending limb, NaCl is actively transported into the medullary extracellular fluid and as water cannot follow due to its relative impermeability, the remaining tubular fluid becomes hypotonic (B). The distal convoluted tubule therefore receives this hypotonic fluid from the loop of Henle (C).

The permeability to water is controlled by antidiuretic hormone (ADH, vasopressin) in the distal convoluted tubule to achieve an isotonic tubular fluid (D).

The distal tubule and collecting ducts are only slightly permeable to urea which means that the concentration of urea increases in this part of the nephron. The collecting ducts near the renal papilla are readily permeable to urea, which allows it to diffuse back into the interstitium and so maintain the high osmolality in this region (E).

11. A False

    B True

    C False

    D True

    E True

Aldosterone is produced in the zona glomerulosa of the adrenal cortex (A), and is the most important mineralocorticoid. The main function of the mineralocorticoids is to regulate the transport of Na^+ and K^+ in the kidney and other organs such as the intestine, gallbladder and salivary glands.

Cholesterol is taken up from the plasma and acts as the precursor to the synthesis of the sex hormones (such as testosterone, progesterone and oestradiol), glucocorticoids (such as cortisol) and the mineralocorticoid aldosterone (B).

The rate of formation and release of aldosterone fluctuates according to the salt intake and time of day. The rate of secretion is highest in the early morning and lowest in the evening (C). This diurnal variation also applies to the renin–angiotensin system as a whole and is thought to also involve changes in posture, stress and melatonin secretion.

Reduced blood volume, hyperkalaemia and hyponatraemia all stimulate the release of aldosterone (D). In response to these stimuli aldosterone causes Na^+ retention and increases K^+ excretion (E). The retained Na^+ results in the secondary retention of water, causing an increase in the extracellular fluid volume, largely via the renin–angiotensin system.

12. A False

    B True

    C True

    D False

    E True

Metabolic acidosis may occur as a result of:

- Failure to excrete the normal acid load in renal failure
- The ingestion of acid
- The excess production of exogenous acid (in diabetes mellitus and starvation where there is incomplete metabolism of fats and ketoacids) (B)
- A high protein intake resulting in increased production of hydrochloric and sulphuric acids (A)
- Loss of HCO_3^- due to diarrhoea or by the kidneys
- The incomplete oxidation of carbohydrate, which occurs in the anaerobic production of lactic acid (C)

Metabolic alkalosis may arise from:

- The increased metabolism of organic anions such as lactate and citrate to CO_2 and H_2O (D)

- Increased intake of alkaline substances
- Persistent vomiting
- Increased renal excretion of H$^+$ ions in K$^+$ deficiency

A diet high in vegetable matter produces a large amount of HCO$_3$$^-$ which is excreted in the urine making it alkaline (E).

13. **A** False

   B False

   C True

   D True

   E False

The oesophagus enters the stomach at the cardia in the fundus. The body, antrum and pylorus make up the rest of the stomach, which leads onto the duodenum.

The size of the stomach is dependent on its contents; as it fills, it is the proximal portion that enlarges (A).

The tubular glands of the stomach mucosa contain chief cells and parietal cells, which produce some of the contents of gastric acid. The gastric mucosa also contains endocrine cells and mucus-producing cells (B).

The rate at which the stomach empties is dependent on signals from the stomach and duodenum (C). The stomach signals are from nervous stimulation caused by distension and the hormone gastrin, which is secreted from the antral mucosa. This increases pyloric pumping force and inhibits the pylorus, thus promoting stomach emptying. The signals from the duodenum, however, depress the pyloric pump and usually increase pyloric tone (D).

Gastrin causes the secretion of acidic gastric juices by the stomach and it has a moderate stimulatory effect on motor functions of the stomach. By enhancing the activity of the pyloric pump gastric emptying is promoted (E).

14. **A** False

   B True

   C True

   D False

   E False

Jaundice, or *icterus*, generally develops when the bilirubin concentration in the plasma is >18 µmol/L (A). It is initially the sclera that takes on the characteristic yellow colour, followed by the skin.

In pre-hepatic jaundice, there is an increased production of bilirubin, e.g. due to excess haemolysis, when increased production far exceeds the liver's capacity to conjugate the bilirubin. Therefore, there is excess unconjugated bilirubin in the plasma (B).

Hepatic jaundice can occur as a result of damaged hepatocytes, inflammation of the liver cells (hepatitis), deficiency of glucuronyl transferase (Gilbert's syndrome), inhibition of glucuronyl transferase (by steroids) or an inborn defect of bilirubin secretion into the bile canaliculi (Dubin–Johnson syndrome) (C). Glucuronyl transferase is the enzyme responsible for conjugation of bilirubin for further metabolism; therefore, a reduction in glucuronyl transferase activity leads to an increase in unconjugated bilirubin levels. Gilbert's syndrome is the single most common form of hereditary hyperbilirubinaemia and is thought to occur in up to 10% of the population.

Only some causes of hepatic jaundice, such as certain forms of hepatocellular damage and Dubin–Johnson syndrome, result in dark urine, although all forms of post-hepatic jaundice do (D). The cause of the dark urine is elevated levels of conjugated, water soluble, bilirubin. It can be seen therefore that a failure in conjugation of bilirubin will not lead to dark urine.

Post-hepatic jaundice usually occurs as a result of obstruction to the bile ducts by stones or tumours, which causes increased levels of conjugated bilirubin in the bloodstream. In post-hepatic jaundice, there is very little bilirubin that enters the intestine. This is where bilirubin is broken down by intestinal bacteria to stercobilinogen, which is then oxidised to stercobilin. Stercobilin is the substance that gives faeces its characteristic brown colour. Lower levels of stercobilinogen in the intestine thus result in pale-coloured stools (E).

15. **A** False

    B True

    C True

    D False

    E True

Many factors influence the control and regulation of hepatic blood flow (see **Table 2.3**). The supine position and food increase blood flow to the liver (A, D).

During hypoxia, blood flow is redistributed from the kidneys and gastrointestinal tract to vital organs such as the heart and brain, thereby reducing hepatic perfusion (B).

Table 2.3 Factors affecting hepatic blood flow	
Decreased blood flow	**Increased blood flow**
Positive pressure ventilation	Food
Hypoxia	Acute hepatitis
Hypercarbia	Supine posture
Abdominal surgery	Enzyme inducing drugs
Ganglion blocking drugs	
Vasopressin	
Volatile anaesthetics	

Positive pressure ventilation causes a reduction in hepatic blood flow as this increases intra-thoracic pressure, which reduces venous return to the heart, thus reducing cardiac output and blood flow to the liver (C).

Volatile anaesthetics also decrease cardiac output which results in decreased hepatic blood flow (E).

16. **A** False

    B False

    C True

    D True

    E False

Fever is an abnormally high body temperature and the most frequent cause is infection by viruses and bacteria. Prostaglandins, released by phagocytes, reset the hypothalamic thermostat at a higher temperature (A). The temperature regulating reflex mechanisms will then act to bring the core body temperature up to this new setting, thus increasing the body temperature.

In heat exhaustion, the body temperature is generally normal and there is profuse perspiration resulting in cool and clammy skin (B). The symptoms of heat exhaustion are dizziness, muscle cramps, vomiting and fainting and are due to the loss of fluids and electrolytes.

Heatstroke can occur when the temperature and relative humidity are high, making it difficult for the body to lose heat by radiation, conduction or evaporation (C). The blood flow to the skin is decreased and perspiration is reduced resulting in the body temperature increasing.

The elderly are more prone to hypothermia as they have a reduced metabolic response to lower temperatures and a reduced perception of cold as well as hot temperatures (D).

Macrophages release interleukins 1 and 6 (IL-1, IL-6) once they become active during inflammation and infection (E). The interleukins promote the synthesis of proteins in the liver that act as pyrogens to generate fever.

17. **A** False

    B True

    C False

    D True

    E True

The secretion of hormones by endocrine glands is stimulated or inhibited by three main mechanisms:

- Signals from the nervous system (A)
- Chemical changes in the blood (B)
- Other hormones (D)

Most hormones are released in short bursts, with little or no secretion in between these episodes (C). At resting states the blood levels of the hormones are low, but when stimulated the glands will release the hormones in bursts and the blood levels will then increase.

Many hormones are regulated by negative and positive feedback mechanisms, but most often it is a negative feedback system maintaining the homeostasis of hormone secretion (E).

In a negative feedback system, the secretion of the hormone is decreased as its levels at the target organ rise. The converse occurs in a positive feedback system; for example, oxytocin is released to stimulate contractions of the uterus and as the uterus contracts more oxytocin is released.

18. A True

B True

C False

D True

E False

The main physiological action of insulin is to decrease the blood glucose concentrations, i.e. to oppose the actions of glucagon. It does this by:

- Increasing the transport of glucose from blood into cells (A)
- Increasing glycogenesis (conversion of glucose into glycogen) (B)
- Increasing lipogenesis (conversion of glucose into fatty acids) (C)
- Decreasing glycogenolysis (breakdown of glycogen to glucose-1-phosphate and glucose)
- Reducing gluconeogenesis (formation of glucose from non-carbohydrate substances such as lactate)
- Increasing protein synthesis

The secretion of insulin is largely under control of a negative feedback mechanism involving blood glucose concentrations. An increase in blood glucose concentrations will stimulate insulin secretion and decreased concentrations inhibit it.

There are also other mechanisms of insulin secretion:

- Increased blood levels of amino acids can stimulate insulin release
- Human growth hormone (hGH) raises plasma glucose concentrations which then stimulate insulin secretion
- Adrenocorticotrophic hormone (ACTH) increases plasma glucose concentrations which then stimulate insulin release (D)
- Somatostatin inhibits the release of insulin
- Increased parasympathetic activity stimulates the release of insulin (E)

19. A False

B True

C False

D False

E True

Cerebral blood flow (CBF) is affected my many factors. Of note, between a $Paco_2$ of 2.7 and 10.7 kPa, there is a linear increase in CBF by approximately 2–4% for each 0.13 kPa (1 mmHg) increase in $Paco_2$ (A). For each degree Celsius decrease in body temperature, there is a 5% decrease in CBF (B). Volatile anaesthetics such as isoflurane increase CBF by a vasodilatory effect, while thiopentone reduces CBF and cerebral oxygen consumption (C, E). Opioids such as fentanyl have no direct effect on CBF when administered as sole agents (D). Other factors affecting CBF are summarised in **Table 2.4.**

Table 2.4 Factors affecting cerebral blood flow (CBF)

Increased CBF	Reduced CBF	No effect
Hypercapnia	Hypocapnia	$Pao_2 > 6.7$ kPa
$Pao_2 < 6.7$ mmHg	Mean arterial pressures < 50 mmHg	Opioids
Mean arterial pressures > 150 mmHg	Sympathetic stimulation	
Parasympathetic stimulation	Thiopentone	
All volatile agents	Propofol	
Ketamine	Benzodiazepines	
Increased blood viscosity	Etomidate	

20. **A** True

   B True

   C False

   D True

   E False

Safe transfusion is dependent on full cross matching. Incompatible blood based on the ABO and Rhesus systems in particular causes agglutination due to antigen–antibody complexes (see **Table 2.5**).

Table 2.5 Blood group genotypes, antigens and antibodies

Blood group	% of population	Genotype	Red cell antigen	Plasma antibody
A	42	AA/AO	A	Anti-B
B	8	BB/BO	B	Anti-A
AB	3	AB	A and B	None
O	47	OO	None	Anti-A and anti-B

21. A True

B True

C False

D True

E False

The hepatic extraction ratio (HER) is the proportion of drug removed by the liver. It is affected by three main factors:

- Hepatic blood flow representing drug delivery (B)
- Free or unbound drug fraction representing the fraction of drug that can interact with hepatic enzymes (A)
- Intrinsic metabolic capacity of enzymes represented by Michaelis–Menton constants, accounting for the intrinsic ability of liver enzymes to metabolise individual substances in the absence of flow or protein-binding restrictions (D)
- pKa and lipid solubility have no direct effects on hepatic extraction ratio (C, E)

The HER can be high, intermediate or low:

- *High HER (>0.7):* 'flow-dependent clearance' – high metabolic capacity for a drug causes rapid removal of free drug from the circulation. This clearance is independent of protein binding, but highly dependent on hepatic blood flow. Examples include propofol, ketamine, morphine and lidocaine.
- *Intermediate HER (0.3–0.7)* – clearance is affected by changes in protein binding, metabolic capacity and hepatic perfusion. Examples include aspirin and codeine.
- *Low HER (<0.3):* 'capacity-limited clearance' – Low metabolic capacity means even if there is low protein binding, enzymes saturate rapidly and a concentration gradient between plasma and hepatocytes is eliminated rapidly. Clearance is independent of hepatic blood flow. Examples include warfarin, phenytoin and diazepam.

22. A False

B False

C True

D True

E False

The time constant, τ, is the time taken for the plasma concentration of a drug to reduce to zero had the original rate of change continued (B). It is inversely proportional to the rate constant (k) and clearance (Cl), but directly proportional to the volume of distribution (V_D) (A), and can be represented by:

$$\tau = \frac{V_D}{Cl}$$

Therefore, as V_D increases, so will τ (D). After one time constant, the plasma concentration will have fallen by 63%; thus, 63% of the process will be complete. After two time constants, the plasma concentration will have fallen by 87%, while after three time constants the plasma concentration will have fallen by 95% (C).

τ is longer than the half-life, irrespective of the drug (E):

$$t_{1/2} = 0.693.\tau$$

23. A False

   B False

   C True

   D False

   E True

Drug elimination is usually an exponential process, meaning the rate of change is proportional to the concentration of the drug at that time. This is also called first-order kinetics. With certain drugs, elimination becomes independent of concentration and is constant, known as zero-order kinetics **(Figure 2.3)**.

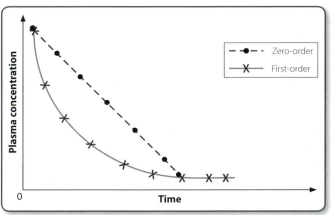

Figure 2.3 First and zero-order kinetics.

Plasma concentrations may not reach a steady state on administration of drug, because as more drug is delivered above the rate of metabolism or excretion, accumulation of the drug will occur. In addition, small increases in dosage may lead to large increases in plasma concentration. These drugs are often described as having a 'narrow therapeutic window,' and may need plasma levels checking to ensure they are within the therapeutic range. Some drugs undergo both first- and zero-order kinetics depending on plasma concentration and enzymatic saturation.

The following drugs undergo zero-order kinetics (**PESTT**):

Phenytoin

Ethanol

Salicylates (C)

Thiopentone

Theophylline (E)

Clonidine, paracetamol and methanol all undergo first-order kinetics (A, B, D).

24. A True

   B False

   C False

   D False

   E False

Drug binding to plasma proteins depends on:

- Free drug concentration
- Drug affinity to protein-binding sites
- Protein concentration

The two most common plasma proteins binding drugs are albumin and α_1-glycoprotein (also called α_1 acid glycoprotein). Albumin is a basic protein thus binds predominantly acidic and neutral drugs such as warfarin, non-steroidal anti-inflammatories, phenytoin, diazepam, thiopentone and propofol (B, C, E). α_1-glycoprotein is acidic therefore binds mainly basic drugs such as morphine, fentanyl, lidocaine and quinine (A). Paracetamol is only minimally protein-bound and would preferentially bind to albumin (D).

25. A False

   B False

   C False

   D True

   E True

Thiobarbiturates and oxybarbiturates display different properties. Thiobarbiturates are generally very lipid soluble, highly protein bound and metabolised in the liver. Oxybarbiturates are usually less lipoid soluble, less protein bound and can be excreted unchanged in the urine (A).

Thiopentone is a highly lipid soluble and protein-bound barbiturate. It is approximately 80% protein bound and is one of the most highly protein-bound barbiturates (B).

Barbiturates are known to increase the duration of opening of GABA-dependent chloride channels in the central nervous system, increasing chloride conductance and resulting in hyperpolarisation of the channels and subsequent neuronal inhibition. Thiobarbiturates are known to only act on the β-subunit of GABA$_A$ receptors (C).

Thiopentone is the sulphur analogue of the oxybarbiturate pentobarbitone (D).

All barbiturates are derived from barbituric acid, which is the condensation product of urea and malonic acid (**Figure 2.4**) (E).

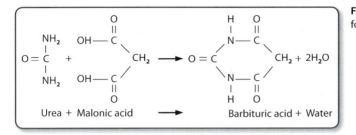

Figure 2.4 Barbituric acid formation.

26. A True

  B False

  C True

  D True

  E False

Ketamine is a phencyclidine derivative. It stimulates the sympathetic nervous system, which is the opposite effect of other induction agents (A). As a result there is an increase in the plasma levels of noradrenaline and adrenaline, causing an increase in heart rate, cardiac output and blood pressure. These cardiovascular changes result in an increase in myocardial oxygen demand (B).

Ketamine can increase the respiratory rate and preserves laryngeal reflexes. It also causes bronchodilatation, so is a useful induction agent for patients with brittle or poorly controlled asthma (C).

Ketamine causes dissociation between the thalamocortical and limbic systems (D). It also acts as a potent analgesic and has amnesic properties. Vivid and unpleasant dreams, hallucinations and delirium can all occur following the use of ketamine, but may be reduced by using opioids or benzodiazepines concurrently. These central nervous system side effects are less common in the extremes of age and in patients who are allowed to wake up in a quiet undisturbed recovery area. There is also an increase in the cerebral blood flow and intracranial pressure.

Nausea and vomiting occur more frequently than with the administration of other intravenous induction agents (E).

27. A False

  B False

  C True

  D True

  E True

The partial pressure of anaesthetic gas in the alveoli is in equilibrium with that in the arterial blood, that is in turn in equilibrium with that in the brain at steady state. The alveolar partial pressure of the anaesthetic gases is therefore an indirect measure of the partial pressure in the brain. There are many factors which can speed up the rise in alveolar partial pressure and hence that in the brain.

Adding nitrous oxide to oxygen will result in a faster rise in the alveolar partial pressure as the nitrous oxide rapidly diffuses across the alveolar capillary membrane, leaving a relatively larger concentration of anaesthetic gas in the alveoli, and hence a more rapid rise in the partial pressure of anaesthetic agent. The nitrous oxide mixture therefore exhibits the concentration effect and second gas effect which is not seen with air/oxygen mixtures (A).

With a high cardiac output, the concentration gradient between the alveoli and pulmonary blood is maintained and as a result the partial pressure of the anaesthetic gases in the alveoli rises slowly. The opposite is true for a low cardiac output (B).

An increase in ventilation will cause a faster rise in the alveolar concentration (C), as does an increase in inspired concentration of volatile anaesthetic (D).

Patients with a small functional residual capacity have a small volume present to dilute the inspired anaesthetic gas, so the rise in alveolar partial pressure is rapid, which results in a faster onset of anaesthesia (E). Conversely, a large functional residual capacity dilutes the inspired concentration, which then slows down the rate of rise in partial pressure.

28. **A** True

    B False

    C False

    D False

    E True

Paracetamol is classed as a non-steroidal anti-inflammatory drug (NSAID) (A) despite having no effect on cyclo-oxygenase (B). It has been included in this group because of its moderate analgesic and anti-pyretic properties.

The exact mechanism of the anti-pyretic effect is unknown, but it is thought to be due to inhibition of prostaglandin synthesis in the central nervous system; it has no effect on the leukotrienes (C).

Paracetamol is metabolised by the liver to glucuronide, sulphate and cysteine conjugates (D). The main metabolites are the glucuronide conjugates that are actively excreted in the urine. One of the metabolites, N-acetyl-p-amino-benzoquinoneimine, is highly toxic but is rapidly conjugated and then excreted. Following toxic doses of paracetamol, this conjugation pathway becomes saturated and the toxic metabolite accumulates causing hepatocellular damage.

Paracetamol is well absorbed from the gut and has an oral bioavailability of 80% (E). It does not cause irritation to the stomach lining unlike the other NSAIDs.

29. **A** False

    B False

    C True

    D False

    E True

An 'opioid' is a substance that includes naturally occurring and synthetic substances that have an affinity for opioid receptors. 'Opiates' are naturally occurring substances with morphine-like properties. There are several subtypes of opioid receptors, and they are found in the central nervous system, spinal cord and peripherally. The classification originally included σ-receptors, which produced mydriasis, tachypnoea and delirium, but have now been excluded as opioid receptors as they are not reversed by naloxone and exhibit a high affinity for ketamine (A).

μ_1-Receptors produce analgesia; μ_2-receptors produce respiratory depression, inhibit gut motility, cause miosis and euphoria and can cause bradycardia (B). κ-receptors cause analgesia, sedation and miosis, and δ-receptors cause analgesia and respiratory depression.

There are thought to be three κ-receptor subtypes (κ_1, κ_2 and κ_3) acting on G_i G-protein-coupled receptors, three μ-receptor subtypes and two δ-receptor subtypes (C).

Opioid receptors are located presynaptically and activate the inhibitory G_i isoform of G-protein-coupled receptors leading to cell membrane hyperpolarisation (D).

Naloxone is a pure opioid antagonist and reverses the opioid effects at μ-, κ- and δ-receptors (E). It does, however, have its highest affinity for μ-receptors.

30. **A** True

   B False

   C True

   D False

   E False

Quinidine is the prototype class Ia agent. It slows phase 0 of the action potential but leaves the resting potential unaltered. Conduction through atrial, ventricular and Purkinje fibres is slowed, whereas atrioventricular nodal conduction may accelerate due to its vagolytic effects. It is active against both atrial and ventricular arrhythmias (A).

Flecainide is a fluorinated aromatic hydrocarbon and is the prototype of class Ic agents. It is used to suppress ventricular arrhythmias. Lignocaine is the first-line drug used for treating ventricular arrhythmias (B).

Disopyramide is a class Ia antiarrhythmic agent, with electrophysiological properties similar to those of quinidine, but with some added class III activity. It is active against both atrial and ventricular ectopics (C).

β-Blockers are class II agents and are of value in the prevention and treatment of supraventricular arrhythmias, especially those due to Wolf–Parkinson–White syndrome (D).

Sotalol is a non-selective β-adrenoceptor antagonist which also prolongs cardiac repolarisation, thus demonstrating both class II and class III properties (E).

31. A False

   B True

   C False

   D True

   E True

Amiodarone is a unique wide-spectrum antiarrhythmic drug. It is mainly a class III agent but also has powerful class I activity and ancillary class II and IV activity (A). It blocks sodium, calcium and repolarising potassium channels.

Amiodarone is effective in atrial fibrillation because of its actions on the superior pulmonary veins and atrioventricular (AV) node (B). Amiodarone prolongs the refractory period of the superior pulmonary veins and inhibits the AV node. It also non-competitively blocks α- and β-adrenergic receptors (class II). The weak class IV (calcium antagonist) effect may explain bradycardia and AV nodal inhibition and the low incidence of Torsades de Pointes.

Amiodarone requires a large oral loading dose as it has a slow onset of action when given orally (C). It has low gastrointestinal absorption of up to 50% bioavailability and is slowly eliminated with a long half-life of up to 6 months. It undergoes extensive hepatic metabolism and is mostly (95%) protein bound. Excretion is largely via the biliary tract and skin.

Intravenous amiodarone is indicated for the treatment and prophylaxis of frequently recurring ventricular fibrillation or destabilising ventricular tachycardia and in those patients refractory to other treatments (D). Intravenous amiodarone can cause hypotension.

The commonest side effect of amiodarone use is sinus bradycardia, especially in the elderly. Other side effects include optic neuritis/neuropathy, skin discoloration, photosensitivity, hypothyroidism, hyperthyroidism, pulmonary fibrosis, peripheral neuropathy and hepatotoxicity (E).

32. A False

   B True

   C False

   D True

   E False

Inodilators are agents which have both inotropic and vasodilator properties. They are able to reduce afterload and preload whist increasing myocardial contractility.

Low-dose dopamine, milrinone and dobutamine are inotropes that belong to this group of drugs.

At low doses, dopamine acts on dopaminergic receptors peripherally which inhibits noradrenaline release and thus causes vasodilatation. It also has inotropic effects by acting on the β-adrenoceptors in the heart. At high doses, dopamine causes α-adrenoceptor stimulation with peripheral vasoconstriction (A).

The phosphodiesterase inhibitors are also inodilators. They are usually reserved for very serious haemodynamic situations such as acute left ventricular (LV) failure with a low cardiac output despite adequate LV filling pressure. Milrinone is an example that inhibits the breakdown of cyclic adenosine monophosphate in cardiac and peripheral vascular smooth muscle, resulting in augmented myocardial contractility and peripheral arterial and venous dilatation (B). The dilator effect helps to conserve myocardial oxygen consumption.

Adrenaline has mixed β_1- and β_2-stimulatory actions with some added a-effects at high doses. A low infusion rate decreases blood pressure (by its vasodilator effect), and a higher dose will increase peripheral resistance and blood pressure (combined inotropic and vasoconstrictor effect) (C).

Dobutamine has potent inotropic effects with β_2-stimulatory actions too, resulting in vasodilation, potentially resulting in hypotension (D).

Sodium nitroprusside is a donor of nitric acid that vasodilates by formation of cyclic guanosine monophosphate in vascular tissue. It has no inotropic action (E).

33. **A** True

  B False

  C False

  D False

  E True

Local anaesthetics are weak bases that must be in the unionised state to penetrate the phospholipid membrane into the cytoplasma, where they become ionised and block sodium channel activity (C).

Potency is related to lipid solubility, where the more lipid soluble, the more potent (A).

Duration of action is directly proportional to protein binding, as drug bound to protein represents a store of drug (B).

Speed of onset is determined by the pKa as this determines the state of ionisation. The pKa is the pH at which there is equilibrium between ionised and unionised states. For weak bases such as local anaesthetic agents, they are more ionised below their pKa, thus the higher the pKa, the more ionised a drug will be at physiological pH (D). Because it is the unionised form that is active, the lower the pKa, the faster the speed of onset (E).

34. **A** False

  B False

  C False

  D False

  E True

Eutectic mixture of local anaesthetic (EMLA) is composed of 2.5% lidocaine with 2.5% prilocaine (A). The term eutectic means that the mixture of two substances produces a third with unique physical properties. In this case, EMLA has a lower melting point than its two constituent substances, thus is an oil at room temperature (B). Once removed from the skin, it may continue to be released from dermal depots, lasting 60–90 minutes (D). The prilocaine within it can be broken down to o-toluidine, not para-aminobenzoic acid (C), a substance that may lead to the development of methaemoglobinaemia (E).

35. A True

   B False

   C True

   D False

   E True

Suxamethonium is a depolarising muscle relaxant that acts by binding to nicotinic acetylcholine receptors and depolarises the membrane, reducing the efficacy of acetylcholine. It has a number of potential adverse effects.

- Hyperkalaemia: depolarisation of muscle cells causes potassium efflux, which can be life-threatening in patients with high potassium or neuromuscular disorders. In normal individuals, serum potassium may increase by up to 0.5 mmol/L
- Arrhythmias: bradycardia may occur, particularly in children or on repeated dosing, due to muscarinic receptor activation at the sinoatrial node (A)
- Raised intraocular pressure: the pressure may be increased by 10 mmHg for minutes, although this can be offset by the use of anaesthetic agents
- Myalgia: post-operative muscle pains occur, predominantly in young women
- Raised intragastric pressure: the pressure increases by 10 cmH$_2$O, but due to an increase in lower oesophageal sphincter tone there is no increased risk of gastric reflux (D)
- Malignant hyperthermia: this is a disorder of the ryanodine receptor causing uncontrolled calcium entry into the cytoplasm leading to increased CO$_2$ production, muscle rigidity, metabolic acidosis, coagulopathy and potentially death. Prompt treatment with dantrolene has reduced the mortality from 70–80% to under 5%
- Suxamethonium apnoea: this condition can be a congenital reduction in plasma cholinesterase activity or acquired in conditions such as renal failure, liver failure, pregnancy and drugs. It leads to a prolonged duration of action of suxamethonium of a number of hours
- Anaphylaxis: suxamethonium is the cause of up to half of all episodes of anaphylaxis due to neuromuscular blocking drugs (E)
- Other effects: suxamethonium may cause rhabdomyolysis and myotonias in patients with neuromuscular disorders (C), as well as masseter spasm

Liver failure is not a recognized complication of suxamethonium use (B).

36. A True

   B True

   C True

   D False

   E False

The anticholinesterases inhibit the enzyme acetylcholinesterase responsible for the hydrolysis of acetylcholine to acetate and choline. The $N(CH_3)_3{}^+$ of acetylcholine binds to the anionic site of the enzyme, while the $=O-OH$ end binds to the esteratic site. Edrophonium is a quaternary amine that weakly binds to acetylcholinesterase with ionic bonds rather than covalent bonds (A). Neostigmine (B) and pyridostigmine (C) are quaternary amines that form carbamylated complexes with the enzyme, while physostigmine is a tertiary amine with a similar mechanism of action (D). Pralidoxime does have a quaternary amine structure, but it is an acetylcholinesterase reactivator rather than inhibitor and is used to treat organophosphorus poisoning (E).

37. **A** False

B False

C True

D False

E True

Antimicrobials are drugs used to either prevent bacterial cell replication (bacteriostatic) or directly kill bacteria (bactericidal). They can be classed based on their molecular structure or qualities as seen in **Table 2.6**.

Table 2.6 Antibiotic classes

Classification	Antimicrobial
Penicillins	Benzylpenicillin
	Penicillin V
	Amoxicillin
	Flucloxacillin
First-generation cephalosporins	Cefalexin
	Cephradine
	Cefuroxime (D)
Second-generation cephalosporins	Cefaclor
	Cefotaxime
Third-generation cephalosporins	Ceftazidime
β-Lactams	Imipenem
	Meropenem (E)
Tetracyclines	Tetracycline
	Doxycycline
Aminoglycosides	Gentamycin (C)
	Neomycin
Macrolides	Erythromycin
	Clarithromycin (B)
4-Quinolones	Ciprofloxacin (A)
	Nalidixic acid

38. A False

  B True

  C False

  D False

  E True

Midazolam is a benzodiazepine acting on the GABA$_A$ receptor demonstrating the physical property of tautomerism. In solution at a pH of 3.5, it is ionised (C) with an open seven-membered diazepine ring, making it water soluble (D). When the surrounding pH is >4, the ring closes and the midazolam is no longer ionised making it more lipid soluble. Its oral bioavailability is <45% (A), with a volume of distribution of 1–1.5 L/kg and a protein binding of 95% (E). It is metabolised in the liver to 1α-hydroxymidazolam which has weak activity, followed by conjugation then urinary excretion (B).

39. A True

  B False

  C False

  D True

  E True

Tricyclic antidepressants, including imipramine, amitriptyline and nortriptyline, exert their effect by preventing noradrenaline and serotonin reuptake into nerve terminals of monoaminergic neurones by competitively inhibiting uptake 1 (A). Some might also inhibit presynaptic α$_2$-adrenoceptors to increase noradrenaline release. Other mechanisms include antimuscarinic, antihistaminergic (H$_1$ receptors), and antiadrenergic (α$_1$-adrenoceptors) effects (B). As well as antidepressant effects, TCAs cause sedation, fatigue and can be proconvulsant. The antimuscarinic effects include constipation, urinary retention, blurred vision and dry mouth (E). Cardiac effects include postural hypotension and arrhythmias, as well as prolonged PR and QT intervals with amitriptyline. Although their pharmacological effects are immediate, their clinically desired effect may take weeks to manifest (D). Phenelzine is a monoamine oxidase inhibitor (C).

40. A False

  B True

  C False

  D True

  E True

Diuretics are a class of drug that stimulate renal urine production and water excretion. They can be classed as:

- Aldosterone antagonists: spironolactone and eplerenone
- Carbonic anhydrase inhibitors: acetazolamide

- Loop diuretics: furosemide (frusemide)
- Osmotic diuretics: mannitol
- Potassium sparing diuretics: amiloride
- Thiazide diuretics: bendroflumethiazide (bendrofluazide)

Their sites of action can be summarised as seen in **Figure 2.5**.

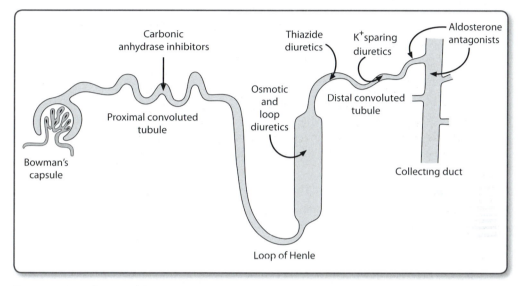

Figure 2.5 Sites of action of diuretics.

41. A True

  B True

  C False

  D False

  E False

Two conductors with a current flowing through them will exert a force on each other. This phenomenon is called magnetism, and the region through which this force is exerted is the magnetic field (A). There is a flow of electrons induced when a magnetic field changes and this results in the production of an electric current (B). The magnetic field strength is defined as the power of the magnetic field in a vacuum, not in air (C). The term magnetic flux is used to describe the magnetic filed present in a material. Diamagnetic materials decrease the magnetic flux, ferromagnetic materials increase it and paramagnetic materials only slightly increase the magnetic flux (D). The unit of magnetic flux is the weber (Wb), and the tesla (T) is the unit of magnetic flux density (E).

42. A False

  B False

C True

D True

E False

Alternating current (AC) is the flow of electrons in one direction and then in the opposite direction, rather like a sine wave if seen graphically. Direct current (DC) is the steady flow of electrons in one direction only. The two can be combined and this results in a current which does not have a steady value but whose electrons generally move in one direction (A).

The unit of current is the ampere which is the flow of 6.24×10^{18} electrons per *second* past a point and it is defined as the electromagnetic force associated with an electric current (B).

In a galvanometer, a current, which is what is being measured, is passed through a coil of wire that is suspended in a magnetic field. As the current flows, the magnetic field makes the coil rotate and this rotational force is proportional to the strength of the current (C).

The potential difference across a conductor is based on energy production and current flow. The unit of potential difference is the volt and this is defined as the potential difference that produces a current of one ampere when the rate of energy dissipated is 1 watt (D).

When a coiled wire has a current passed through it, the magnetic field it produces is strongest within the core of the coil. This can be further increased by placing a ferromagnetic material into the core (E).

43. A False

   B False

   C True

   D False

   E True

The high voltage electricity from power stations is supplied to substations, where the voltage is reduced using transformers (A). This electricity is then transported to the hospital via two wires, one live and one neutral wire. The neutral wire is earthed at the substation, not the live wire (B). At the hospital, the mains sockets have live, neutral and earthed conductors. The current density and the size of the current flowing through the person will determine the effect of the electric shock (C). The flow of current is dependent on the resistance, or impedance, to the flow of electricity through the body. The impedance of skin and tissues is relatively small, which means electricity will flow if an electric circuit is formed when someone is in contact with faulty equipment (D). This is partly why antistatic shoes are worn in the theatre environment. Antistatic shoes provide a high enough impedance to protect against electric shock, but also allow the safe dissipation of electrostatic charges that may build up on the person's clothing (E). The impedance of such shoes should be up to $10\,M\Omega$.

44. A True

 B True

 C False

 D True

 E False

Using the principles of Dalton's law, if a cylinder of air had a pressure of 100 kPa, as 21% of the gas in the cylinder will be oxygen, the partial pressure exerted by oxygen would be 21 kPa (A). Entonox is a 50:50 mixture of nitrous oxide and oxygen, so again using Dalton's law, the pressure exerted by nitrous oxide would be half of the total pressure, 50 kPa (B). Avogadro's hypothesis states that equal volumes of gases at the same temperature and pressure will contain an equal number of molecules. Therefore, two identical cylinders with different gases will contain the same number of molecules (C).

100 kPa is approximately equivalent to:

- 1 bar
- 750 mmHg (D)
- 750 torr
- 14.5 psi
- 1020 cmH$_2$O

The critical temperature of a gas is the temperature above which a gas cannot be liquefied by pressure alone. The critical temperature for oxygen is −119°C, so no matter how much pressure is applied to the oxygen in the cylinder, it would not be possible to liquefy the oxygen at room temperature (E).

45. A True

 B False

 C False

 D True

 E False

'Wash-in' curves are exponential curves (see **Figure 2.6**) and can be seen upon using constant rate infusions of drugs (A).

Figure 2.6 Wash-in curve.

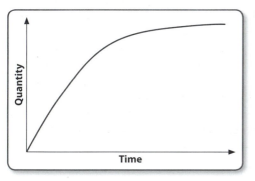

The build-up exponential curve is an inverted negative exponential. An example of this is the curve generated by a constant pressure generator ventilator. When volume is plotted against time, a build-up exponential curve is seen as in **Figure 2.7**. It is similar to a wash-in curve.

A plot of volume against time for inspiration in a patient on a constant flow generator will produce a linear curve, as the rate of filling of the lungs is constant due to the constant flow (see **Figure 2.8**). This is a linear, non-exponential process (B).

The curve produced when the multiplication of cancer cells is plotted against time is an example of a positive exponential curve (C). Another example of this process is the uninhibited multiplication of bacteria (see **Figure 2.9**).

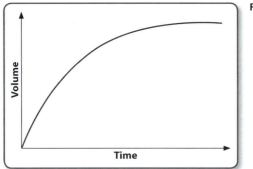

Figure 2.7 Build-up exponential.

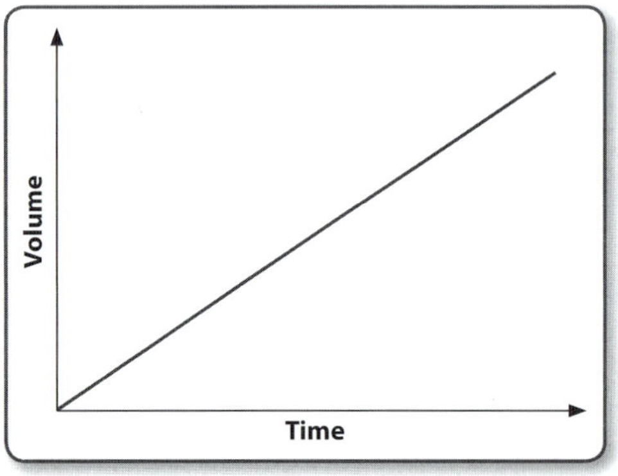

Figure 2.8 Constant flow generator.

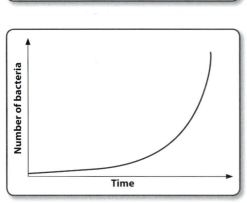

Figure 2.9 Bacterial multiplication.

The expiration of gases from the lungs produces an exponential curve called a 'wash-out' curve (D). This is because the rate of emptying is initially fast then slows down (see **Figure 2.10**).

The wash-out curve seen with the plot of dye concentration against time for the dye dilution technique of measuring cardiac output is an exponential curve, but there is recirculation of dye; therefore, a second curve is seen (see **Figure 2.11**). For the thermodilution technique, a plot of temperature against time shows an exponential wash-out curve, without a second curve (E) (see **Figure 2.12**).

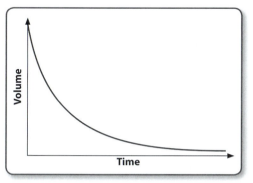

Figure 2.10 Wash-out curve.

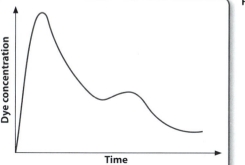

Figure 2.11 Dye dilution curve.

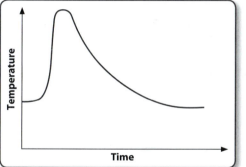

Figure 2.12 Thermodilution curve

46. **A** True

B False

C True

D True

E True

The Système International (SI) of units was established in 1960 and is now the recognised system of measurement communication, which avoids the confusion that used to occur when different systems of units were used.

In medicine, most physical quantities are measured in SI units, but there are a few non-SI units still in use, such as millimetre of mercury (mmHg) and partial gas pressures.

There are base or fundamental SI units (see **Table 2.7**) and derived SI units (see **Table 2.8**).

Table 2.7 Fundamental SI units	
Physical quantity	**SI unit and symbol**
Length	Meter, m
Mass	Kilogram, kg
Time	Second, s
Electric current	Ampere, A
Amount of substance	Mole, mol
Temperature	Kelvin, K
Luminous intensity	Candela, cd

Table 2.8 Derived SI units	
Physical quantity	**Derived SI unit and symbol**
Frequency	Hertz, Hz
Force	Newton, N
Pressure	Pascal, Pa
Energy, work	Joule, J
Power	Watt, W
Electric charge	Coulomb, C
Electric potential	Volt, V
Absorbed dose	Gray, Gy
Temperature	Degrees Celsius, °C

47. A False

   B True

   C False

   D True

   E False

The critical temperature is defined as the temperature above which a substance cannot be liquefied, irrespective of how much pressure is applied (A). The critical pressure is the vapour pressure of a substance at its critical temperature (B).

Dalton's law of partial pressure states that in a mixture of gases the pressure exerted by each gas is the same as that which it would exert if it alone occupied the container (C).

Avogadro's hypothesis states that equal volumes of gases at the same temperature and pressure contain equal numbers of molecules (D). This lends to the ideal gas constant, stating that:

$$\frac{p_1 \times V_1}{T_1 \times n_1} = \frac{p_2 \times V_2}{T_2 \times n_2} = \text{constant}$$

where p is pressure of the gas, V is volume of the gas, T is temperature in kelvin of the gas, and n is number of molecules.

The pseudocritical temperature is the temperature at which a gas mixture will separate out into its constituent parts, and is dependent on the pressure (E).

48. A True

   B True

   C False

   D True

   E False

During the normal breathing process, inspired gases are brought to body temperature and 100% relative humidity by the upper respiratory tract by the time the gases reach the alveoli (A). Essentially the upper respiratory tract acts as a heat and moisture exchanger.

Heat and moisture exchangers are disposable devices that can have a hydrophobic or hygroscopic membrane incorporated within them (B). The hydrophobic membrane has a large surface area and offers low resistance to the flow of gas. The membrane has a low thermal conductivity that can generate a temperature gradient, allowing water vapour from expired gases to condensate on the surface (C). The subsequent inspired breath is then humidified and heated by this condensed water vapour on the membrane mesh. Composite hygroscopic filters are made up of a hygroscopic layer plus a polarised fibre membrane. They work in a similar way to hydrophobic filters, but are more efficient.

During low-flow anaesthesia, heated breathing tubes will increase the humidity of inspired gases (D).

Both pneumatic and ultrasonic nebuliser humidifiers can be heated (E). As well as providing humidification of the inspired gases, they can also be used to deliver drugs to the breathing circuit. Pneumatic nebulisers require a jet of high-pressure gas, whereas ultrasonic nebulisers do not need a driving gas. Ultrasonic nebulisers create smaller and finer droplets compared with pneumatic nebulisers.

49. A True

　　B True

　　C False

　　D True

　　E False

The central core of the human body is maintained at a constant temperature, whereas the surface layer is at a lower temperature that is variable. Core temperature is regulated within very narrow limits of about 37°C ± 0.5°C, surface temperature can range from 32°C to 35°C, depending on physiological factors. This ensures optimal enzymatic activity throughout the core compartments. The anterior hypothalamic nucleus is responsible for thermoregulation in humans (C). The tissues and organs within the core compartment are well perfused and include the brain, thorax and abdominal organs (A) and some of the deep tissues of the limbs with relatively uniform temperatures (D).

The core tissues contribute 60–75% of the thermal input to the thermoregulatory system (E).

50. A True

　　B False

　　C True

　　D False

　　E False

Reynold's number is used to determine whether the flow in a tube will be laminar or turbulent (A). If the calculated number, which is a dimensionless figure, is low then the flow pattern will be laminar, as the viscous forces will dampen any irregularities (B). A high number means that any eddies or vortices present will dominate and this will create turbulent flow. A number <2000 will indicate laminar flow through a tube is most likely, between 2000 and 4000 the flow will be a mixture of laminar and turbulent and >4000 will indicate turbulent flow is most likely (C).

To calculate Reynold's number, the following formula is applied (D, E):

$$Re = \frac{\rho v d}{\eta}$$

where v is the mean flow velocity, d is the characteristic dimension or diameter, ρ is the fluid density, η is the viscosity.

51. A True

   B False

   C False

   D False

   E False

A current of 50–100 µA or more may cause ventricular fibrillation if applied directly to the heart due to high current density (A). This is called microshock. However, a current of 100 mA may cause ventricular fibrillation when applied to the body surface.

Alternating current (AC) requires a lower current than direct current (DC) to cause ventricular fibrillation, although this can occur with both AC and DC (B).

An increase in frequency will reduce the stimulation effect yet increase the heating effect (C). The higher the frequency, the less risk to the patient. A frequency of 50 Hz, which is that of mains current, is the most dangerous.

Ohm's law states that current is indirectly proportional to impedance but directly proportional to potential difference (voltage) (D).

Water reduces the resistive path of a current, in particular if it contains electrolytes. The main impedance is skin resistance that can be up to 1 million ohms which is reduced when wet (E).

52. A False

   B False

   C False

   D True

   E False

Oxygen is stored as a gas in cylinders of molybdenum steel with a black body and white shoulders at a pressure of 137 bar (13700 kPa) (B, C). The pin index system is a safety mechanism designed to prevent incorrect connection of gas cylinders to cylinder yokes, and has pins in positions 2 and 5 for oxygen (A). For larger oxygen cylinders, bull-nosed cylinder connectors with specific internal threads reduce the risk of incorrect cylinder connection.

In a cylinder manifold, size J cylinders are used with a capacity of 6800 L, while size E cylinders are used on anaesthetic machines with a capacity of 680 L of oxygen (D).

Because oxygen is stored in cylinders as a gas above its critical temperature (–118°C), Boyle's law may be applied. This states that at a constant temperature, the volume of a fixed mass of a perfect gas varies inversely with the pressure. Thus, the decrease in pressure is a linear one with progressive use of oxygen within the cylinder (E).

53. A False

   B False

C False

D True

E True

Entonox is a mixture of 50% oxygen and 50% nitrous oxide (N_2O) by volume that is used to provide analgesia without disruption of consciousness. Its analgesic effects take 30 seconds and continue for approximately 1 minute after cessation. It is stored as a gas in cylinders with French blue bodies and white and blue quartered shoulders at 13,700 kPa (B). The pseudocritical temperature is the temperature at which a gas mixture may separate out into its constituent components, and is −5.5°C for Entonox (A). This separation is called the Poynting effect, and when it occurs the cylinder contents include a liquid mixture of nitrous oxide with a gas mixture of predominantly oxygen above it. Thus, when used there will be an initial high concentration of oxygen which is used up first followed by a hypoxic mixture of nitrous oxide (C). By storing cylinders horizontally at temperatures above −5.5°C and mixing the cylinders before use, this potentially hazardous effect can be avoided (see **Figure 2.13**) (D).

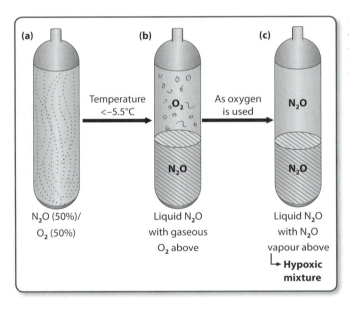

Figure 2.13 Entonox separates out into nitrous oxide liquid and oxygen gas leading to the potential delivery of a hypoxic gas mixture.

Entonox is delivered on demand by a two-stage pressure demand regulator mouthpiece, most commonly the Carnét demand valve (E). The first stage of the valve contains two chambers to reduce the inlet pressure, while the second-stage chamber delivers the gas on inspiration by the patient at ambient pressure.

54. A True

B True

C True

D True

E True

Flow is the quantity of fluid passing a given point per unit time, where fluid can be gas or liquid. Methods for measurement in gases or liquids include:

- Rotameters: constant pressure, variable orifice devices in anaesthetic machines
- Pneumotachographs: constant orifice, variable pressure devices using variable pressure transduces and laminar resistors
- Pitot tubes: variation of pneumotachographs with two tubes facing opposite directions attached to differential pressure transducers (see **Figure 2.14**) (D)

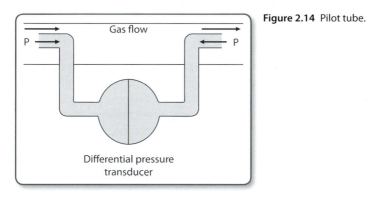

Figure 2.14 Pilot tube.

- Electromagnetic flowmeter: change in temperature of thermistors is proportional to gas flow (A)
- Wright respirometer: constant pressure, variable orifice relying on a rotating vane based on expiratory flow rates (C)
- Bourdon gauge
- Ultrasonic flowmeters: turbulence in a rod causes oscillations which may be measured by a Doppler probe, the frequency of oscillations being proportional to gas flow (B)
- Fick principle
- Benedict Roth spirometers

Methods for flow measurement only in liquids include:

- Visual observation
- Infrared drip counters (E)
- Pumps: Infusion or volumetric

55. A True

B False

C False

D False

E True

The Tec Mark 6 is a vapouriser specifically designed for use with desflurane because the agent has characteristic physical properties. Firstly, the saturated vapour pressure is 89.2 kPa at 20°C meaning traditional plenum vapourisers would be unable to deliver safe concentrations without very high fresh gas flow rates. In addition, the boiling point of desflurane is 23.5°C which is very close to room temperature. This would lead to significant variation in concentrations of vapour that are delivered.

To optimise desflurane delivery despite these physical properties, the Tec Mark 6 vapouriser electrically heats desflurane to 39°C at a pressure of 194 kPa (nearly 2 atmospheres), after which the gaseous desflurane is directly added to the fresh gas flow (A, E). The amount of vapour added to the fresh gas flow must therefore be proportional to the fresh gas flow rate which is achieved using a flow restrictor to the fresh gas flow causing increased back pressure that is detected by differential pressure transducers altering vapour delivery (D).

The mechanics are different to conventional plenum vapourisers, such as the Tec Mark 5, which pass the fresh gas flow directly into the vapourising chamber and maximise saturation using wicks and baffles (B). Tec Mark 5 and older vapourisers are also temperature compensated using bimetallic strips or aneroid bellows, are temperature stabilised with a heat sink enclosure with high specific heat capacity and thermal conductivity (C).

56. **A** True

    B False

    C True

    D True

    E True

Scavenging systems can either be passive or active. Passive scavenging systems are simple and cheap, require no external energy supply (D), and comprise of:

- A collecting and transfer system: 30 mm connectors are used to avoid accidental connection to breathing circuits that have connectors sized 15 and 22 mm (B). The collecting tubing is attached to expiratory valves or adjustable pressure-limiting (APL) valves and is driven by patient expiration or the ventilator (C)
- A receiving system: this may use reservoir bags. These contain pressure relief valves to avoid positive pressures of >1000 Pa (1 kPa) and negative pressures <−50 Pa (A)
- A disposal system: this comprises wide-bore tubing to the roof of the building or theatre ventilation system. It uses wind to entrain expired gases. Because this is a ventile system, excessive pressures caused by wind may lead to reversal of flow and inefficient scavenging (E).

57. **A** False

    B True

    C False

D True

E False

The Bain breathing system is a coaxial Mapleson D arrangement in which the inner 14 mm tube is connected to the fresh gas flow, and the outer 30 mm tube leads to the reservoir bag and adjustable pressure-limiting (APL) valve at the machine end (B). It is the most efficient breathing system for controlled ventilation, with its efficiency not being affected by the length of the tubing (A). It is commonly used in anaesthetic practice due to its compactness at the patient end (C). The Bain breathing system can be attached to the Penlon Nuffield 200 ventilator and must have an internal volume of >500 mL (E).

The internal tube can become disconnected or kink leading to failed oxygenation, despite apparent movement of the reservoir bag. To check the patency of the internal tubing, the Pethick Test can be applied. This entails occluding the end of the circuit and filling it with oxygen from the emergency oxygen flush with the APL valve closed, then releasing the occlusion and pressing the emergency oxygen flush once again. Because of the Venturi effect, a patent inner tube will cause the reservoir bag to collapse as the air within the larger tube becomes entrained (D).

58. A True

   B True

   C True

   D False

   E True

Pulse oximetry utilises spectrophotometric principles of absorption of radiation through a sample (C). Beer's law relates the absorption of radiation through a solution to its concentration, while Lambert's law relates the absorption of radiation to the thickness of the layers it passes through (A). At least two light-emitting diodes (LEDs) emit light at the red wavelength of 660 nm at which deoxyhaemoglobin is better absorbed and infrared wavelengths of 940 nm where oxyhaemoglobin is better absorbed (B, D). Each LED may be on or off, with a sequence cycling up to 30 times a second.

Both constant absorption (due to venous blood, tissue and bone) and non-constant absorption due to arterial blood occurs, with only the non-constant absorption being interpreted and analysed by microprocessors (E).

59. A True

   B True

   C False

   D True

   E True

Severinghaus electrodes are designed to indirectly measure partial pressure of carbon dioxide in a sample. They are a modification of the pH electrode, containing a carbon dioxide permeable membrane separating the sample and a thin film of sodium bicarbonate solution in contact with hydrogen ion sensitive glass (A, E). As the carbon dioxide diffuses into the solution, it then reacts with the water to generate hydrogen ions that are sensed by the glass. There is also a silver/silver chloride reference electrode in contact with the electrolyte solution (C).

Because carbon dioxide must diffuse across the membrane to produce a response, it means that this electrode is a slow response device, taking 2–3 minutes for a result (B). In addition, it must be temperature controlled at 37°C and regularly calibrated (D).

60. A True

B True

C False

D False

E True

Non-invasive blood pressure measurement may be continuous or intermittent (**Table 2.9**).

Table 2.9 Methods of non-invasive blood pressure measurement	
Continuous	**Intermittent**
Finapres (Peñaz technique)	Manual (e.g. sphygmomanometer)
Doppler ultrasound	von Recklinghausen oscillotonometer
	Automated oscillometry

The use of cuffs for blood pressure measurement may potentially lead to inaccuracies. Over-reading may occur if the cuff is too small and too tight in obese patients, and may also occur if the systolic pressure is <60 mmHg (A, B, E). Under-reading may be seen with large cuffs and high systolic pressures. They may be inaccurate in atrial fibrillation and arrhythmias or with external compression (C). Shivering may lead to failure of measurement or inaccurate measurement (D).

Answers: SBAs

61. D Pulmonary artery

Pulmonary artery catheters, although diminishing in use, allow cardiac output monitoring as well as demonstrating useful physiological principles. It is inserted via an internal jugular or subclavian vein sheath, then the balloon tip is inflated with 1–1.5 mL of air allowing the catheter to be 'floated' through the tricuspid valve, right ventricle, pulmonary valve, pulmonary artery and then wedged in pulmonary capillaries. The pressure waveform varies depending on the location of the catheter tip as demonstrated by the pressure waveform seen in **Figure 2.15**.

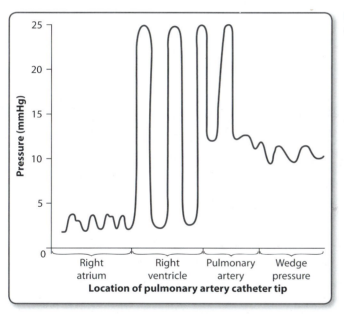

Figure 2.15 Pulmonary artery catheter pressure waveforms.

The pressures seen in the waveforms include:

- Right atrium: 0–5 mmHg
- Right ventricle: 20–25/0–5 mmHg
- Pulmonary artery: 20–25/10–15 mmHg
- Pulmonary artery wedge pressure: 6–12 mmHg (end expiratory)

Thus, a pressure of 24/14 probably corresponds with pulmonary arterial pressure.

Cross M, Plunkett E. Physics, pharmacology and physiology for anaesthetists – key concepts for the FRCA. Cambridge: Cambridge University Press; 2008.

62. A Reduced interstitial hydrostatic pressure

The clinical features described suggest development of acute negative pressure pulmonary oedema, a recognised risk with prolonged laryngospasm and airway obstruction. Because of occlusion of upper airways, highly negative intrathoracic pressures are generated, thereby allowing in-drawing of fluid from the pulmonary vasculature into the interstitium due to Starling forces:

$$\dot{Q} = K\,[(P_c - P_i) - \sigma\,(\pi_c - \pi_i)]$$

where $\dot{Q}$ is the net fluid flow, K is the capillary filtration coefficient, P_c and P_i are the hydrostatic pressures in capillaries and interstitium respectively, σ is the reflection coefficient, representing membrane permeability, and π_c and π_i are the oncotic pressures in capillaries and interstitium respectively.

The reduced interstitial hydrostatic pressure (P_i) compared to the capillary hydrostatic pressure (P_c) would encourage fluid to flow from the latter to the former in this patient.

There is no evidence of excessive fluid administration, capillary hydrostatic pressure is unlikely to increase significantly and oncotic pressure would remain unchanged. The interstitial hydrostatic pressure, as mentioned, will reduce.

McConkey PP. Postobstructive pulmonary oedema: A case series and review. Anaesth Intensive Care 2000; 28:72–76.

63. D 10 mL of 0.25% bupivacaine

In paediatric practice, caudal blocks are commonly performed with patients under general anaesthesia. The dosing follows the Armitage regimen, whereby 0.25% bupivacaine is used at a volume of 0.5 mL/kg for a lumbosacral block up to L1, 1 mL/kg for a thoracolumbar T10 block and 1.25 mL/kg for a T6 block. Although the other regimes quoted are within accepted dosing maximums, the most suitable regime for this patient would be 10 mL of 0.25% bupivacaine.

Brown TCK, Eyres RJ, McDougall RJ. Local and regional anaesthesia in children. Br J Anaesth 1999; 83:65–77.

64. C Beriplex (prothrombin complex concentrate)

Warfarin acts by inhibition of vitamin K epoxide reductase, the enzyme responsible for oxidising vitamin K after carboxylation of clotting factors II (prothrombin), VII (proconvertin), IX (Christmas factor) and X (Stuart–Prower factor). Reversal of the effects of this vitamin K antagonist is dependent on severity of coagulopathy and urgency of reversal.

Vitamin K: this should be given intravenously for major or life-threatening bleeding at a dose of 5 mg, or 1–2 mg if the patient is not compromised. A single intravenous dose of vitamin K may reverse the effects of warfarin within 12–24 hours.

NovoSeven (recombinant factor VIIa): this is a serine protease drug that is indicated for use in haemophilias but can be used in the setting of massive haemorrhage. However, due to the high risk of arterial thrombosis, use of NovoSeven has been restricted.

Beriplex (prothrombin complex concentrate): this contains clotting factors I, VII, IX, X as well as proteins C and S. It is rapidly prepared and administered intravenously, with dosing dependent on the international normalised ratio. It is recommended for use in massive haemorrhage or patients with or without haemodynamic compromise due to vitamin K antagonists. In the above clinical scenario, it would be first line along with 5–10 mg of intravenous vitamin K.

Fresh frozen plasma: this is the plasma component of blood, containing factors II, V, VII, IX, X and XI among other substances and requiring ABO-compatibility prior to use. It is administered in doses of 12–15 mL/kg. It may be associated with fluid overload, transfusion reactions and metabolic disturbances. As it is not available immediately, in the above scenario it would not be as valuable as Beriplex.

Cryoprecipitate: this is the fraction of plasma that contains factors VIII and XIII, fibrinogen and von Willebrand factor. It is indicated in disseminated intravascular coagulation, massive blood transfusions and haemophilias. In the scenario presented here, it would not reverse an elevated INR.

Stanworth SJ. The evidence-based use of FFP and cryoprecipitate for abnormalities of coagulation tests and clinical coagulopathy. Hematology/American Society of Hematology Education Program 2007;179–186.

65. D Plasma osmolality is 310 mOsm/kg

This patient has acute kidney injury most likely due to contrast-induced nephropathy (CIN) on a background of diabetes and gout. His confusion is most likely due to uraemic encephalopathy that may occur in either acute or chronic renal failure, but is unlikely due to the normal chloride of 106 mmol/L.

The anion gap is the difference between measured cations and anions, the size of the difference contributing to diagnosis of the underlying cause of a metabolic acidosis:

$$([Na^+] + [K^+]) - ([Cl^-] + [HCO_3^-]).$$

In this patient therefore:

$$(142 + 5.3) - (106 + 19.3) = 22 \text{ mmol/L}.$$

The normal range is variably quoted but should be in the range of 10–18 mmol/L. The most likely causes of a metabolic acidosis with a high anion gap are lactic acidosis, ketoacidosis, uraemia and toxins such as methanol, salicylates and biguanides.

There is no significant difference in administering prophylactic N-acetylcysteine (NAC), intravenous fluids or sodium bicarbonate to a patient prior to receiving contrast, although the evidence base is variable. There is, however, no evidence base for NAC in the *treatment* of established CIN.

The plasma osmolality is normally 290 mOsm/kg and can be measured using an osmometer or estimated with the following equation:

$$(2 \times [Na^+]) + [urea] + [glucose]$$

Thus, in this patient the osmolality is:

$$(2 \times 142) + 18 + 8 = 310 \text{ mOsm/kg}$$

The most common cause of a hyperosmolar state is hyperosmolar non-ketotic coma secondary to type II diabetes, but may also be due to dehydration, uraemia and drugs such as mannitol or ethanol.

There may be some indication for initiation of renal placement therapy in this patient because of symptomatic uraemia; however, haemofiltration or haemodiafiltration is the most commonly used method in the intensive care setting rather than haemodialysis. Other indications for RRT include refractory hyperkalaemia, refractory acidosis, fluid overload, anuria or oliguria, sepsis and clearance of toxins.

Pannu N, Manns B, Lee H, Tonelli M. Systematic review of the impact of N-acetylcysteine on contrast nephropathy. Kidney Int 2004; 65:1366–1374.
Webb ST, Allen JSD. Perioperative renal protection. Contin Educ Anaesth Crit Care Pain 2008; 8176–180.
Hall NA, Fox AJ. Renal replacement therapies in critical care. Contin Educ Anaesth Crit Care Pain 2006; 6:197–202.

66. A Increased minute ventilation

The most important physiological mechanism for high-altitude acclimatisation is hyperventilation. This can be demonstrated by the alveolar gas equation in this patient, where the atmospheric pressure at 6 km is approximately half than at sea level, assuming a Pa_{CO_2} of 5.3 kPa:

$$PA_{O_2} = PI_{O_2} - \frac{Pa_{CO_2}}{R}$$

where PA_{O_2} is the alveolar partial pressure of oxygen in kPa, PI_{O_2} is the inspired partial pressure of oxygen in kPa, $PI_{O_2} = FI_{O_2} \times$ (Atmospheric pressure – Humidification) in kPa, Pa_{CO_2} is the arterial partial pressure of carbon dioxide in kPa, R is the respiratory quotient and is normally approximately 0.8.

$$PA_{O_2} = [0.21 \times (50 - 6.3)] - \frac{5.3}{0.8} = 2.5 \text{ kPa.}$$

If the minute volume is increased fivefold, then Pa_{CO_2} will reduce fivefold from 5.3 kPa to approximately 1 kPa:

$$PA_{O_2} = [0.21 \times (50 - 6.3)] - \frac{1}{0.8} = 7.9 \text{ kPa.}$$

Hyperventilation is stimulated by hypoxaemia, thus predominantly *peripheral* chemoreceptors in the carotid body rather than central chemoreceptors. The alkaline pH is then corrected by renal excretion of bicarbonate, but this does not itself acclimatise a patient.

Hypoxaemia also stimulates an increase in erythropoietin production of haemoglobin in an attempt to increase the oxygen-carrying capacity of the blood. However, this is a more chronic change and is only of limited benefit as increased haemoglobin concentrations can have adverse effects.

At moderate altitudes, there is an increased production of 2,3-diphosphoglycerate causing a rightward shift of the oxyhaemoglobin dissociation curve, while higher altitudes demonstrate a leftward shift due to respiratory alkalosis.

West JB. Respiratory physiology: The essentials, 9th edn. Baltimore: Lippincott Williams & Wilkins; 2012.

67. B Hydration

This patient is likely to be suffering from post-dual puncture headache (PDPH). The risk factors can be patient factors or anaesthetic factors as seen in **Table 2.10**.

Table 2.10 PDPH risk factors	
Patient factors	**Anaesthetic factors**
Female	Needle used
Obesity	Multiple attempts
Previous PDPH	Insertion technique

The clinical features include positional bilateral temporal or frontal headache, neck ache, photophobia, nausea and vomiting and cranial nerve palsies.

The gold standard therapy for PDPH is performing an epidural blood patch; however, if this is performed within 24 hours, then there is a 70% failure rate that reduces to 4% if performed *after* 24 hours. Simple analgesia with paracetamol and non-steroidal anti-inflammatory drugs should be routinely prescribed; however, codeine might increase the risk of constipation that may worsen symptoms.

Hydration is a vital treatment modality; although oral hydration is sufficient, the role of intravenous hydration remains debatable. This is the best option for the current patient, particularly because the symptoms have been present for <24 hours.

Oral caffeine, sumatriptan, adrenocorticotrophic hormone (ACTH) and epidural infusions of saline have a large disparity in the evidence base for their use. Bed rest is recommended, although there is a limited evidence base for this.

Macintyre PE, Schug SA, Scott DA, et al, and APM:SE Working Group of the Australian and New Zealand College of Anaesthetists and Faculty of Pain Medicine. Acute pain management: Scientific evidence, 3rd edn. Melbourne: ANZCA & FPM; 2010.

68. C Forced air warmer

Perioperative hypothermia is defined as a core body temperature <36.0°C from 1 hour before induction of anaesthesia to 24 hours after entry to recovery area. Hypothermic patients, patients at risk of hypothermia or patients undergoing anaesthesia for longer than 30 minutes should have forced air warming as this has been shown to be the most effective method of rewarming or preventing heat loss.

The first four causes of intraoperative hypothermia can be remembered by the mnemonic 'Royal College Exam Room':

- Radiation (40%): use forced air warmers and warmed intravenous fluids
- Convection (30%): maintain warm theatre temperature
- Evaporation (20%): avoid skin and tissue exposure
- Respiration (8%): use heat and moisture exchange filters
- Conduction (2%): minimise contact with cold surfaces
- Anaesthesia: monitoring, awareness and active warming

Forced air warmers such as the Bair Hugger system reduce the radiant heat losses from patients and can provide effective warming to hypothermic patients, and would be the most effective method in the example given above.

National Institute for Clinical Excellence (NICE). CG65: Perioperative hypothermia (inadvertent). London: NICE; 2008.

69. D 14 gauge peripheral cannula

The patient exhibits features of class III/IV haemorrhagic shock (see **Table 2.11**) and will require warmed IV fluids and blood transfusion as part of the acute treatment. Intravenous access allowing for the highest flow rates is best achieved using wide-bore peripheral cannulae as determined by the Hagen–Poiseuille equation for laminar flow:

$$\text{Flow} = \frac{\Delta P \pi r^4}{8\eta l}$$

where r is radius of the tube, η is fluid viscosity, l is length of the tube, ΔP is pressure gradient along the tube.

It can be seen that short, wide-bore intravenous access devices would allow for the greatest flow rates, while a device that is rapidly inserted and secured will also aid speed of delivery of fluids.

A 20-gauge cannula will allow up to 80 mL/min of crystalloid, while a 14-gauge will allow up to 360 mL/min of crystalloid.

An intraosseous cannula may be used in patients with difficulty in obtaining intravenous, and fluids and blood products may be administered. However, due to the high venous resistance, high pressures would be required to administer fluids at a fast rate.

A central venous catheter has a wider lumen than a 14-gauge peripheral cannula; however, the lumen is segmented in to multiple smaller lumens. In addition, central venous catheters are longer and therefore it can be seen according to the Hagen–Poiseuille equation that higher flow rates would be achieved with the peripheral cannula.

Table 2.11 Classes of haemorrhagic shock depending on clinical presentation

	Class I	Class II	Class III	Class IV
Blood loss	0–15%	15–30%	30–40%	>40%
Heart rate	<100	100–120	120–140	>140
Blood pressure	Normal	Normal, decreased pulse pressure	Low	Low
Respiratory rate	14–20	20–30	30–40	>35
Urine output	>30	20–30	5–15	Minimal
Mental status	Unchanged/ anxious	Anxious	Anxious/ confused	Confused/ obtunded

Peripherally inserted central catheter lines are inserted predominantly for long-term administration of intravenous drugs such as antibiotics, chemotherapeutic agents and parenteral nutrition. The have narrow and long lumens that begin at a peripheral vein, usually in the arm, and are passed to sit in the superior vena cava or right atrium. They serve no role in the acute setting, and high flow rates are difficult to achieve.

American College of Surgeons Committee on Trauma. ATLS® student course manual, 9th edn. Chicago. 2012.

70. D Elasticity of the arterial wall is analogous to resistors

For blood to flow around the body, it has to be pumped by the heart. In this hydraulic system, the blood flow is analogous to electrical current, the pulsatile blood pressure to voltage (alternating current) and the vascular resistance to electrical impedance. Some parts of the circulatory system have the ability to store blood and these would be analogous to capacitors and inductors. The elasticity of the arterial wall acts as capacitance, and it is the thin-walled non-elastic vessels which act as resistors.

Zamir M. The physics of coronary blood flow. New York: Springer; 2005.

71. D Use of a heat and moisture exchanger filter (HME filter)

There are various methods used to reduce pollution in theatres. Adequate ventilation and the frequent changing of circulating air is the most important. This reduces the amount of anaesthetic gases and vapours present in the theatre air, and when compared with unventilated theatres, there is a fourfold reduction in the gases contaminating air. Low-flow anaesthesia reduces the amount of vapour wasted and vented to the atmosphere. Scavenging collects waste anaesthetic gases and discards them away from theatre air. This can be done passively or actively. Using total intravenous anaesthesia results in an overall reduction in the amount of vapour used, thereby reducing theatre pollution.

Heat and moisture exchange filters do not reduce theatre pollution; they humidify and heat inspired gases.

Al-Shaikh B, Stacey S. Essentials of anaesthetic equipment, 3rd edn. Oxford: Churchill Livingstone; 2007.

72. C Ulnar nerve

When performing an ultrasound-guided axillary brachial plexus block, the median, radial, ulnar and musculocutaneous nerves are all visualised and blocked under direct vision. The intercostobrachial nerve is not visualised but is also blocked.

In this case, the ulnar nerve does not need to be blocked as its sensory supply is to the ulnar one and half fingers on the palmar surface (via the palmar cutaneous branch), the dorsal aspect of the little finger and the medial side of the ring finger (via the dorsal branch). These areas are not part of the region of the laceration, so do not need to be blocked.

The radial nerve supplies the lateral three and a half fingers on the dorsal surface of the hand, and the median nerve supplies the lateral three and a half fingers on the palmar surface; therefore, both these nerves need to be blocked to cover the area of surgery.

The musculocutaneous nerve needs to be blocked not only because of its sensory innervation, but also because it supplies the biceps, coracobrachialis and brachialis muscles, which elicit ischaemic pain when a tourniquet is inflated for surgery. Thus, this nerve needs to be blocked to reduce the effects of tourniquet pain, which will be inflated to allow the surgeon to have a bloodless operating field.

The intercostobrachial nerve supplies sensation to the upper inner aspect of the arm. When the tourniquet is inflated, the patient may experience a 'pinching' sensation, especially over the medial aspect of the upper arm, which is why this nerve is also blocked.

Brown DL. Atlas of regional anesthesia, 4th edn. Philadelphia: Saunders; 2010.

73. D High-frequency jet ventilation

The best way to achieve adequate ventilation and allow surgical access in this case would be through high-frequency jet ventilation. This could be achieved using either the supraglottic or subglottic routes. Attaching the high-frequency jet ventilator to a metal cannula on the suspension laryngoscope allows oxygen to be jetted into the trachea and allows the surgeon to operate at the same time. Subglottic jet ventilation is achieved either through a jet catheter which can be passed under direct vision into the trachea or via a cricothyroidotomy cannula.

Potential complications of this technique include barotrauma, surgical emphysema, gas trapping, pneumomediastinum and mucosal desiccation as a result of inadequate humidification.

Spontaneous ventilation for such a long procedure in an adult is difficult to achieve as the patient may cough or develop laryngospasm as a result of instrumentation of the trachea.

Endotracheal intubation or laryngeal mask airway is not option as it would not allow surgical access.

A tracheostomy may be an option, depending on the location of the papillomas in the trachea, but it is likely to affect surgical access and is a drastic choice of airway management that most patients would rather avoid.

English J, Norris A, Bedforth N. Anaesthesia for airway surgery. Contin Educ Anaesth Crit Care Pain 2006; 6:28–31.
Evans E, Biro P, Bedforth N. Jet ventilation. Contin Educ Anaesth Crit Care Pain 2007; 7:2–5.

74. E Beveled tip

Tracheal tubes can be cuffed or uncuffed. In this case, the patient has a cuffed tube in place that is leaking, which suggests that the cuff is not functioning appropriately.

Tracheostomy tubes have an introducer to aid insertion, which is then removed. They have flanges to allow the tube to be fixed in place by ribbons tied around the patients neck or by sutures. Inner cannulas are inserted to prevent the whole tracheostomy tube requiring replacing when secretions accumulate and dry out causing obstruction of the lumen. The inner tube can simply be changed, while the tracheostomy tube remains in place. The inner cannula does, however, reduce the internal diameter of the tube.

A 15 mm connector is attached to allow the tracheostomy tube to be attached to a breathing circuit for ventilator support.

The tips of tracheostomy tubes are square cut and not beveled; this is to reduce the risk of obstructing the tube if the tip happens to rest against the wall of the trachea.

Regan K, Hunt K. Tracheostomy management. Contin Educ Anaesth Crit Care Pain 2008; 8:31–35.

75. A Methaemoglobinaemia

The pulse oximetry reading is a false low reading, and of all the options the only ones that can cause this are methaemaglobinaemia and methylene blue. As there is no mention of the administration of methylene blue, then the more likely explanation is a congenital cause for methaemaglobinaemia. This is an increase in circulating haemoglobin where the iron atom in the haem moiety is in the ferric form (normally this should be <1%) and not the usual reduced ferrous form.

Patients can have a congenital deficiency of the reducing enzymes which normally convert methaemaglobin to haemoglobin. It can also be acquired by drugs and chemicals such as prilocaine, quinones and sulphonamides.

With methaemoglobinaemia, the measured arterial oxygen saturation tends towards 85% as both the oxygenated and deoxygenated forms absorb light equally at 660 and 940 nm. It also causes the oxygen dissociation curve of the unaffected haemoglobin to shift to the left, causing a reduction in oxygen delivery to the tissues.

Hypoperfusion and severe vasoconstriction will give inaccurate and inconsistent readings, but would not explain the above discrepancy. Hyperbilirubinaemia has no effect on the pulse oximeter reading.

Al-Shaikh B, Stacey S. Essentials of anaesthetic equipment, 3rd edn. Oxford: Churchill Livingstone; 2007.

76. B Single burst twitch response

Peripheral nerve stimulators are used to monitor transmission across the neuromuscular junction. The least precise method of assessing a partial neuromuscular block is the twitch response to a single burst. This is where a short duration stimulus of low frequency (0.1–1 Hz) is applied to a peripheral nerve.

A tetanic stimulation is where a 50–100 Hz stimulus is applied to a peripheral nerve and any residual neuromuscular block is detected. Sustained tetanic contraction with post-tetanic potentiation is seen with normal neuromuscular function.

The ratio of the fourth to the first twitch in a train-of-four (ToF) stimulation is called the ToF ratio. The ToF stimulation consists of four twitches of 2 Hz applied over 2 seconds. When fully relaxed, there are no twitches elicited, but on recovery the first twitch appears first, then the second, the third and the fourth. The ToF ratio is the response of the fourth twitch divided by the response of the first.

Double-burst stimulation is the application of two short tetanic stimulations of 50 Hz for 60 ms, 750 ms apart. In non-depolarising blockade, the second response is weaker than the first; it also allows a more accurate visual assessment.

Post-tetanic potentiation is used to assess more profound degrees of neuromuscular block. With normal neuromuscular function following a sustained tetanic contraction, post-tetanic potentiation is seen. With neuromuscular blockade, no post-tetanic stimulation is seen.

McGrath CD, Hunter JM. Monitoring of neuromuscular block. Contin Educ Anaesth Crit Care Pain 2006; 6:7–12.

77. E Ethylene oxide gas

Ethylene oxide gas is used to sterilise instruments that can withstand temperatures of 50–60°C. It should be used under carefully controlled conditions as it is extremely toxic and explosive. It can be used for heat-labile equipment, fluids and rubber.

All the other methods described are forms of high-level disinfection. This can be achieved by boiling, moist heat or chemically.

Sabir N, Ramachandra V. Decontamination of anaesthetic equipment. Contin Educ Anaesth Crit Care Pain 2004; 4:103–106.

78. C Dryness of mouth

Dryness of mouth is an anticholinergic side effect that is not elicited by metoclopramide, whereas cyclizine has this effect.

The extra-pyramidal side effects, such as acathisia and oculogyric crises, occur more frequently in higher doses, in patients with renal impairment and the elderly.

Metoclopramide increases the tone of the lower oesophageal sphincter by about 17 mmHg, accelerates gastric emptying, enhancing the amplitude of gastric contractions and accelerates small intestinal transit time.

Sasada M, Smith S. Drugs in anaesthesia and intensive care, 4th edn. Oxford: Oxford University Press; 2011.

79. A Transfusion related graft-vs-host disease

This patient is having an early complication of blood transfusion. Symptoms usually appear soon after starting the transfusion and include headache, chest and flank pain, fever, chills, flushing, rigors, nausea and vomiting, urticaria, dyspneoa and hypotension.

Transfusion-related graft-vs-host disease is rare, but it can occur after simple blood transfusions in patients who are immunocompromised. It is a late complication and occurs as a result of the donor-derived immune cells mounting an immune response against the host tissue. Clinical features include a maculopapular rash, abdominal pain and diarrhoea.

The following is a list of *early* complications of blood transfusion:

- Haemolytic reaction
- Non-haemolytic febrile reaction
- Allergic reaction to proteins
- Transfusion-related acute lung injury
- Reaction secondary to bacterial contamination
- Circulatory overload
- Air embolism
- Citrate toxicity

Maxwell MJ, Wilson MJA. Complications of blood transfusion. Contin Educ Anaesth Crit Care Pain 2006; 6:225–229.

80. D Noradrenaline

Following a heart transplant, both sympathetic and parasympathetic innervations are lost to the transplanted heart. Because of the loss of parasympathetic tone, the resting heart rate is higher than normal at about 90–100 beats per minute. The transplanted heart rate is dependent on donor sinus node activity.

Indirectly acting sympathomimetic drugs will have no effect on the heart rate, so administration of atropine, glycopyrrolate, cyclizine or glyceryl trinitrate will not have an effect.

Only direct acting β-agonist agents such as adrenaline, isoprenaline and noradrenaline will have the desired chronotropic effect.

Morgan-Hughes NJ, Hood G. Anaesthesia for a patient with a cardiac transplant. BJA CEPD Reviews 2002; 2:74–78.

81. B Hypoglossal nerve

Death is defined as an irreversible loss of consciousness and the ability to breathe. Brainstem death, also called death by neurological criteria, occurs when there is irreversible damage to the brainstem, while the heart continues to beat and the ventilation is maintained artificially.

Brainstem death testing begins by fulfilment of preconditions (deeply unconscious, apnoeic and ventilated) with no doubt that the underlying brain damage is irreversible. Reversible causes must be excluded, such as drugs, cardiovascular causes, electrolyte and endocrine abnormalities. Finally, formal testing may take place. The assessment of cranial nerves along with demonstration of apnoea is performed, testing for the following cranial nerves (**Table 2.12**).

Table 2.12 Cranial nerves tested during brainstem death testing

Test performed	Sensory cranial nerve	Motor cranial nerve
Pupillary light reflex	Optic (II)	Oculomotor (III)
Corneal blink reflex	Trigeminal (V)	Facial (VII)
Vestibulo-ocular reflex	Vestibulocochlear (VIII)	Oculomotor (III), trochlear (IV), abducens (VI)
Pain response	Trigeminal (V)	Facial (VII)
Gag reflex	Glossopharyngeal (IX)	Vagus (X)
Cough reflex	Vagus (X)	Vagus (X)

Thus, the olfactory (I), accessory (XI) and hypoglossal (XII) nerves are not tested for as they do not form part of a reflex arc.

Oram J, Murphy P. Diagnosis of death. Contin Educ Anaesth Crit Care Pain 2011; 11:77–81.

82. B Partial right recurrent laryngeal nerve palsy (Figure 2.16B)

Unilateral complete palsy: the vocal fold on the affected side assumes a slightly lateral position midway between abduction and adduction. Speech is not greatly affected because the other fold compensates, moving towards the affected one.

Bilateral complete: both folds are midway between abduction and adduction. Breathing is impaired because the rima glottidis is partially closed; speech is lost.

Unilateral partial: abductors are more paralysed than adductors. The affected fold assumes the adducted midline position. It is thought either that abductors receive more nerve fibres than adductors, so relatively more abductor fibres are damaged, or fibres to abductors are more exposed and prone to injury.

Bilateral partial: bilateral paralysis of abductors and drawing together of folds. Acute dyspnoea and stridor follow; cricothyroidotomy or tracheostomy is necessary.

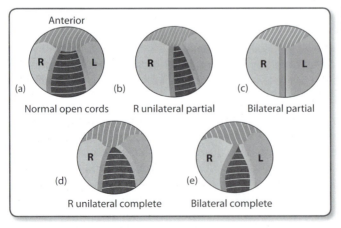

Figure 2.16 Palsy of the recurrent laryngeal nerve.

Malhotra S, Sodhi V. Anaesthesia for thyroid and parathyroid surgery. Contin Educ Anaesth Crit Care Pain 2007; 7:55–58.

83. A 6 mg adenosine

Supraventricular tachycardia is usually a benign condition and can be associated with either a structurally normal or structurally abnormal heart. Adverse features of adult tachyarrhythmias, including hypotension, syncope, heart failure or chest pain, warrant synchronised direct current cardioversion.

In the absence of instability, patients with supraventricular tachycardia may be treated first with vagal manoeuvres such as the Valsalva manoeuvre or carotid sinus massage. If this fails then a rapid bolus of 6 mg adenosine may be given, followed by two further boluses of 12 mg if no response is seen. If there is no improvement following adenosine, or there is a contraindication to adenosine, then 2.5–5 mg verapamil may be used. If there is still no improvement, then a discussion with the cardiologists is indicated and either sotalol or amiodarone may be used.

Resuscitation Council (UK). Advanced life support, 6th edn. London: Resuscitation Council (UK), 2011.

84. C Systolic blood pressure < 90 mmHg

The systemic inflammatory response syndrome (SIRS) is present in any patient with two of the following four:

- Heart rate >90 beats per minute
- Respiratory rate >20 breaths per minute
- Temperature >38°C or <36°C
- White blood cell count of $>12 \times 10^9$ or $<4.0 \times 10^9$

Sepsis is the presence of SIRS triggered by an infective agent. Severe sepsis is sepsis associated with end-organ dysfunction, hypoperfusion, or hypotension. Septic shock is sepsis with refractory hypotension despite adequate fluid resuscitation. Thus, the diagnosis of sepsis does not require the presence of hypotension; however, severe sepsis and septic shock do.

Dellinger RP, Levy MM, Carlet, JM, et al. Surviving sepsis campaign: International guidelines for management of severe sepsis and septic shock. Crit Care Med 2008; 36:296–327.

85. C Sevoflurane

Uterine atony is one of the most common causes of post-partum haemorrhage. The most likely anaesthetic cause of uterine atony is the use of volatile anaesthetic agents that cause a dose-dependent relaxant effect on the uterus. Although the minimum alveolar concentration (MAC) reduces in pregnancy, obstetric general anaesthesia results in a relatively high risk of awareness. Therefore, it is still important to achieve MAC values of up to 1.0 from induction to delivery, which may be reduced to 0.75 following delivery to minimise uterine atony and blood loss. Often nitrous oxide is administered in combination with volatile agents such as sevoflurane to increase the MAC delivered with a reduced requirement for volatile agents.

Nitrous oxide, opioid analgesics and ketamine do not suppress uterine tone. Thiopentone does not reduce uterine tone but it may suppress uterine contractions when administered at high dose. Both depolarising and non-depolarising neuromuscular blocking drugs have no effect on uterine tone.

Banks A, Norris A. Massive haemorrhage in pregnancy. Contin Educ Anaesth Crit Care Pain 2005; 5(6):195–198.

86. B Flecainide

The mechanism of action of the drug described is a Vaughan Williams class Ic agent (see **Table 2.13**), which includes flecainide and propafenone. These drugs act on both supraventricular and ventricular tachycardias. In Wolff–Parkinson–White (WPW) syndrome, they act by slowing conduction in the accessory pathway (see **Figure 2.17**).

Table 2.13 Modified Vaughan Williams classification

Class	Mechanism of action	Drugs
Ia	Block Na+ channels, prolong refractory period	Disopyramide, procainamide, quinidine
Ib	Block Na+ channels, shorten refractory period	Lidocaine, mexiletine, phenytoin
Ic	Block Na+ channels, no effect on refractory period	Flecainide, propafenone
II	β-adrenoceptor blockade	Atenolol, propranolol
III	K+ channel blockade	Amiodarone, bretylium, sotalol
IV	Ca2+ channel blockade	Diltiazem, verapamil
V*	Miscellaneous	Adenosine, digoxin, magnesium sulphate

*Antiarrhythmic agents that do not fit into any of the original classes described by Vaughan Williams in 1970 were later classified into class V.

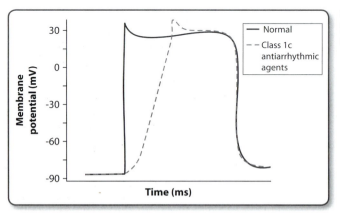

Figure 2.17 A Effect of class Ic antiarrhythmic agents on cardiac action potentials.

Peck TE, Hill, SA, Williams M. Pharmacology for anaesthesia and intensive care, 3rd edn. Cambridge: Cambridge University Press; 2008.

87. C Blood from the inferior vena cava mainly passes through the foramen ovale

The fetal circulation varies from the adult circulation anatomically and physiologically. Gas exchange occurs at the placenta rather than the lungs, and oxygenated blood is preferentially directed to the heart and brain.

Oxygenated blood from the placenta passing into the umbilical vein is 80% saturated (Po_2 of 4.7 kPa), half of which bypasses the hepatic circulation in the ductus venosus to the inferior vena cava. Blood with a saturation of 65% enters the inferior vena cava; up to 70% this bypasses the right ventricle and passes through the foramen ovale into the left atrium, left ventricle and into the ascending aorta. This ensures that the heart, brain and upper extremities receive the most saturated blood possible.

Venous blood entering the right atrium from the superior vena cava is only 25% saturated, and it passes through the right ventricle and the pulmonary artery. The high pulmonary vascular resistance means that only 10% of the cardiac output enters the pulmonary circulation; therefore, blood from the pulmonary artery is shunted via the ductus arteriosus into the descending aorta. This provides saturation of 55% to the descending aorta and lower body.

The fetal oxyhaemoglobin-dissociation curve is shifted to the left to allow for greater uptake of oxygen at the placental unit.

Murphy PJ. The fetal circulation. Contin Educ Anaesth Crit Care Pain 2005;5(4):107–112.

88. E Reduced systemic vascular resistance

There are many physiological changes in pregnancy. Systemic vascular resistance (SVR) is reduced which may be significantly compounded by sepsis causing further reduction in SVR, particularly in gram-negative sepsis. Therefore, this is the most likely cause of haemodynamic collapse.

In pregnancy, stroke volume and cardiac output increase by up to 60%, while left ventricular mass increases as well. Aortocaval compression occurs from approximately 20 weeks gestation, while there is an increase in plasma volume by up to 50% at term. Although red blood cell mass increases, the plasma volume increases to a greater extent causing a physiological anaemia. Serum albumin decreases, increasing the free portion of drug administered but also reducing the colloid osmotic pressure leaving women at greater risk of pulmonary oedema.

There is increased minute ventilation, and a respiratory alkalosis ensues as pregnancy progresses. However, this leaves little scope for respiratory compensation of metabolic acidosis due to sepsis in pregnancy. An increase in oxygen consumption of up to 60% leaves women at an even greater risk of hypoxaemia in the event of hypoventilation.

The most recent Centre for Maternal and Child Enquiries report for 2006–2008 revealed that the most common direct cause of maternal death was sepsis; thus, there has been a renewed drive to detect and treat sepsis early in the parturient.

Centre for Maternal and Child Enquiries (CMACE). Saving Mothers' Lives: reviewing maternal deaths to make motherhood safer: 2006–2008. The Eighth Report on Confidential Enquiries into Maternal Deaths in the United Kingdom. BJOG 2011; 118(suppl 1):1–203.
Cormack C. Diagnosis and management of maternal sepsis and septic shock. Anaesthesia Tutorial of the Week 2011;235.

89. B Tachycardia in phase 1

The Valsalva manoeuvre is 10 seconds of forced expiration of 40 mmHg against a closed glottis. It is used as a bedside test to diagnose autonomic neuropathy, to terminate supraventricular tachycardia, as well as intraoperative assessment of bleeding points in head and neck surgery. There are four phases to the manoeuvre (see **Figure 2.18**).

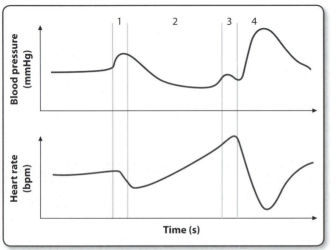

Figure 2.18 The Valsalva response.

- Phase 1: increased intrathoracic pressure increases venous return, thereby causing an increase in blood pressure and a reflex reduction in heart rate
- Phase 2: continued increased intrathoracic pressure reduces venous return, activating the baroreceptor reflex leading to tachycardia and vasoconstriction to restore the fall in blood pressure
- Phase 3: release of intrathoracic pressure causes pooling of blood in the pulmonary vasculature leading to a reduced blood pressure
- Phase 4: continued compensatory mechanisms with continued venous return leading to overshoot of blood pressure and bradycardia until a return to baseline

Smith T, Pinnock C, Lin T. Fundamentals of anaesthesia, 3rd edn. Cambridge: Cambridge University Press; 2009.

90. A Cardiogenic shock

Hypoxia can be due to insufficient tissue oxygen supply or an inability of cellular oxygen utilisation (see **Table 2.14**). The causes of hypoxia can be classified as:

Hypoxic hypoxia: Arterial Po_2 of <12 kPa, reduced venous Po_2

- Hypoventilation
- Diffusion impairment such as in pulmonary oedema
- Shunt such as atelectasis
- Ventilation/perfusion mismatch such as asthma or pneumonia

Anaemic hypoxia: Normal arterial Po_2, reduced venous Po_2

- Low haemoglobin concentration or ability of haemoglobin to carry oxygen (e.g. carbon monoxide poisoning)
- Increased oxygen extraction from the tissues thus low venous Po_2

Stagnant hypoxia: Normal arterial Po_2, normal venous Po_2

- Oxygen-carrying capacity is unchanged but there is a reduction in tissue perfusion (e.g. cardiogenic shock)

Histotoxic hypoxic: Normal arterial Po_2, high venous Po_2

- Oxygen-carrying capacity and tissue perfusion are normal, but there is a failure of cellular oxygen utilisation.
- Reduced oxygen extraction therefore leads to an increased venous Po_2.

In this clinical scenario, stagnant hypoxia is the apparent feature. Cardiogenic shock is the only option demonstrating stagnant hypoxia.

Table 2.14 Arterial and venous Po_2 in different aetiologies of hypoxia

Condition	Arterial Po_2 (100% saturation, P_{75})	Venous Po_2 (75% saturation, P_{75})
Normal	>12 kPa, normal	5.3 kPa, normal
Hypoxic hypoxia	<12 kPa, low	<5.3 kPa, low
Anaemic hypoxia	>12 kPa, normal	<5.3 kPa, low
Stagnant hypoxia	>12 kPa, normal	5.3 kPa, normal
Histotoxic hypoxia	>12 kPa, normal	>5.3 kPa, high

West JB. Respiratory physiology: The essentials, 9th edn. Baltimore: Lippincott Williams & Wilkins; 2012.

Chapter 3

Mock paper 3

60 MTFs and 30 SBAs to be answered in three hours

Questions: MTFs

Answer each stem 'True' or 'False'.

1. **The following statements regarding heart sounds are true:**
   A   In a healthy person, heart sounds are due to the opening and closing of the heart valves
   B   The second heart sound comes immediately after a pause
   C   The mitral and tricuspid valves close simultaneously
   D   Splitting of the second heart sound suggests valvular abnormality
   E   Third and fourth heart sounds are difficult to hear due to their high frequency

2. **With regard to the mechanism of cardiac muscle contraction:**
   A   In the resting state, the actin-binding sites are blocked by troponin
   B   Contraction is initiated by a rise in intracellular potassium
   C   The myosin head attaches to the actin-binding site to initiate contraction
   D   Energy for cross-bridge cycling is provided by adenosine diphosphate
   E   The force of contraction is independent of the number of cross-bridges formed.

3. **Regarding baroreceptors:**
   A   They are mainly located in the carotid sinus and ascending aorta
   B   The carotid sinus is found in the external carotid artery
   C   Afferent fibres from the carotid sinus travel via the vagus nerve
   D   They respond to stretch and not pressure
   E   Baroreceptors in the carotid sinus are sensitive to mean arterial pressure and pulse pressure

4. **The following statements regarding the effects on vascular smooth muscle are correct:**
   A   Acidosis causes vasoconstriction
   B   Adenosine causes vasodilatation
   C   Prostaglandin F causes vasodilatation
   D   Prostacyclins cause vasodilatation
   E   Serotonin causes vasoconstriction

5. **The following are true regarding oxygen consumption by the kidneys:**
    A   It is about 100 mL of oxygen per minute
    B   The arteriovenous difference for oxygen is similar to the heart
    C   Oxygen consumption in the cortex is 20 times greater than in the medulla
    D   In the medulla energy metabolism is mainly anaerobic
    E   Renal oxygen consumption can be calculated using the Fick principle

6. **Regarding the tubular transport of substances in the nephron:**
    A   The initial process is filtration
    B   Hydrogen ions are actively reabsorbed with water
    C   It includes the passive transcellular excretion of the endogenous products of metabolism
    D   Exogenous substances are actively secreted
    E   Products of metabolism from tubular cells undergo active and passive cellular secretion into the tubular lumen

7. **Regarding the hormonal control of salt and water excretion:**
    A   Antidiuretic hormone (ADH) is secreted from the hypothalamus
    B   Atrial stretch receptors cause direct release of ADH
    C   ADH causes an increase in water reabsorption by the kidneys
    D   Salt excess results in release of ADH and aldosterone
    E   Atrial natriuretic peptide increases the renal reabsorption of sodium ions

8. **Regarding acid/base balance:**
    A   pH is the logarithmic measure of the effective hydrogen ion concentration
    B   Buffers act by fully neutralising acids and bases
    C   Haemoglobin is an important buffer
    D   Plasma proteins act as buffers in the blood
    E   Bicarbonate levels are controlled primarily by the lungs

9. **Regarding lung compliance, which of the following are true:**
    A   It varies with different lung volumes
    B   The pressure volume loop is sigmoid shaped during normal tidal volume
    C   It is increased in the elderly
    D   It is less during inflation than deflation when measured dynamically
    E   It requires knowledge of intrapleural pressures to calculate

10. **Functional residual capacity:**
    A   May be calculated using helium dilution methods
    B   Is reduced by positive end-expiratory pressure
    C   Is reduced during general anaesthesia
    D   Is approximately 1.5 L in adults
    E   Is the sum of residual volume and the inspiratory reserve volume

11. **Regarding the alveolar–arterial oxygen tension difference:**
    A   It is increased under general anaesthesia
    B   It is normally 0.5–1 kPa with room air

C   In the elderly it is greater
D   It is reduced by sevoflurane
E   May be decreased by right-to-left intracardiac shunts

12. **Pulmonary vascular resistance:**
    A   Is calculated using Fick principle
    B   Requires knowledge of the right atrial pressure to calculate
    C   Is lowest at functional residual capacity
    D   Increases with pulmonary embolism
    E   Reduces with exercise

13. **Regarding the chemical composition of hormones:**
    A   The peptide hormones have a benzene ring attached to an amino acid chain
    B   Steroid hormones all consist of a four-ring structure
    C   Amine hormones have an alpha amino group on a benzene ring
    D   All steroids are derived from cholesterol
    E   Peptide hormones may have carbohydrate groups attached to them

14. **Regarding hormones secreted by the thyroid gland:**
    A   The follicular cells secrete thyroxine and calcitonin
    B   The thyroid gland is the only endocrine gland that stores its hormones in large quantities
    C   Peroxidase oxidises iodine to iodide to enable the iodination of tyrosine
    D   99% of T3 & T4 is bound to transport proteins in the blood
    E   T3 is more potent and secreted in larger quantities than T4

15. **Regarding hormones secreted from the adrenal medulla:**
    A   Dopamine is one of the catecholamines secreted
    B   They are all derived from tyrosine
    C   Dopamine is a precursor of adrenaline and noradrenaline
    D   The rate limiting step for their synthesis is phenylalanine hydroxylase dependent
    E   They are metabolised by hydroxylation and decarboxylation

16. **The lower oesophageal sphincter:**
    A   Is found in the oesophagus about 2–5 cm above the cardia
    B   Is anatomically the same as the rest of the oesophagus
    C   Is normally relaxed
    D   Relaxes when the peristaltic wave passes down the oesophagus
    E   Is functionally normal in achalasia of the cardia

17. **Regarding the pancreas, which of the following are true:**
    A   It secretes about 2 L of pancreatic juice per day
    B   Secretion is under the control of gastrin and secretin
    C   The stimulus for hormone secretion is a high pH and fat in the gastrointestinal tract
    D   The bicarbonate in pancreatic juices activates pancreatic enzymes
    E   Trypsin and chymotrypsin are pancreatic enzymes

18. **Cerebrospinal fluid:**
    A   Has a volume of 150 mL
    B   Is more acidic than plasma
    C   Is secreted from the arachnoid villi
    D   Contains 2 g/L of albumin
    E   Glucose concentration is less than one third than that of the serum

19. **The sympathetic nervous system:**
    A   Unmyelinated preganglionic efferent fibres have a thoracolumbar outflow
    B   Provides fibres to the facial nerve
    C   Has acetylcholine as a neurotransmitter
    D   Stimulates renin secretion
    E   Causes pupillary constriction

20. **Regarding red blood cells, the following are true:**
    A   Their circulating lifespan is 20 days
    B   Production is reduced in response to increased circulating red blood cells
    C   Mean corpuscular volume increases in iron deficiency
    D   They are multinucleated
    E   They contain enzymes for glycolysis

21. **Regarding mammillary three-compartment models:**
    A   The initial plasma concentration decline is due to metabolism
    B   The second and third compartments have an equilibrium constant of k23
    C   Distribution into the second compartment is faster than the third compartment
    D   Drug elimination is a linear process
    E   Drug clearance is out of either the central or second compartments

22. **The following drugs need dose adjustment in renal failure:**
    A   Hydralazine
    B   Enoximone
    C   Tramadol
    D   Phenytoin
    E   Atracurium

23. **Regarding phase II metabolic processes:**
    A   They include acetylation
    B   They aim to reduce water solubility of a drug
    C   They always render drugs inactive
    D   They only occur in the liver
    E   They may precede a phase I metabolic process

24. **Regarding structural isomers:**
    A   They include enantiomers
    B   Codeine phosphate and dobutamine are examples
    C   Tautomer is an example
    D   They include morphine
    E   They contain a chiral centre

25. **Regarding drug–receptor interactions, which of the following are true:**

    A   Potency relates to how well a drug binds to a receptor
    B   Antagonists have an intrinsic activity of 0
    C   Efficacy is same as intrinsic activity
    D   Partial agonists may have maximal efficacy
    E   Agonists have a high receptor affinity

26. **Bupivacaine:**

    A   Has a toxic plasma concentration of 1.5 μg/mL
    B   Is more lipid soluble than lidocaine
    C   Has a pKa of 7.9
    D   Is less cardiotoxic than ropivacaine
    E   Is an enantiopure preparation

27. **The following drugs undergo ester hydrolysis:**

    A   Amethocaine
    B   Esmolol
    C   Lorazepam
    D   Phenytoin
    E   Mivacurium

28. **Methohexitone:**

    A   Is a methylated thiobarbiturate
    B   Causes a less intense excitatory phase than thiopentone
    C   Should be avoided in patients with epilepsy
    D   Produces fewer complications than thiopentone following inadvertent arterial injection
    E   Has a lower incidence of hypersensitivity compared with thiopentone

29. **Which of the following pharmacokinetic properties are true:**

    A   Thiopentone undergoes hepatic oxidation to inactive metabolites
    B   Ketamine is highly protein bound
    C   Propofol is conjugated and metabolised by the liver
    D   Etomidate is metabolised by the liver to quinol and glucuronide
    E   Most of the unbound thiopentone is in the ionised form

30. **Volatile anaesthetics are associated with which of the following:**

    A   Isoflurane depresses minute volume and increases Pa_{CO_2}
    B   Sevoflurane causes breath holding
    C   Halothane decreases cerebral blood flow
    D   Desflurane sensitises the heart to catecholamines
    E   Enflurane can cause seizure activity in patients with epilepsy

31. **Which of the following non-steroidal anti-inflammatory drugs are correctly classified:**

    A   Tenoxicam is an acetic acid derivative
    B   Ibuprofen is a propionic acid
    C   Paracetamol is a para-aminophenol

    D   Diclofenac is an anthranilic acid derivative

    E   Ketorolac is an acetic acid derivative

32. Regarding the pharmacokinetic properties of morphine, which of the following is correct:

    A   It is a weak base

    B   It is well absorbed from the stomach

    C   It is highly lipid soluble

    D   It is only metabolised in the liver

    E   It is mostly metabolised to the active morphine-6-glucuronide

33. Which of the following prolongs the action of neuromuscular blocking drugs:

    A   Respiratory acidosis

    B   Hyperkalaemia

    C   Gentamicin

    D   Lidocaine

    E   Temperature of 38.4°C

34. Atracurium:

    A   Is a chiral mixture of three stereoisomers

    B   Should be avoided in renal failure

    C   Causes histamine release

    D   Has pro-convulsant breakdown products

    E   Is stable at a temperature of 36.5°C

35. Sugammadex:

    A   Is a δ-cyclodextrin

    B   Has no effect on vecuronium

    C   Has no active metabolites

    D   Is minimally plasma protein bound

    E   Is faster acting than neostigmine

36. Which of the following drugs act on GABA receptors:

    A   Ketamine

    B   Isoflurane

    C   Baclofen

    D   Lorazepam

    E   Naloxone

37. Lithium:

    A   Has 100% oral bioavailability

    B   Is not bound to plasma proteins

    C   Prolongs depolarising and non-depolarising neuromuscular blockade

    D   Undergoes mainly hepatic metabolism

    E   Can cause thyroid dysfunction

38. Calcium channel antagonists:

A   Interfere with the inward displacement of Ca^{2+} ions
B   Depress phases III and IV of the cardiac action potential
C   Are useful for treating ventricular arrhythmias
D   Undergo minimal first-pass metabolism
E   Increase smooth muscle contractility and peripheral resistance

39. The following are correctly classified:

A   Furosemide is a loop diuretic
B   Amiloride is a loop diuretic
C   Bumetanide is a thiazide diuretic
D   Acetazolamide is an aldosterone antagonist
E   Metolazone is a thiazide diuretic

40. The following are true regarding antimicrobial drugs:

A   Penicillins are bacteriostatic
B   Cephalosporins contain a β-lactam ring
C   Tetracyclines inhibit bacterial protein synthesis
D   Aminoglycosides are ineffective against gram-negative organisms
E   Macrolides are bactericidal and inhibit DNA synthesis

41. The following are true regarding electrical safety:

A   Alternating currents cannot pass through a capacitor
B   Class II equipment is earthed
C   The resistance of a capacitor is proportional to the frequency of an alternating current
D   Class I electrical equipment is of low voltage
E   Class II equipment is double-insulated

42. Regarding electrodes used to detect biological signals:

A   They are coated with silver chloride
B   They typically have a high impedance to minimise mains interference
C   Needle electrodes usually deliver better signals than electrode pads
D   Movement artefacts are reduced by using a gel-covered foam pad on the electrode surface
E   Skin impedance is reduced by wiping with alcohol solution

43. Regarding different modes of surgical diathermy:

A   The most efficient cutting waveform is a continuous sine wave
B   Coagulation is best achieved with a continuous waveform at lower voltages that are required for cutting
C   Desiccation is the destructive charring of tissue by arcing
D   Cutting diathermy causes boiling of intracellular fluid
E   Bipolar diathermy is better at coagulation than cutting

44. **Concerning the principles of laser:**
    A   Laser is an acronym for light amplification by stimulated emission of radiation
    B   Laser controls the way that energised atoms release electrons
    C   Light or electricity is used to create excited atoms
    D   Photons are released as the excited atoms relax
    E   Photons are of varying wavelengths

45. **The following are derived from SI units:**
    A   Ampere
    B   Watt
    C   Newton
    D   Mole
    E   Pascal

46. **Regarding the principles of measurement:**
    A   Extrapolation is measurement within the range over which an instrument has been calibrated
    B   Calibration of an instrument removes the chances of a systemic error
    C   An accurate measurement is precise and unbiased
    D   An exponential relationship cannot be changed into a linear one
    E   Calibration may use a reference such as standard measurement of length or weight

47. **The following are disadvantages of humidification methods:**
    A   Ultrasonic nebulisers deposit water in the breathing circuit
    B   Bubble humidifiers increase the work of breathing
    C   Humidifiers can cause bacterial contamination of the circuit
    D   Heat and moisture exchangers increase dead space
    E   Heated humidifiers can cause over-hydration

48. **Concerning non-electrical techniques of temperature measurement, which of the following are true:**
    A   Mercury thermometers are more suitable than alcohol thermometers at very high temperatures
    B   Alcohol thermometers have a linear scale
    C   Alcohol freezes at –39°C
    D   A Bourdon gauge is a type of dial thermometer
    E   A bimetallic strip thermometer works on the principles of heat capacity

49. **Regarding the storage of oxygen in hospitals, which of the following are true:**
    A   It is stored in liquid form
    B   The critical temperature of oxygen is –160°C
    C   At –150°C, oxygen is a liquid
    D   The oxygen pipeline pressure is kept at about 7 bar
    E   A refrigeration unit is needed to keep the storage vessel cool

50. **Regarding non-invasive blood pressure measurement, which of the following are true:**

   A   When using oscillotonometry, diastolic pressure values are prone to inaccuracies

   B   Too large a cuff overestimates and too small a cuff underestimates blood pressure measurement

   C   Oscillometry requires the use of a double cuff

   D   In oscillometry, the maximum amplitude detected as the cuff is deflated is the systolic pressure

   E   Automated devices such as the DINAMAP (device for indirect non-invasive automatic mean arterial pressure) use oscillotonometry to measure the blood pressure

51. **Regarding electrical shock:**

   A   Pain is felt at 5 mA

   B   The severity does not depend on the current density

   C   Ventricular fibrillation is more likely if the current reaches the heart during repolarisation

   D   Antistatic shoes prevents the current from passing to the earth

   E   50 mA is sufficient to cause tonic myocardial contraction

52. **Safety mechanisms on anaesthetic machines which minimise the risk of delivering unsafe gas mixtures include:**

   A   Emergency oxygen flush

   B   Chain-link mechanism

   C   Schrader valves

   D   Paramagnetic analysers

   E   Pressure reducing valves

53. **Tec Mark 5 vapourisers:**

   A   Have a bypass stream fully saturated with vapour

   B   Contain bimetallic strips in the vapourising chamber

   C   Are coded blue for desflurane

   D   Have wicks and baffles to maximise vapour saturation

   E   Contain copper heat sinks

54. **The following airway devices have oesophageal drainage ports:**

   A   i-gel

   B   LMA ProSeal

   C   LMA Supreme

   D   Combitube

   E   Intubating LMA

55. **Examples of a T-piece breathing system include:**

   A   Mapleson A

   B   Mapleson C

C   Mapleson D
D   Mapleson E
E   Mapleson F

56. **Oxygen in its gaseous form can be measured with:**
A   Galvanic cells
B   Diamagnetism
C   Raman scattering
D   Polarography
E   Infrared spectroscopy

57. **Regarding filters, which of the following are true:**
A   Epidural filters have a pore size of 0.2 microns
B   Blood giving set filters have a pore size of 2–18 microns
C   Platelets can be administered through blood giving set filters
D   A pore size of 25 microns filters most micro-organisms
E   They may remove microaggregates

58. **Concerning capnography, which of the following are true:**
A   End-tidal carbon dioxide can be higher than arterial carbon dioxide
B   Absorption of infrared light is in the wavelength of 42.8 μm
C   The rise time is the time for the sample to reach the analyser
D   They contain glass windows in the sample chamber
E   Collision broadening reduces the measured amount of carbon dioxide

59. **Regarding the DINAMAP (device for indirect non-invasive automatic mean arterial pressure), which of the following are true:**
A   It has a proximal occluding cuff
B   It is accurate to +/– 0.5%
C   The cuff bladder should be 40% of the arm circumference
D   It utilises the principle of oscillometry
E   Cuff deflation is at a rate of 6 mmHg per second

60. **Defibrillators:**
A   Have 5000 V between capacitor plates
B   Contain a diode
C   Should be set to deliver an external unsynchronised shock of 4 J/kg in children
D   Discharge alternating current from capacitors
E   Have three switches

Questions: SBAs

For each question, select the single best answer from the five options listed.

61. You have anaesthetised a fit 30-year-old, 70 kg, man for a laparoscopic appendectomy. You have intubated his trachea with a size 8 endotracheal tube secured at 22 cm at the lips and are ventilating his lungs via a circle system at a rate of 12 breaths per minute with tidal volumes of 500 mL and positive end-expiratory pressure (PEEP) of 5 cmH$_2$O.

    Which one of the following manoeuvres is least likely to affect dead space?

    A   Reducing the amount of tubing in the circuit
    B   Reducing tidal volume to 350 mL
    C   Removing PEEP
    D   Advancing the endotracheal tube to 24 cm at the lips
    E   Administering 200 µg of atropine sulphate

62. A 48-year-old woman is having a laparoscopic ovarian cystectomy when the surgeon says they think the patient is bleeding. Her oxygen saturations is 96%, blood pressure 85/62 and heart rate 112 beats per minute.

    What is the most appropriate immediate action?

    A   Perform an arterial blood gas sample
    B   Order one unit of blood
    C   Observe for changes
    D   Give a fluid challenge
    E   Tell the surgeons to end the case

63. A 34-year-old man presents with polyuria, polydipsia and confusion. His arterial blood gas shows pH 7.14; $Paco_2$ 3.5 kPa; Pao_2 12.4 kPa; HCO$_3^-$ 14.6 mmol/L; lactate 4.7 mmol/L; glucose 27.3 mmol/L.

    What is the most likely underlying pathogenesis?

    A   Hyperosmolar non-ketotic coma
    B   Diabetes insipidus
    C   Diabetic ketoacidosis
    D   Salicylate toxicity
    E   Decompensated liver failure

64. A 6-year-old, 20 kg, girl presents with a 2-day history of vomiting and right iliac fossa pain. She is estimated to be severely dehydrated with a deficit of 10%.

    What fluid regimen is most suitable to replace her fluid deficit?

    A   1000 mL 0.9% NaCl in 6 hours
    B   2000 mL 0.18% NaCl/4% glucose in 12 hours
    C   400 mL Hartmann's solution in 12 hours
    D   1000 mL 15% glucose in 24 hours
    E   2000 mL 0.9% NaCl in 24 hours

65. When floating a pulmonary artery catheter in a 75-year-old man, the pressure reading from the tip of the catheter is 25/2 mmHg.

    The most likely position for the catheter would be?

    A   Right atrium
    B   Right ventricle
    C   Pulmonary artery
    D   Right internal jugular vein
    E   Left atrium

66. When using a cardiac catheter with incorporated electrodes, it must be designated to a type of electrical safety.

    Which electrical safety class or type is the cardiac catheter most likely to belong to?

    A   Class 1
    B   Type B
    C   Class 3
    D   Type BF
    E   Type CF

67. You are performing a rapid sequence intubation in a 45-year-old woman for an emergency laparotomy. You have failed to intubate her after three attempts.

    The next step should be?

    A   Releasing cricoid pressure
    B   Commence face mask ventilation
    C   Insertion of a laryngeal mask airway
    D   Another attempt at direct laryngoscopy
    E   Insertion of an intubating laryngeal mask airway

68. A 63-year-old man with severe left ventricular failure requires immediate cardiovascular support. He is in a local district general hospital where the cardiologist has asked for your help.

    Which of the following would be the most appropriate next step?

    A   Adrenaline infusion
    B   Urgent coronary artery bypass graft
    C   Insertion of an intra-aortic balloon pump
    D   Heart transplant
    E   Milrinone infusion

69. A 75-year-old man is having a laparotomy for excision of a large bowel carcinoma. He has a thoracic epidural in place and is being actively warmed by using a warm air blanket and infusion of warm fluids.

    Which of the following is *least* likely to be a consequence of mild peri-operative hypothermia?

    A   Increased risk of myocardial ischaemia

B Increased analgesia requirements
C Increased surgical wound infection
D Longer duration of neuromuscular blockade
E Longer hospital stay

70. You are performing a lumbar plexus block on a patient undergoing elective total hip replacement

   Which of the following nerves is least likely to be blocked with a successful lumbar plexus block?

   A Sciatic nerve
   B Femoral nerve
   C Ilioinguinal nerve
   D Obturator nerve
   E Genitofemoral nerve

71. A 65-year-old woman is having an MRI scan of her head for unexplained severe headaches.

   Which of the following implanted devices is an absolute contraindication for performing the scan?

   A Joint prosthesis
   B Artificial heart valve
   C Sternal wires
   D Cochlear implant
   E Breast implant

72. You are anaesthetising a morbidly obese patient for bariatric surgery who weighs 180 kg and you need to calculate the appropriate drug doses for some of the intravenous drugs you will be administering.

   Which of the following drugs does *not* have a significant change in volume of distribution when administered in morbidly obese patients?

   A Thiopentone
   B Midazolam
   C Remifentanil
   D Paracetamol
   E Etomidate

73. You are performing a rapid sequence induction on a patient having a laparotomy. The patient is being administered 100% oxygen at a flow rate of 7 L/minute.

   What is the most efficient breathing system to use for pre-oxygenating this patient?

   A Mapleson A
   B Mapleson B
   C Mapleson C
   D Mapleson D
   E Mapleson E

74. A 45-year-old presents to the intensive care unit with a left-sided bronchopleural fistula and requires intubation.

Which is the best device to use for lung isolation?

A   White tube
B   Left-sided double-lumen tube
C   Endobronchial blocker
D   Right-sided double-lumen tube
E   Carlens tube

75. A 34-year-old Chinese lady has had an open reduction and internal fixation of her ankle fracture 3 days ago. She is taking 1g of paracetamol every 4–6 hours, 50 mg diclofenac three times a day and 60 mg of codeine phosphate four times a day. She still has significant pain.

What is the most likely pharmacological reason for her inadequate pain control?

A   Defective CYP2D6 isoenzyme
B   Treatment with metronidazole
C   Inadequate drug dosing
D   Co-administration of phenytoin
E   Defective CYP3A5 isoenzyme

76. A 57-year-old man with chronic liver failure presents with a dislocated shoulder. He has been given 10 mg of intravenous morphine in the emergency department and 90 minutes later his respiratory rate is 6 breaths per minute, oxygen saturations are 92% on 2 L of oxygen and his consciousness level has decreased.

What is the most likely underlying mechanism for his clinical deterioration?

A   Reduced phase I metabolism
B   Increased volume of distribution
C   Decreased plasma protein levels
D   Reduced phase II metabolism
E   Decreased bioavailability

77. A 27-year-old, 70 kg, man is having an abscess drained under local anaesthetic. The surgeon infiltrates the area with 30 mL of 2% lidocaine with 1:200,000 adrenaline. Upon insertion of the scalpel, the patient experiences significant pain.

What physicochemical property best explains this?

A   There is reduced protein binding
B   Lidocaine is less potent in infected tissue
C   Acidic pH denatures the lidocaine
D   There is increased local perfusion removing the drug
E   Lidocaine is more ionised in infected tissue

78. A 35-year-old woman has a rapid sequence induction for an incision and drainage of an axillary abscess. The procedure lasts 10 minutes, but she is not yet breathing spontaneously, with a heart rate of 110 beats per minute and a blood pressure of 142/86 mmHg.

What is the *least likely* cause for her ongoing apnoea?

A   Pregnancy
B   Thyrotoxicosis
C   Serum potassium of 3.3 mmol/L
D   Dibucaine number of 20
E   Plasma cholinesterase genotype of Es:Es

79. A 52-year-old man presents for an elective hernia repair. He has a background history of schizophrenia, for which he receives 20 mg of chlorpromazine three times a day.

Which receptor does chlorpromazine *not* antagonise?

A   Nicotinic
B   Dopaminergic
C   Histaminergic
D   Muscarinic
E   Noradrenergic

80. A 86-year-old woman with diabetes mellitus and hypertension has a spinal anaesthetic for a dynamic hip screw. Her blood pressure decreases to 64/36 mmHg with a heart rate of 68 beats per minute, despite having full sensation to her chest wall.

What is the most likely underlying pathophysiology?

A   Autonomic neuropathy
B   High spinal blockade
C   Hypovolaemia
D   Myocardial ischaemia
E   Reduced ventricular compliance

81. A 34-year-old woman presents with a massive post-partum haemorrhage of more than 2 L blood loss. She is short of breath and tachycardic. A bedside analysis gives a haemoglobin value of 5.8 g/dL. Her blood group is known to be A$^+$.

What is the most appropriate infusion to administer?

A   O$^-$ blood
B   500 mL Gelofusine
C   A$^+$ crossmatched blood
D   1 L Hartmann's solution
E   AB$^-$ crossmatched blood

82. Fetal development requires a rich oxygen supply from the mother.

Which of the following is *least* likely to contribute to this?

   A   The double Bohr effect
   B   Increased fetal haemoglobin
   C   High uterine blood flow
   D   Low fetal 2,3-diphosphoglycerate (2,3-DPG)
   E   The Haldane effect

83. A 38-year-old obese woman undergoes a laparoscopic salpingectomy under a general anaesthetic with a laryngeal mask airway. In the recovery room, she has a respiratory rate of 34 breaths per minute, saturations of 91% on 5 L of oxygen administered via a face mask and a heart rate of 108 beats per minute. She has reduced airway entry on her right side with unilateral crackles.

    What is the most likely diagnosis?

   A   Pulmonary oedema
   B   Pneumonia
   C   Pneumothorax
   D   Aspiration pneumonitis
   E   Venous thromboembolism

84. A 86-year-old woman presents with acute severe central abdominal pain with no guarding, a respiratory rate of 32 breaths per minute, heart rate of 142 beats per minute irregularly irregular and a blood pressure of 86/52 mmHg. A diagnosis of acute mesenteric ischaemia (ischaemic gut) is suspected.

    What arterial blood gas result would most strongly support this diagnosis?

   A   Mixed respiratory and metabolic acidosis
   B   Metabolic acidosis with a large anion gap
   C   Ketoacidosis
   D   Respiratory alkalosis
   E   Metabolic acidosis with a normal anion gap

85. A 76-year-old man is undergoing a left thoracoscopy. You have intubated him with a left-sided double-lumen tube.

    What is the best method for confirming correct placement of the tube?

   A   Auscultation
   B   Inspection of the chest
   C   Direct laryngoscopy
   D   Fibreoptic examination
   E   Capnography

86. A 65-year-old man presents having been rescued from a house fire. He has a cherry-red complexion to his skin, complains of a headache, nausea and of feeling weak. His heart rate is 122 beats per minute with a blood pressure of 92/58 mmHg.

    Which of the following is most in keeping with the likely diagnosis?

   A P_{50} of the oxyhaemoglobin dissociation curve is 2.8 kPa
   B   Pulse oximetry saturation is 85%

C   Peripheral neuropathy
D   Reduced arterial Pao_2
E   Increased cardiac output

87. A 26-year-old woman who is 36 weeks pregnant feels generally unwell. She has oxygen saturations of 97% on 15 L of oxygen via a non-rebreathing mask, a heart rate of 130 beats per minute and a blood pressure of 88/55 mmHg.

What is the most important intervention to perform next on this patient?

A   Send a group and save blood sample
B   Perform arterial blood gas sampling
C   Obtain intravenous access
D   Perform a left lateral tilt
E   Intubate and ventilate

88. A 51-year-old woman presents for a laparoscopic excision of a phaeochromocytoma. She has been started on a drug acting at the adrenoceptors 4 weeks previously.

Which drug is this most likely to be?

A   Yohimbine
B   Isoprenaline
C   Labetalol
D   Propranolol
E   Phenoxybenzamine

89. A 36-year-old man presents with status epilepticus and has been started on a phenytoin infusion. He has been transferred to the intensive care unit where you have had to write the prescription chart.

Which of the following statements regarding phenytoin is *least likely* to be true?

A   It undergoes first-order kinetics
B   It is highly protein bound
C   It undergoes zero-order kinetics
D   Dialysis may reduce plasma concentrations
E   May increase dose requirements for lorazepam

90. A 52-year-old man is on the intensive care unit with sepsis and multiorgan failure. He is ventilated, receiving a noradrenaline infusion and is having continuous veno-venous haemofiltration. Upon discussion with the microbiologists, he is to be started on systemic antimicrobial agents.

Which one of the following antibiotics is *least likely* to require dose modification?

A   Flucloxacillin
B   Co-amoxiclav
C   Gentamicin
D   Tazocin (pipericillin/tazobactam)
E   Cefuroxime

Answers: MTFs

1. A False
    B False
    C True
    D False
    E False

    When the heart valves close the cusps balloon back as they stop blood from refluxing. The sudden tension in the cusps sets up a brief vibration, which is transmitted through the walls of the heart and arteries to the chest wall, where it can be heard. In normal heart valves, it is only closure that is audible while the opening is silent (A).

    Two heart sounds are normally clearly audible per beat, the first and second sounds, followed by a pause; the first heart sound occurs immediately after the pause (B).

    The mitral and tricuspid valves close simultaneously and it is the closure of these valves that is responsible for the first heart sound (C).

    The second heart sound can be 'split' in healthy young individuals (D). There could be an initial aortic component followed by a fractionally delayed pulmonary component. Splitting of this sound is common during inspiration. Inspiration increases stroke volume by increasing filling of the right ventricle, which prolongs the right ventricular ejection time, so delaying pulmonary valve closure.

    The third and fourth heart sounds are of low frequency so are difficult to hear, especially to untrained ears (E). The third heart sound is caused by blood flowing rapidly into the relaxing ventricles during early diastole, essentially during ventricular filling. The fourth sound is caused by atrial systole and occurs just before the first heart sound; it is due to atrial contraction occurring under pressure with forceful ventricular distension and may occur in aortic stenosis and hypertension (see **Figure 3.1**).

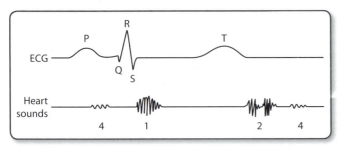

Figure 3.1 Heart sounds and their relationship to the ECG.

2. A False
    B False

C True

D False

E False

Contraction of the myocyte is caused by shortening of its sarcomeres. The actin-binding site is blocked by tropomyosin and in the resting state the myosin heads are disengaged (A).

Contraction is initiated by a sudden rise in free intracellular calcium, which binds to troponin C, which is a component of the troponin complex (B). This displaces the tropomyosin molecule and exposes actin-binding sites for the myosin molecules, which are now able to bind to actin.

The myosin head attaches to the exposed myosin-binding site on the actin molecule (**Figure 3.2**), and a change in the angle of this cross-bridge allows the thin filaments to be moved towards the Z line, causing muscle contraction (C).

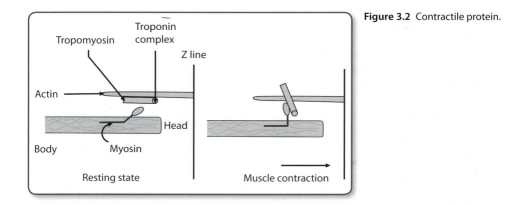

Figure 3.2 Contractile protein.

The energy is provided by adenosine triphosphate (ATP), which is broken down by the enzyme ATPase (found on the myosin head) to adenosine diphosphate (D). ATP is formed in mitochondria by oxidative phosphorylation, which is why the myocyte contains a large number of mitochondria.

The force of contraction depends directly on the number of cross-bridges formed and therefore the concentration of free calcium ions within the myocyte (E).

3. **A** False

B False

C False

D True

E True

The baroreceptors are stretch receptors located in the walls of blood vessels and the heart chambers, and they respond to distension of the walls as a result of increased pressure (A).

The main location of the baroreceptors is in the carotid sinus and arch of the aorta (B). The baroreceptors are non-encapsulated nerve endings found in the adventitial layer. Other locations for the baroreceptors are in the atria, ventricles, lungs and coronary arteries.

The carotid sinus is a thin-walled dilatation at the proximal end of the internal carotid artery.

The afferent fibres for the carotid sinus ascend in the glossopharyngeal (IXth cranial) nerve to the petrous ganglion, where the parent cells are located (C). The aortic baroreceptor afferents ascend in the vagus (Xth cranial) nerve and terminate in the nucleus tractus solitarius.

The baroreceptors are actually mechanoreceptors and respond to stretch rather than pressure. A rise in arterial pressure causes arterial distension and this is what stimulates the mechanoreceptors (D).

The carotid baroreceptors are sensitive to both mean arterial pressure and pulse pressure (E). The greater the oscillation in pressure around the mean, the greater the activity in the nerve trunk and the greater the reflex. This is partly due to the dynamic sensitivity of the receptors.

4.   **A**   False

    B   True

    C   False

    D   True

    E   True

The tunica media layer of the blood vessels contains smooth muscles arranged circumferentially around the vessel wall. It is the active tension of these cells that controls the radius of the vessels. There are many chemical by-products of metabolism and these are intrinsic acids produced by the body called autoacids that affect the tone of the vascular smooth muscle.

Acidosis causes vasodilatation due to the release of endothelium-derived relaxing factor and inactivates membrane calcium channels (A). This is an example of metabolic vasodilatation; other metabolic vasodilators are hypoxia, acidosis (due to the local release of carbon dioxide and lactic acid) and potassium ions released by contracting muscles.

The dilator effect of adenosine is endothelium independent; it inhibits neurotransmitter release by a pre-junctional effect and reduces calcium influx across the vascular smooth muscle membrane (B).

The prostaglandin F-series are mainly vasoconstrictors, while prostacyclin and prostaglandin E are vasodilators (C). They contribute to inflammatory vasodilatation and reactive hyperaemia. Prostaglandins are vasoactive agents causing vasodilatation and are synthesised from the fatty acid pre-cursor, arachidonic acid, and are produced in macrophages, leucocytes and endothelium (D).

Serotonin (5-hydroxytryptamine) is a derivative of the amino acid tryptophan and is found in platelets, the intestine wall and central nervous system. It is released from platelets during clotting and has vasoconstrictor effects to aid haemostasis (E).

5. A False

    B False

    C True

    D True

    E False

The oxygen consumption in the kidney is about 18 mL/minute. The arteriovenous oxygen difference for the whole kidney is only 14 mL/L of blood, compared with 62 mL/L for the brain and 114 mL/L for the heart (A). The arteriovenous difference for oxygen is therefore relatively small in the kidney, as little oxygen is extracted from the blood and this is due to the relatively high renal blood flow (B).

The main function of the renal cortex is filtration of large volumes of blood through the glomeruli, because there is active transport and more energy expenditure, it has a large oxygen consumption compared with the medulla (C).

The blood flow to the medulla is relatively low, as is oxygen utilisation and the main substrate is glucose (D). The Po_2 of the medulla is only about 15 mmHg (it is about 50 mmHg in the cortex). Due to the counter current exchange between the arterial and venous circulations, the partial pressure of O_2 in the renal tissue is low.

The Fick principle states that the rate of removal of a substance from an organ equals the rate entering it minus the rate leaving it. If this is applied to the kidneys, renal plasma flow equals the rate of removal divided by the arterial minus venous concentration. The Fick principle would be used to measure the renal plasma flow and the renal blood flow, but would not be an appropriate way of measuring the renal oxygen consumption (E). The kidney uses oxygen mainly to generate potential energy for tubular re-absorption. The oxygen tension in the kidney is determined by the filtration fraction, as most of the work of reabsorption is closely tied to sodium transport. Renal oxygen consumption is calculated by multiplying renal blood flow by the difference between arterial and venous blood (renal oxygen extraction):

$$\text{Renal oxygen consumption} = \text{renal blood flow} \times (AO_2 - VO_2).$$

6. A True

    B False

    C False

    D True

    E True

Filtration occurs at the glomerulus and approximately a fifth of plasma water is filtered off (A). The glomerular filter also allows the free passage of small dissolved substances, but larger substances such as plasma proteins cannot pass. Some low-molecular substances bind to large plasma proteins, which make them non-filterable.

After filtration, water and other substances are resorbed back into the blood. Electrolytes, amino acids, uric acid, lactate and glucose are examples of substances that are reabsorbed. H^+ ions are actively secreted (B).

The endogenous products of metabolism, such as uric acid, sulphates and glucuronides are actively secreted into the tubular lumen, not passively (C).

The active transcellular secretion of exogenous substances such as antibiotics, diuretics and para-amino hippuric acid (PAH) occurs throughout the nephron (D).

The products of metabolism from tubular cells such as ammonium (NH_4^+), H^+ ions and hippurate undergo cellular secretion into the tubular lumen. NH_4^+ diffuses passively in its ionic form (NH_3), whereas H^+ ions are actively secreted. Therefore, these metabolic products from tubular cells are actively and passively secreted (E).

7. **A** False

    B True

    C True

    D False

    E False

Osmoreceptors in the hypothalamus stimulate the release of antidiuretic hormone (ADH) from the posterior lobe of the pituitary gland when there is a rise in the osmolality of the extracellular fluid (A).

When there is a water deficit, the reduced volume causes a reduction of pressure in the atria, resulting in the stretch receptors sending signals directly to the hypothalamus with a resultant release of ADH (B).

ADH increases the permeability of the collecting ducts to water, resulting in increased water reabsorption at times when there is a water deficit (C).

Salt excess increases the plasma osmolality, which results in an increase in the release of ADH, which in turn increases the extracellular volume (ECV) by increasing water retention and stimulating thirst (D). The increase in ECV also causes an increase in the plasma volume, which inhibits the renin-angiotensin II-aldosterone mechanism.

Atrial natriuretic peptide is released from vesicles in the atrial wall when there is increased stretching of the wall, resulting in increased excretion of sodium ions by the kidneys (E).

8. **A** True

    B False

C True

D True

E False

pH is the negative logarithm to base 10 of the hydrogen ion concentration (the 'p' in pH is the symbol for $-\log_{10}$) (A).

The pH value of the blood is about 7.4, which is equal to a H^+ ion activity of about 40 nmol/L. It is important to maintain a constant pH for effective enzyme function and metabolism to occur. Buffers act by partially neutralising the acids and bases that exist in the body as a result of metabolism (B). Haemoglobin is a very important buffer in the erythrocytes (C):

$$HbH \rightleftharpoons Hb^- + H^+$$

$$HbO_2H \rightleftharpoons HbO_2^- + H^+$$

Apart from haemoglobin, there are other important buffers in the blood including plasma proteins and the organic and inorganic phosphates (D).

The CO_2/HCO_3^- buffer is one of the main buffer systems of the body,

$$CO_2 + H_2O \rightleftharpoons H_2CO_3 \rightleftharpoons HCO_3^- + H^+$$

It has the added advantage that both sides of the buffer can be controlled independently by different organs. The CO_2 partial pressure in the blood is primarily controlled by the lungs, with variations in ventilation keeping the levels constant (E). The kidneys, with some contribution from the liver, control HCO_3^- levels.

9. A True

    B False

    C True

    D True

    E True

When plotted on a pressure/volume curve, the slope of the graph determines the lung compliance. Because the curve is sigmoid shaped, therefore the lung compliance is variable depending on the lung volume (see Figure 1.9) (A). When plotted in normal tidal volume breathing, the lung compliance is roughly linear (B). There are a number of factors affecting the compliance of the lungs (see Table 2.1) and old age does result in increased lung compliance (C). On the pressure/volume curves for inspiration and expiration, there is a greater pressure required at any volume to expand the lung in inspiration than expiration (D). This is due to the forces required to overcome surface tension and is called hysteresis. Therefore, the lungs are less compliant during inspiration than expiration. Calculation of lung compliance requires measurement of intrapleural pressures using an oesophageal balloon (E).

10. A True

    B False

C True

D False

E False

The functional residual capacity is the volume of air left in the lungs at the end of a normal expiration. It is the sum of the residual volume and expiratory reserve volume and is usually approximately 2.5–3 L (D, E). It can be measured by:

- Helium dilution: at the end of a normal expiration, air with a known concentration of helium (which is non-soluble in blood) is inspired while CO_2 is absorbed and O_2 replaced (A). This continues until equilibrium is reached, and thus the total amount of helium in the closed circuit is:
  = Initial concentration × volume of apparatus
  = New concentration × volume of (lungs + apparatus)
- Nitrogen washout: the subject breathes 100% oxygen at the end of normal expiration while expired gas volume is analysed for N_2 which is 79% if it comes from the functional residual capacity (FRC). This allows the FRC to be derived
- Body plethysmography: the subject breathes through a mouthpiece in an enclosed chamber. After a normal expiration, the mouthpiece is occluded. The subject tries to expand their lungs in the enclosed chamber and the pressure and volume can be derived using Boyle's law as can be seen in **Table 3.1**. The functional residual capacity is reduced during general anaesthesia and by increased positive end expiratory pressure (PEEP).

Table 3.1 Factors affecting functional residual capacity (FRC)

Reduced FRC	Increased FRC
Supine position	Upright position
Obesity	Increased airway resistance
Pregnancy	Asthma
General anaesthesia and intermittent positive pressure ventilation (IPPV)	PEEP and continuous positive airway pressure (CPAP)
Restrictive lung disease	Exercise

11. A True

B False

C True

D False

E False

The alveolar-arterial (A-a) oxygen tension difference is a measure of $\dot{V}/\dot{Q}$ mismatch or shunt. The alveolar Po_2 is calculated with the alveolar gas equation, while the arterial Po_2 is measured. When breathing room air, it is normally 1.5–2.0 kPa, but this increases to up to 15 kPa when breathing 100% O_2 as there is no correction for shunt (B). In the elderly, it is usually 4–5 kPa in room air (C). There are a number of factors that increase the A-a gradient:

- Ventilation defect: general anaesthesia, reduced functional residual capacity (FRC), dead-space ventilation (A)
- Perfusion defect: shunt, reduced cardiac output, hypovolaemia, anaemia
- Diffusion defect: exercise, emphysema
- Hormones: liver failure, pregnancy
- Drugs: volatile anaesthetics, vasodilators (D)
- Right-to-left shunt (E)

12. **A** False

   B False

   C True

   D True

   E True

Pulmonary vascular resistance (PVR) is the equivalent of systemic vascular resistance and its calculation is based on the principle of Ohm's law, measured in $dynes.s/cm^5$ with a conversion factor of 80 (A, B):

$$PVR = \frac{\text{Mean pulmonary artery pressure} - \text{Left atrial pressure}}{\text{Cardiac output}} \times 80$$

At low lung volumes, the pulmonary vessels are compressed, while at high lung volumes they are over stretched, which also increases the resistance. PVR is therefore lowest at functional residual capacity (C). It is affected by a number of factors (see **Table 3.2**).

Table 3.2 Factors affecting pulmonary vascular resistance (PVR)

Increased PVR	Decreased PVR
Decreased pH	Increased pH
Decreased Pao_2	Increased Pao_2
Increased $Paco_2$	Decreased $Paco_2$
Adrenaline	Acetylcholine
Noradrenaline	Prostacyclin
5-Hydroxytryptamine	Nitric oxide
Histamine	Increased cardiac output
Thromboxane A_2, angiotensin	Increased peak airway pressures
High/low lung volumes	Volatile anaesthetics
Pulmonary embolism, atelectasis, effusion (D)	Exercise (E)

13. A False

   B True

   C True

   D True

   E True

Hormones are the chemical messengers of the body. They transmit information which is necessary for the regulation of the functions of many organs and cells in the body. All hormones have chemical structures derived from peptides, glycoproteins, steroids or the amino acid tyrosine.

The peptide and protein hormones are made up of amino acid chains, which vary in length. They are synthesised on rough endoplasmic reticulum. Some have carbohydrate groups attached to them and are called glycoproteins; an example is thyroid-stimulating hormone (A, E).

All steroid hormones are derived from cholesterol and have a four-ring structure (B, D). They are synthesised on the smooth endoplasmic reticulum, and small differences in the side groups attached to the rings allow for the diversity of function of the steroids.

The amine hormones are the simplest hormone molecules and most are derived from the amino acid tyrosine. The exceptions are histamine, which is derived from the amino acid histidine and serotonin and melatonin, which are derived from tryptophan. They all retain an a-amino group on a benzene ring (C).

14. A False

   B True

   C False

   D True

   E False

The thyroid gland is mostly made up of spherical sacs called thyroid follicles, which are made up of follicular cells which manufacture thyroxine (T4) and triiodothyronine (T3). It is the parafollicular cells which produce calcitonin (A).

The thyroid gland is the only endocrine gland that stores its secretory product in large quantity, about 100 days worth is stored (B).

T3 and T4 are synthesised by attaching iodine to tyrosine and storing this in the gland. This is then secreted into the blood, under the control of thyroid-stimulating hormone. The process initially involves the trapping of iodide by the thyroid follicular cells, which is then oxidised to iodine, catalysed by the enzyme peroxidase (C). Negatively charged iodide (I^-) cannot bind to tyrosine, so these anions have to undergo this oxidation process. As soon as iodine is formed it attaches to tyrosine amino acids, which are part of the thyroglobulin molecules in the colloid.

Binding of one iodine forms monoiodotyrosine (T1) and a second iodination forms diiodotyrosine (T2). These then couple to form T3 and T4.

Both T3 and T4 are lipid soluble, so they diffuse through the plasma membrane and into the blood. More than 99% of T3 and T4 is attached to the transport protein thyroxine-binding globulin (D).

T4 is secreted in greater quantity than T3, but T3 is much more potent (E). Most of T4 is converted to T3 as it enters the cells from the blood, by removal of one iodine molecule.

15. A True

 B True

 C True

 D False

 E False

Adrenaline, noradrenaline and dopamine are all secreted from the adrenal medulla (A). They are stored in granules and their secretion is initiated by acetylcholine released from the preganglionic neurons that innervate the secretory cells.

The three principal catecholamines are formed by the hydroxylation and decarboxylation of the amino acid tyrosine (B). Most of the tyrosine is of dietary origin, but some is formed from phenylalanine.

Tyrosine is formed from phenylalanine by the enzyme phenylalanine hydroxylase (found mainly in the liver). Tyrosine is then converted to DOPA (dihydroxyphenylalanine) by tyrosine hydroxylase in the cytoplasm of the cells in the adrenal medulla (C). This is the rate-determining step of the whole process, as it is subject to feedback inhibition by dopamine and noradrenaline (D). Dopamine is then formed from DOPA, by the actions of DOPA decarboxylase. The dopamine then enters granulated vesicles, where it is converted to noradrenaline by dopamine β-hydroxylase. Noradrenaline can then be converted to adrenaline (see **Figure 3.3**).

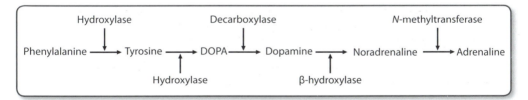

Figure 3.3 Adrenaline synthesis.

Adrenaline and noradrenaline are catabolised to biologically inert products by oxidation and methylation; these reactions are catalysed by monoamine oxidase (MAO) and catechol-O-methyl-transferase (COMT) respectively (E). MAO is found on the surface of mitochondria, particularly in neurons. COMT is found in the liver, kidneys and smooth muscle.

16. A True

   B True

   C False

   D True

   E False

The oesophageal circular muscle, about 2–5 cm above the junction with the stomach, is slightly thickened, although anatomically the same as the rest of the oesophagus, functions as the lower oesophageal sphincter (A). It is tonically constricted, whereas the rest of the oesophagus is completely relaxed (C).

In order to allow the easy passage of food from the oesophagus into the stomach, the lower oesophageal sphincter relaxes ahead of the peristaltic wave (B, D).

In achalasia, the lower oesophageal sphincter does not relax sufficiently, resulting in food accumulating above the cardia causing dilation of the oesophagus (E).

17. A True

   B False

   C False

   D False

   E True

The pancreas secretes approximately 2 L of pancreatic juices daily into the duodenum (A). The juice contains bicarbonate and digestive enzymes. Secretion is under neural and hormonal control. Neural control is via the vagus nerve and hormonal control is via secretin and cholecystokinin (CCK). The stimulus for secretin secretion is a low pH and fat (C). Secretin increases the volume of pancreatic juices and raises the bicarbonate level (B).

The bicarbonate in the pancreatic juices neutralises the gastric acid and does not activate the enzymes (D).

The fat content of the chyme also stimulates the release of CCK, which has the role of increasing the enzyme content of pancreatic juice.

Trypsin and chymotrypsin are proteolytic enzymes present in pancreatic juices (E). They are initially secreted as the inactive precursors, trypsinogen and chymotrypsinogen, then activated by enteropeptidase.

18. A True

   B True

   C False

   D False

   E False

The brain is bathed in cerebrospinal fluid, which is a nutritive and protective fluid. It also fills the ventricles of the central nervous system.

70% of the cerebrospinal fluid (CSF) is produced by the choroid plexus (which is a collection of blood vessels and tissues), while the remaining 30% is produced in the endothelium of cerebral capillaries (C). It has a volume of 150 mL and is reabsorbed from the arachnoid villi into the dural venous sinuses (A). The choroid plexus secretes approximately 650 mL of CSF daily.

CSF has a pH of 7.28–7.32 and contains only 0.2–0.4 g/dL of protein (B, D). The glucose concentration is usually one half to two thirds than that of the serum, and in pathological conditions such as bacterial meningitis this can be reduced (E).

The exchange of substances between the blood and CSF is strictly controlled across the blood–CSF and blood–brain barrier. Substances such as glucose and amino acids are transported by special mechanisms but proteins are unable to cross the barrier.

19. A False

B True

C True

D True

E False

The sympathetic nervous system is responsible for 'fight or flight' responses of the autonomic nervous system. Preganglionic fibres are myelinated, and they have a thoracolumbar outflow from T1 to L2 (A). The sympathetic trunk consists of a bilateral chain of ganglia including the cervical (3), thoracic (12), lumbar (4) and sacral (4) ganglia. The cervical ganglia also supplies sympathetic supply to the facial nerve (VII), the glossopharyngeal (IX), vagus (X) and hypoglossal (XII) nerves (B). The neurotransmitter at the ganglia and adrenal medulla is acetylcholine, while the neurotransmitter at the postganglionic nerve endings is noradrenaline (C). Renin release is influenced by β-adrenergic stimulation and responds to circulating adrenaline. Effects of sympathetic stimulation include:

- Eyes: pupillary dilation; ciliary muscle relaxation (E)
- Cardiovascular: tachycardia, increased contractility; vasoconstriction via α-adrenoceptors; vasodilatation via β-adrenoceptors
- Pulmonary: bronchodilatation; reduced secretions
- Gastrointestinal: reduced motility and secretions; sphincteric contraction
- Metabolic: increased insulin and glucagon via β-adrenoceptors, decreased by α-adrenoceptors
- Genitourinary: detrusor muscle relaxation, sphincteric contraction; renin secretion (D)

20. A False

B True

C False

D False

E True

Red blood cells (erythrocytes) are formed in the bone marrow by erythropoiesis in response primarily to erythropoietin (EPO). EPO release from the kidney and liver is in response to hypoxia, increased metabolism and haemorrhage, with a reduced production due to increased erythrocytes (B).

Erythrocytes are highly specialised cells with no nucleus or organelles and comprising 95% haemoglobin with the remainder including enzymes for glycolysis (D, E). They have a circulating survival of approximately 120 days after which they are removed by the reticuloendothelial system (A).

The normal mean corpuscular volume (MCV) is 80–100 fL, which increases due to reticulocytosis, alcohol consumption, vitamin B_{12} and folate deficiency (C). The MCV decreases in iron deficiency and atypical haemoglobin.

21. A False

   B False

   C True

   D False

   E False

A mammillary three-compartment model is composed of a central compartment, one well-perfused peripheral compartment (the second compartment) and one poorly perfused peripheral compartment (the third compartment). The capacity of each compartment represents a drug reservoir, and the total volume of distribution is equal to the volume of the three compartments. The second and third compartments come to equilibrium with the central compartment, but do not directly communicate (see **Figure 3.4**) (B).

Upon drug administration into the central compartment, normally representing the plasma, there is an exponential decline in concentration due to redistribution

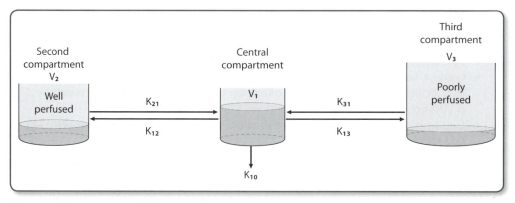

Figure 3.4 Compartment models.

initially to the well-perfused second compartment, followed by the third compartment (A, C, D). Drug clearance only occurs via the central compartment at a slower exponential rate than drug redistribution (E).

22. **A** True

    B True

    C True

    D False

    E False

Renal excretion of drugs depends on glomerular filtration, tubular secretion and tubular diffusion.

- Filtration: substances with a low molecular weight (<7000 Da) are freely filtered, while the upper limit is approximately 70,000 Da. Other factors reducing filtration include high protein binding, high lipid solubility and high ionic charge
- Secretion: energy-dependent carrier systems for acidic or basic drugs can actively secrete substances against concentration gradients and achieve maximal drug clearance, despite high protein binding. Acidic drugs being pumped this way compete with each other, as do basic drugs with each other
- Diffusion: a concentration gradient at the distal tubules causes passive diffusion of substances. Highly polar drugs such as digoxin or gentamicin diffuse across and become trapped in the tubules. Additionally, acidic drugs may become more ionised in alkaline urine, thereby increasing their excretion, e.g. salicylates

In renal failure, drugs that are dependent on renal excretion by any of the above mechanisms may need dose modification. These include hydralazine (A) (an antihypertensive used predominantly in pregnancy), enoximone (B) (a phosphodiesterase III inhibitor with inodilator properties) and tramadol (C). Because phenytoin is extensively metabolised by the liver to predominantly inactive metabolites, its dosing is independent of renal function (D). Atracurium is metabolised by Hoffman degradation as well as non-specific esterases, thus does not require dose readjustment in renal impairment (E).

23. **A** True

    B False

    C False

    D False

    E False

The aim of metabolism is to either activate an inactive drug or inactivate an active drug. Inactivation is generally achieved by making the drug water soluble to allow excretion either in the urine or in the bile. This can be achieved by either phase I or phase II metabolism.

Phase I metabolism includes oxidation, reduction or hydrolysis, taking place predominantly in the liver, although may also occur at extrahepatic sites. It is usually catalysed by cytochrome P450 enzymes in the smooth endoplasmic reticulum, and usually precedes phase II. Phase I reactions not dependent on P450 enzymes include metabolism of ethanol by alcohol dehydrogenase to acetaldehyde, as well as monoamine oxidase inactivation of noradrenaline, adrenaline and dopamine.

Phase II metabolism increases water solubility and reduce lipid solubility in order to allow drug excretion in the urine or bile, while inactivating the drug (B). It does not precede phase I metabolism, but often occurs following phase I metabolism (E). It involves synthetic processes of conjugation, including acetylation, glucuronidation, methylation and sulphation (A). It usually occurs in the liver but may take place in the kidneys, lungs or spleen (D). Very rarely, phase II reactions can lead to active drug properties, but most commonly inactivate drugs (C).

24. A False

    B False

    C True

    D True

    E False

Isomers are molecules with the same atomic formulae but different structural arrangements (**Table 3.3**). Structural isomers have the same chemical formulae but different border of atomic bonds. This includes chain isomers (carbon skeleton changes but functional group remains in the same position), positional isomers (carbon skeleton unchanged, functional group position varies), functional isomers (changed functional group) and tautomers (change in molecular structure depending on environment) (C). Examples include dihydrocodeine and dobutamine, enflurane and isoflurane, and morphine (tautomerism) (B, D).

Table 3.3 Classification of isomers	
Structural isomers	**Stereoisomers**
Chain isomers	Enantiomers (optical isomers)
Positional isomers	Diastereoisomers (optical isomers)
Functional isomers	*Cis*-trans isomers (geometric isomers)
Tautomers	

Stereoisomers have the same chemical composition but different three-dimensional configuration. They can be optical isomers containing a single chiral centre (enantiomers) or two or more chiral centres (diastereoisomers) (A). A chiral centre is a central atom bound by four dissimilar groups (E). Alternatively, they can be geometric isomers where two atoms have dissimilar groups and are linked by a ring structure or double bond reducing the mobility molecule.

25. A False

  B True

  C True

  D False

  E True

- Potency: indicates quantity of drug required to achieve a maximal effect (A)
- Efficacy: the magnitude of effect of bound drug, same as intrinsic activity (IA), which can be between 0 (no effect) and 1 (full effect) (C)
- Affinity: how well a drug binds to a receptor
- Agonist: high receptor affinity and IA (=1) (E)
- Antagonist: high receptor affinity but no intrinsic activity (=0) (B)
- Partial agonist: high receptor affinity with partial intrinsic activity (>0; <1) (D)

26. A True

  B True

  C False

  D False

  E False

Bupivacaine is an amide local anaesthetic agent with a moderate onset time and a prolonged duration of action due to high protein binding to α_1-glycoprotein of 95%. It is the most lipid soluble local anaesthetic agent giving it a high relative potency (B). With a pKa of 8.1, it is only 15% unionised at a pH of 7.4 (C). Of all the local anaesthetic agents, it is the most cardiotoxic because it binds to specific myocardial proteins, as well as reducing systemic vascular resistance and myocardial contractility (D). It has a toxic plasma concentration of 1. 5 µg/mL and a maximum safe dose of 2 mg/kg with or without adrenaline (A). It is a racemic mixture, but the S(−) enantiomer of levobupivacaine demonstrates less cardiovascular and neurological toxicity, with a reduction in motor blockade (E).

27. A True

  B True

  C False

  D False

  E True

Amethocaine is an ester local anaesthetic agent that is metabolised predominantly in the plasma by esterases producing the metabolite para-aminobenzoic acid PABA, and is excreted in the kidneys (A).

Esmolol is a short-acting β-blocker that undergoes ester hydrolysis by red cell esterases, producing methanol and an acidic metabolite with weak β-blocking activity (B).

Lorazepam is benzodiazepine with an oral bioavailability of 90%, plasma protein binding of 95% and an intermediate duration of action. It is metabolised by hepatic glucuronidation to inactive water-soluble metabolites (C).

Phenytoin is a hydantoin-derived anticonvulsant that is hydroxylated then glucuronated in the liver (D).

Mivacurium is a short-acting non-depolarising muscle relaxant that is hydrolysed by plasma cholinesterase to largely inactive metabolites (E).

28. A False

B False

C True

D True

E False

Methohexitone is a methylated oxybarbiturate (A). It is formulated as the sodium salt with sodium carbonate which is readily soluble in water and forms an alkaline solution with a pH of 11. Its pKa is 7.9 and at physiological pH approximately 75% of the unbound drug is unionised.

It may cause an excitatory phase before anaesthesia is induced. Muscle twitching, hiccup and increased tone can occur as a result. This is more marked than with thiopentone (B).

Convulsions may be precipitated in patients with a history of epilepsy, so should be avoided in this group of patients (C).

With inadvertent intra-arterial injection, methohexitone produces fewer complications as compared to thiopentone, which causes severe pain due to arterial spasm (D). With accidental subcutaneous injection, methohexitone also produces less tissue damage than thiopentone; this is thought to be due simply to the lower concentration of methohexitone (1% solution), while thiopentone is prepared as a 2.5% solution.

Methohexitone is associated with a higher incidence hypersensitivity reactions compared to thiopentone, which is partly why its use has declined over the years (E).

29. A True

B False

C True

D False

E False

Thiopentone undergoes a triexponential decline after a single bolus dose, resulting in rapid emergence. The initial decline is due to distribution to well-perfused organs such as the liver. The second phase of decline is due to redistribution to muscle and skin. The final decline is due to hepatic oxidation to form inactive metabolites (A).

Ketamine is only 25% protein bound, so has the least percentage of protein binding of all of the intravenous anaesthetic agents (B). It is demethylated to the active metabolite norketamine by hepatic P450 enzymes. This is then metabolised to inactive glucuronide metabolites and excreted in the urine.

Propofol is highly protein bound and has the largest volume of distribution of all of the intravenous anaesthetic agents. It is mainly metabolised in the liver with approximately 60% metabolised to quinol and the remainder being conjugated to glucuronide (C). These are inactive metabolites which are excreted in the urine.

Etomidate is approximately 75% protein bound. It is rapidly redistributed into tissues with a good blood supply. Non-specific hepatic esterases and plasma cholinesterase hydrolyse it to ethyl alcohol and carboxylic acid, which is then excreted in the urine (D).

At physiological pH, thiopentone is mostly protein bound, with only about 10% being unbound to protein and in the unionised form (E). The free unbound drug is 60% unionised and this is the active component. The onset of action of thiopentone is very rapid due to it being highly lipid soluble.

30. **A** True

   B False

   C False

   D False

   E True

All of the volatile anaesthetic agents depress ventilation, but to differing degrees. Isoflurane depresses ventilation more than halothane and sevoflurane but less than enflurane (A), see **Table 3.4**.

Sevoflurane has a pleasant odour and a low blood:gas partition coefficient so is suitable for gas induction; it does not cause breath holding and is not irritant to the upper airways (B). Desflurane has a pungent odour that causes coughing and breath holding; it is therefore not suitable for gas induction. Isoflurane has a pungent smell that can also cause upper airway irritability, coughing and breath holding.

Halothane increases the cerebral blood flow more than any other volatile anaesthetic agent (C). As a result, it will increase intracranial pressure and so should be avoided in patients with intracranial pathology, see **Table 3.5**.

Desflurane does not sensitise the heart to catecholamines. Halothane does and this may lead to arrhythmias (D), see **Table 3.6**.

Enflurane in high concentrations produces 3 Hz spike and wave pattern which is consistent with grand mal seizure activity (E). As a result it is avoided in epileptic patients. It also causes an increase in the cerebral blood flow, less than that seen with halothane, but more than with isoflurane.

Table 3.4 Respiratory effects of volatile anaesthetics

Effect	Halothane	Enflurane	Isoflurane	Sevoflurane	Desflurane
Respiratory rate	↑	↑↑	↑↑	↑↑	↑↑
$Paco_2$	-	↑↑↑	↑↑	↑	↑↑
Tidal volume	↓	↓↓↓	↓↓	↓	↓↓

Table 3.5 Central nervous system effects of volatile anaesthetics

Effect	Halothane	Enflurane	Isoflurane	Sevoflurane	Desflurane
Cerebral blood flow	↑↑↑	↑	↑	↑	↑
Cerebral oxygen requirement	↓	↓	↓	↓	↓
EEG	Burst suppression	Epileptiform activity	Burst suppression	Burst suppression	Burst suppression

Table 3.6 Cardiovascular effects of volatile anaesthetics

Effect	Halothane	Enflurane	Isoflurane	Sevoflurane	Desflurane
Contractility	↓	↓	↓	↓	-
Heart rate	↓↓	↑	↑↑	-	↑
Systemic vascular resistance	↓	↓	↓↓	↓	↓↓
Blood pressure	↓↓	↓↓	↓↓	↓	↓↓
Sensitises to catecholamines	↑↑↑	↑	-	-	-

31. **A** False

B True

C True

D False

E True

Non-steroidal anti-inflammatory drugs can be classified as shown in **Table 3.7**.

32. **A** True

B False

C False

Table 3.7 Classification of non-steroidal anti-inflammatory drugs (NSAIDs)

	Class	Drugs
Non-specific COX* inhibitors	Salicylates	Aspirin
	Para-aminophenols	Paracetamol
	Acetic acid derivatives	Diclofenac, ketorolac, indomethacin
	Propionic acids	Ibuprofen, naproxen
	Anthranilic acids	Mefanamic acid
	Pyrazolones	Phenylbutazone
	Oxicams	Piroxicam
COX-2 inhibitors	Oxicams	Meloxicam
	Pyrazoles	Celecoxib

*Cyclo-oxygenase.

D False

E False

Morphine is a weak base with a pKa of 8.0; therefore, it is ionised when in the acidic environment of the stomach, resulting in poor absorption here (A, B). When it reaches the relatively alkaline environment of the small bowel, it becomes more unionised and then absorption is increased. Morphine undergoes extensive first-pass metabolism and about 25% reaches the systemic circulation following oral administration.

Morphine has a low lipid solubility which can explain some of its effects, such as delayed respiratory depression after intrathecal administration (C).

Morphine is metabolised in the liver and kidneys, although the majority is in the liver (D). About 70% is metabolised to morphine 3-glucuronide and a much smaller proportion to morphine 6-glucuronide (E). The latter is 13 times as potent as morphine and has a similar duration of action. Both are excreted in the urine, so may accumulate in renal failure and result in a prolonged duration of action.

33. **A** True

    B False

    C True

    D True

    E False

Neuromuscular blocking drugs can have a prolonged duration of action because of either congenital (suxamethonium apnoea) or acquired causes (**Table 3.8**).

Table 3.8 Causes of prolonged action of neuromuscular blocking drugs		
Pharmacological	**Pathological**	**Physiological**
Local anaesthetics	Renal failure[*]	Hypothermia
Aminoglycosides	Liver failure[*]	Hypokalaemia
Lithium	Cardiac failure[*]	Hypermagnesaemia
Calcium channel blockers	Thyrotoxicosis[*]	Hypocalcaemia
Volatile anaesthetics	Acidosis	Pregnancy[*]
Oral contraceptive pill[*]	Malignancy[*]	
*Relates to a prolonged block with suxamethonium and mivacurium only.		

34. **A** False

    B False

    C True

    D True

    E False

Atracurium is benzyl isoquinolinium non-depolarising muscle relaxant that is a racemic mixture of 10 stereoisomers (A). It is stable when stored at 4–10°C and is administered at a dose of 0.5 mg/kg, acting within 120 seconds of administration (E). It is 15% protein bound with a volume of distribution of 0.15 L/kg. Atracurium becomes unstable at body temperature and 40% undergoes Hofmann's degradation, which is the spontaneous breakdown to a quaternary monoacrylate and laudanosine. Laudanosine has been shown to be pro-convulsant; however, at concentrations of <17 µg/mL this is highly unlikely (D). The remaining 60% undergoes hydrolysis by non-specific plasma esterases producing laudanosine, a quaternary alcohol and acid. Because of this metabolic pathway, it is the muscle relaxant of choice in patients with hepatic and renal impairment (B). Atracurium may cause bronchospasm due to histamine release (C).

35. **A** False

    B False

    C True

    D True

    E True

Sugammadex (Bridion) is a modified γ-cyclodextrin and is classified as a selective relaxant-binding agent (A). It allows very rapid reversal of neuromuscular blockade from any depth of block due to rocuronium and to a lesser extent vecuronium, being faster acting than neostigmine (B, E). It acts by forming a complex with rocuronium or vecuronium in a 1:1 ratio, thereby reducing their potential for binding to nicotinic acetylcholine receptors. The water-soluble complex generates a concentration gradient for the neuromuscular blocking drug to diffuse away from the neuromuscular junction into the plasma.

Sugammadex is not significantly bound to plasma proteins and undergoes minimal metabolism having no active metabolites, before excretion in the urine, either isolated or bound to rocuronium (C, D).

36. A False

B True

C True

D True

E False

γ-aminobutyric acid (GABA) acts via $GABA_A$ or $GABA_B$ receptors as the predominant inhibitory neurotransmitters of the central nervous system, followed closely by glycine. The $GABA_A$ receptors (see **Figure 3.5**) are ligand-gated, where activation opens a central chloride (Cl^-) channel causing hyperpolarisation of post-synaptic neuronal membranes. Propofol, thiopentone, R-etomidate, isoflurane and all benzodiazepines act on this receptor. The $GABA_B$ receptor is a metabotropic receptor linked to potassium channels via G-proteins, the most recognised agonist being baclofen.

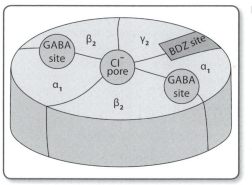

Figure 3.5 $GABA_A$ receptor.

37. A True

B True

C True

D False

E True

Lithium is a basic metal presented in its chloride or carbonated form that is used in treatment of psychiatric disorders, chronic pain states and cardiac output monitoring. The mechanism of action is unclear, but it is thought to increase presynaptic uptake of noradrenaline and induce activity of monoamine oxidase. It has 100% oral bioavailability, with a volume of distribution equalling total body water and is not bound to plasma proteins (A, B). It undergoes minimal metabolism before being excreted by the kidneys as it is a small ion that is freely filtered (D). With a narrow therapeutic index, it may cause thyroid dysfunction including goitre formation or hypothyroidism, as wall as cause nephrogenic diabetes insipidus (E). Electrocardiogram (ECG) changes and arrhythmias may also be present following chronic administration. Lithium has been shown to have a synergistic effect with non-depolarising neuromuscular blockers and an additive effect with suxamethonium (C). It is thought to reduce minimum alveolar concentration requirements and be associated with ECG changes under anaesthesia. Lithium crosses the placenta and is found in breast milk.

38. A True

   B False

   C False

   D False

   E False

Calcium channel blockers interfere with the inward displacement of calcium ions through the slow channels of active cell membranes (see **Figure 3.6**) (A).

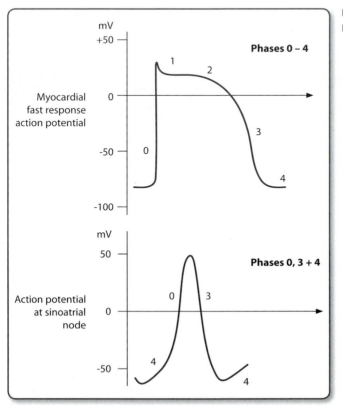

Figure 3.6 Cardiac action potential.

This effect depresses phases II and III of the action potential of the ventricular myofibril, so it prolongs the plateau phase which occurs as a result of the slow inward flux of calcium ions (B).

Re-entry circuits can occur in the atrioventricular node so the actions of calcium channel blockers are particularly useful here. They depress sinoatrial node automaticity and slow atrioventricular node conduction so are used in the treatment of supraventricular arrhythmias (C).

They are all well absorbed from the gut, but undergo extensive first-pass metabolism, so their bioavailablilties range from 10% to 50% (D). They are highly protein bound and mainly eliminated by the liver.

Increased free intracellular calcium increases smooth muscle contractility, peripheral resistance and blood pressure, so calcium channel blockers have the opposite effect (E).

39. A True

  B False

  C False

  D False

  E True

Diuretics can be classified as shown in **Table 3.9** and based on site of location (see question 2.40):

Table 3.9 Diuretic classification	
Class of diuretic	**Drug**
Loop	Furosemide, bumetanide
Thiazide	Bendrofluazide, metolazone
Potassium sparing	Amiloride
Aldosterone antagonists	Spironolactone
Carbonic anhydrase inhibitors	Acetazolamide
Osmotic	Mannitol

40. A False

  B True

  C True

  D False

  E False

The penicillins are bactericidal and inhibit cell wall synthesis by combining with transpeptidases used to cross-link cell wall peptidoglycan (A). Their mechanism of action is dependent on an intact β-lactam ring, which if split open by β-lactamase render them ineffective.

The cephalosporins contain a β-lactam ring structure and are bactericidal like the penicillins (B). They work by combining with the transpeptidase used to cross-link bacterial cell wall peptidoglycan. Its ring is more stable than the penicillins so it is less susceptible to β-lactamase.

The tetracyclines are bacteriostatic and inhibit the protein synthesis of bacterial organisms by binding to the ribosome subunits (C). This prevents tRNA binding to the ribosome so that there is no further binding of amino acids to the peptide chain.

Aminoglycosides are effective against gram-positive and gram-negative organisms (D). They are bactericidal and block protein synthesis by binding to the ribosome subunit in a similar manner to the tetracyclines.

The macrolides inhibit bacterial protein synthesis by binding to ribosomal subunits and inhibit translocation (E). They have a similar range of activity to the penicillins.

41. **A** False

    B False

    C False

    D False

    E True

Alternating current can freely pass through a capacitor. Direct current, however, cannot pass as the resistance of a capacitor is inversely proportional to the frequency of the alternating current (A, C).

Three classes of electrical insulation exist to minimise the risk of electrocution to the patient and anaesthetist.

Class I equipment is fully earthed and all exposed conductive parts are connected to earth; if there is a short circuit, then the current will flow to earth and the fuse will blow (D).

Class II equipment is double insulated and are not earthed (B, E). Their power cables only have neutral and live conductors and their casings are normally made of non-conductive material.

Class III equipment rely on a low-voltage power supply produced from a secondary transformer, which is usually situated well away from the device itself.

42. **A** True

    B False

    C False

    D True

    E True

Electrode pads contain silver and are coated electrolytically with a thin layer of silver chloride (A). In order to minimise interference from mains supply, they have low and stable impedance (B). Needle electrodes deliver poor electrical performance compared with electrode pads and are much more sensitive to movement (C). A foam pad covered with electrolyte gel will greatly reduce movement artefacts, which can change the impedance and electrical potential of the electrode (D). Wiping the skin with alcohol solution will remove grease from the skin surface and this will reduce skin impedance once the electrodes are attached and improve adhesion of the pad (E).

43. **A** True

B False

C False

D True

E True

When high-frequency voltage is passed across the body via suitable electrodes, a current will flow as the body becomes part of the circuit. At frequencies over 100 kHz, the effect of this current is heating of the tissues (diathermy). Rapid heating of tissue over a very small area will produce a high-density arc from the active electrode that will cause boiling of the intracellular fluid (D). The most efficient cutting waveform is a continuous sine waveform (A). This type is excellent for cutting, but not coagulation. Coagulation is achieved by fulguration and desiccation. Fulguration (lightening) is the destructive charring of tissue by arcing, and this is usually achieved by using a flat spatula-shaped electrode tip. Desiccation (drying) is the heating of tissue by direct contact of the tissue with the tip of the electrode (C). The intense heat at the tip causes intracellular water to steam off and the tissue desiccates.

The waveforms for coagulation are continuous and require higher voltages than for cutting diathermy (B). Bipolar diathermy is more effective at coagulation than cutting (E).

44. **A** True

B False

C True

D True

E False

A **laser** (**l**ight **a**mplification by the **s**timulated **e**mission of **r**adiation) is a device that controls the way energised atoms release protons (A, B). The atoms are energised by applying energy supplied by heat, light or electricity (C). This causes them to leave the ground state energy level (or resting state) and reach an excited state. In the excited state, the electrons move to higher energy orbits, but eventually they want to return to the ground state, and when this happens photons are released (D). The released photons are of a specific wavelength or colour (E).

Laser radiation is used to cause tissue destruction by producing intense local heat, and the effects of the laser beam on tissue depend on the wavelength, e.g. CO_2 lasers are used for precise surgical cutting and argon laser is used for photocoagulation in ophthalmology.

45. A False

B True

C True

D False

E True

The Système International (SI) of units is the internationally recognised system of measurement communication. From the base quantities, there are derived quantities, which are shown in Table 2.8. The basic units are combined by multiplication and/or division to form the derived units.

46. A False

B False

C True

D False

E True

Extrapolation is the measurement outside a validated range, and interpolation is the measurement within the range over which the instrument has been calibrated (A).

Calibrating medical instruments used for measurement is done to reduce the systemic error as much as possible, but does not necessarily completely remove the chance of this happening (B). The measurement may not be exact, but it will be within the range of accuracy that the clinical situation requires.

Calibration is the process used to ensure that a measurement made is accurate. It can be done by using samples of known concentration such as air or pure gas when calibrating gas concentration metres, for example. It can also use a reference such as the standard unit of length (metre) or weight (kilogram) (E).

An accurate measurement is unbiased and precise (C). An unbiased measurement is one where the mean of the value is close to the true value and a precise measurement is where repeated measurements are close together.

An exponential relationship can be transformed into a linear relationship by using a natural logarithmic conversion (D).

47. A True

B True

C True

D True

E True

Ultrasonic nebulisers require electricity to function, therefore may present electrical hazards. They can also deposit water into the breathing circuit, which requires drainage and can block the tubing (A). For spontaneous breathing, a bubble humidifier may increase the resistance to inspiration and therefore increase the work of breathing (B). Most heated humidifiers pass a stream of gas over water or across a wick which is dipped in water. This water reservoir can become contaminated with bacterial growth, and therefore cause contamination of the breathing circuit, this is especially true for the cascade type of humidifiers (C).

The heat and moisture exchanger humidifiers are usually placed in between the patient and the breathing circuit; therefore, they can increase dead space and result in rebreathing, especially with small tidal volumes (D). This is more likely to occur in paediatric patients.

A positive water balance can occur with the use of a humidifier, as a result of absorbed fluid from the airways (E). This is not usually a problem in adults, but is more likely with paediatric patients undergoing long anaesthetics.

48. A True

B False

C False

D True

E False

Alcohol thermometers are more suitable than mercury thermometers at very low temperatures, as mercury solidifies at −39°C, while alcohol freezes at −114°C (A, C). But at higher temperatures alcohol thermometers are unsuitable as alcohol has a boiling point of 78.5°C. Mercury thermometers tend to follow a linear scale, but alcohol thermometers have a less linear scale (B).

Both bimetallic strip and Bourdon gauge-type thermometers are dial thermometers (D). The Bourdon gauge-type actually measures pressure, but its properties can be used to measure temperature. Changes in temperature of the sensing elements cause a change in the pressure or volume, which is proportional to the temperature and this can be recorded on a calibrated dial.

A bimetallic strip thermometer has a sensing element that is made up of two dissimilar metals fixed together, usually as a coil. As the temperature changes, the different coefficients of thermal expansion of the two metals result in a winding or unwinding of the coil and movement of the lever on a calibrated scale to indicate the temperature (E).

49. A True

B False

C True

D False

E False

In hospitals, oxygen is usually stored in large storage vessels in liquid form (A). The critical temperature of oxygen is –119°C, so it cannot exist as a liquid when above this temperature (B). At –150°C, oxygen is a liquid because it is below its critical temperature (C). In the storage vessels, oxygen is stored at a temperature of about –160°C and a pressure of about 7 bar (D). As oxygen leaves the container, it needs to be heated by passing it through super heater coils and then it passes through a pressure regulator to keep the pipeline pressure at about 4 bar.

The storage vessel consists of a vacuum container, which is very efficient so no refrigeration unit is required (E). As the oxygen vapourises, it takes the latent heat of vapourisation from the remaining liquid, which also contributes to the cooling of the container (see **Figure 3.7**).

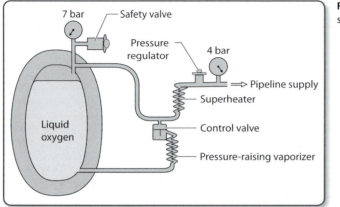

Figure 3.7 Liquid oxygen supply.

50. **A** True

   B False

   C False

   D False

   E False

Non-invasive methods of blood pressure measurement include palpation, auscultation, plethysmography, oscillotonometry and oscillometry. Oscillotonometry requires a double cuff, a narrow upper and wider lower cuff. As the upper cuff is inflated and deflated, the lower cuff detects arterial pulsations. The blood pressure readings using this method are prone to interpretation, especially for the diastolic pressure, so may be inaccurate (A).

When using the auscultation method, errors can occur when the wrong size cuff is used. Too small a cuff overestimates the pressure and too large a cuff underestimates the pressure (B).

Oscillometry uses a single cuff, which compresses and detects the pulsations (C). This is the method used by the standard non-invasive blood pressure measurement automated devices such as the device for indirect non-invasive automatic mean arterial pressure (DINAMAP) (E). As the pressure of the cuff is inflated above systolic blood pressure, then deflated slowly and continuously; the first pulsations detected on the cuff are the systolic pressure. When the pulsations reach maximum amplitude, this represents the mean arterial pressure (D). When these pulsations diminish and disappear, it represents the diastolic pressure.

51. **A** True

B False

C True

D False

E False

Effects of electrocution depend on the current density and occur in the following manner (B):

- 1 mA – tingling
- 5 mA – pain (A)
- 15 mA – tonic muscle contraction; 'can't let go'
- 50 mA – respiratory arrest (E)
- 100 mA – ventricular fibrillation
- 5 A – tonic myocardial contraction; defibrillation amplitudes

The most dangerous time for a current to reach the myocardium is during re-polarisation, which is why direct current cardioversion should always be synchronised with myocardial depolarisation (C).

Antistatic shoes increase the impedance, thereby reducing current flow (D). However, this allows current to dissipate to earth, preventing electrostatic build-up.

52. **A** False

B True

C True

D True

E False

Reducing the risk of delivery of hypoxic gas mixtures can be by either minimising the risk of incorrect gas delivery or minimising oxygen delivery failure.

Minimising incorrect gas delivery

- Colour-coded cylinders and pipelines
- Schrader valves at piped gas outlet (C)
- Pin index system for cylinders
- Non-interchangeable screw thread (NIST) for pipeline connections
- Colour-coded pressure gauges and flowmeters
- Geometrically unique flowmeter knob for oxygen always in the same position
- Oxygen is the last gas added to fresh gas flow mixture

- Chain-link mechanism between oxygen and nitrous oxide rotameters ensuring at least 25% oxygen delivery (B)
- Paramagnetic oxygen concentration analyser (D)

Minimising oxygen delivery failure:

- Oxygen pressure gauge
- Oxygen failure warning alarm, allowing room air to be inspired

Other safety features:

- Avoiding excess pressure delivery: adjustable pressure-limiting (APL) valve and distensible reservoir bag (E)
- Colour-coded vapourisers with key filling systems
- Emergency oxygen flush (A)

53. A False

   B False

   C False

   D True

   E True

Tec Mark 5 plenum vapourisers are temperature compensated (Tec) devices that split fresh gas flow to two separate streams that combine at the outlet port.

The first stream of fresh gas enters the vapourising chamber, where it is fully saturated with vapour (A). This is achieved by increasing the surface area of gas exposed to vapour with wicks, baffles or bubbling the gas through the vapour (D). A control dial then alters the amount of saturated gases that joins the fresh gas flow at the outlet port. The vapourisers also contain copper heat sinks (E).

The second stream is the bypass channel, which joins with the vapourised channel at the inlet port. The ratio of gas entering the bypass channel is called the splitting ratio and is temperature controlled (B). This is achieved by:

- Bimetallic strip: two metals with differing coefficients of thermal expansion bend depending on the temperature, thus adjusting the splitting ratio
- Bellows: fluid with a high coefficient of thermal expansion is contained within the bellows causing them to rise or fall depending on a temperature-dependent fashion
- Metal rods: metallic expansion or contraction adjusts the splitting ratio (see Figure 3.8)

Although desflurane is colour coded as blue, it can only be safely used in Tec Mark 6 vapourisers specifically designed for desflurane (C). This is due to the high-saturated vapour pressure of 89.2 kPa at 20°C and the low boiling point of 23.5°C.

54. A True

   B True

   C True

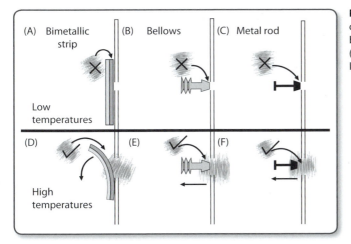

Figure 3.8 The mechanism of temperature control for bimetallic strips (A, D), Bellows (B, E) and Metal rods (C, F) at low and high temperatures.

D True

E False

Supraglottic airway devices (SADs) can be either first-generation such as the classic laryngeal mask airway (LMA) or reinforced LMA, or second-generation SADs. These are defined by having a lower aspiration risk and improved ventilatory efficacy, having been recommended for use in the National Audit Project (NAP4) by the Royal College of Anaesthetists.

The i-gel (Intersurgical) contains an oesophageal drainage tube as well as an integral bite block. It is single-use device and cuffless and allows insertion of fibreoptic bronchoscope through it (A).

The LMA ProSeal (Intavent Direct) also contains an oesophageal drainage tube and bite block, but also a posterior inflatable cuff and is reinforced (B).

The LMA Supreme (Intavent Direct) is a preformed tube with an oesophageal drainage tube and integral bite block as well, but has limited use in difficult airway scenarios (C).

The Combitube is a double-lumen tube that may be inserted either into the oesophagus or trachea, and contains two balloons that isolate the distal oesophagus and allows gastric aspiration (D).

The intubating LMA does not have any suction ports, but allows fibreoptic bronchoscopy or blind intubation through it (E).

55. **A** False

   B False

   C True

   D True

   E True

A T-piece breathing system is one in which the inspired fresh gas flow is closest to the patient end of the circuit with no valves or reservoir bags between fresh gas flow and patient. The Ayre's T-piece Mapleson E is an unmodified T-piece breathing system, while the Jackson-Rees modification (Mapleson F) simply adds an open-ended bag to the expiratory limb. The Mapleson D breathing circuit adds a bag and a valve on the expiratory limb of the T-piece circuit but remains a T-piece in essence.

56. A True

   B False

   C True

   D True

   E False

There are a number of methods for measuring oxygen gas:

Paramagnetic analysers: oxygen has unpaired electrons in its outer shell and is attracted to magnetic field, called paramagnetism. Paramagnetic analysers utilise differential pressure transducers or null-deflection dumb bell devices to give rapid, breath-by-breath, accurate oxygen concentrations (B).

Polarographic (Clark) electrode: a silver/silver chloride anode and platinum cathode have a voltage of 0.6 V within a potassium chloride solution. The cathode donates electrons which react with oxygen and water-generating hydroxy ions, with the voltage produced being proportional to the partial pressure of oxygen in the sample (D).

Galvanic fuel cells: a lead anode and a gold mesh cathode sit in a potassium chloride electrolyte solution. Lead (Pb) reacts with hydroxide ions to liberate electrons which then react with oxygen to further generate hydroxide ions, thereby generating an electrical current that is proportional to the partial pressure of oxygen in the mixture (A).

Mass spectrometry: by firing an electron at a gas sample, some atoms become charged and accelerate through a magnetic field at a detector. The degree deflection indicates the mass of the substance involved, while the amplitude of the signal indicates the number of ions detected.

Raman spectroscopy: electromagnetic radiation is fired at a gas sample, causing energy to be transferred to the sample. This leads to a vibration of atoms in the sample that is released as particular wavelengths which are detected at a photodetector (C).

Infrared spectroscopy: the principle applied to measurement of substances with two or more dissimilar atoms including carbon dioxide, nitrous oxide and the volatile anaesthetic agents, but will not work with oxygen or nitrogen (E).

57. A True

   B False

C True

D False

E True

Filters are devices used to reduce risks of administration of undesirable material to patients such as bacteria, viruses, foreign bodies or biological by-products. They can be attached to breathing systems, such as heat and moisture exchange filters, to fluid giving sets such as blood filters or total parenteral nutrition filters and to catheters such as epidural filters and atmospheric air filters.

Viruses generally have a size of less than 0.1 μm, including human immunodeficiency virus and cytomegalovirus, while bacteria are usually 1 μm or under in size. Filters with pore sizes significantly larger would thus be unable to filter micro-organisms; however, filters with slightly larger pore sizes may still intercept these micro-organisms due to inertial impaction or diffusional interception (D).

Epidural filters are 0.22 microns in size and are generally able to filter bacteria, foreign bodies as well as viruses (A). They have an internal volume of 0.7 mL and Luer connectors.

Standard blood filters have pore sizes of 170–200 microns, thus do not significantly filter bacteria or viruses but remove gross debris and clots (B). They can be used for administration of platelets, fresh frozen plasma, granulocytes or cryoprecipitate (C). Second-generation blood filters have smaller pore sizes of 20–40 microns and can filter microaggregates (E).

58. A False

B False

C False

D False

E False

Capnographs operate on the principles of infrared absorption spectroscopy: Substances containing two or more different atoms absorb infrared radiation at specific wavelengths, 4.3 μm for carbon dioxide (B). A continuous measure of inspired and expired carbon dioxide concentration is performed, thereby giving information on respiratory, cardiovascular, neuromuscular and equipment parameters.

The device has an infrared light source passing through a filter and crystal window into the sample chamber. The crystal is required because glass would absorb the radiation (D). In the sample chamber, carbon dioxide absorbs infrared radiation proportional to the partial pressure of carbon dioxide within the chamber. The radiation then falls onto a thermopile detector that then produces an electrical output. Because nitrous oxide has a similar absorption spectrum of infrared light to carbon dioxide, it may potentially be misinterpreted as carbon dioxide, leading to falsely high readings (E).

The end-tidal carbon dioxide ($ETCO_2$) is the partial pressure of carbon dioxide at the end of expiration. This must always be less than arterial carbon dioxide to allow for a concentration gradient to exist (A). The difference between $ETCO_2$ and arterial CO_2 is usually 0.3–0.6 kPa. Capnographic response depends on the transit time and the rise time. The transit time is the time required for the sample to reach the analyser, and the rise time signifies the time required for the analyser to respond to that sample (C).

59. A False

B False

C True

D True

E False

The device for indirect non-invasive automatic mean arterial pressure (DINAMAP) uses the principles of oscillometry to measure and calculate the systolic, mean arterial and diastolic pressures (see **Figure 3.9**) (D). Most commonly, a single cuff is used that inflates and transmits pressure fluctuations to a pressure transducer connected to a microprocessing unit that has an accuracy of +/−2% (A, B). The onset of oscillatory signals indicates the systolic blood pressure, the maximal amplitude of oscillation is the mean arterial pressure (MAP) and when the signal disappears this corresponds to the diastolic blood pressure (DBP) (see **Figure 3.9**). In addition, the DBP can be derived from:

$$MAP = DBP + \frac{\text{Pulse pressure}}{3}.$$

The cuff deflates at a rate of 2–3 mmHg per second, and the cuff should have a bladder that is 40% the circumference of the arm which should cover two-thirds of the upper arm (C, E).

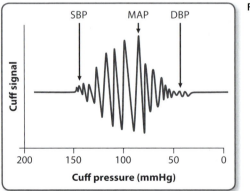

Figure 3.9 DINAMAP.

60. A True

   B False

   C True

   D False

   E True

Defibrillator circuits (see **Figure 3.10**) contain a capacitor to store charge, usually between 5000 and 8000 V that delivers energy as direct current rather than alternating current (A, D). The inductor in the circuit optimises the duration and shape of the current delivered and three switches control the charging and discharging of the capacitor. When the circuit is discharging energy to the patient, either monophasic or biphasic waveforms can be used. Biphasic waveforms deliver lower energy but are more effective at terminating fibrillation and are used in modern defibrillator machines. Thoracic impedance decreases with each subsequent shock delivered, and is normally between 50 and 150 ohms. The energy required for paediatric defibrillation is 4 joules/kg for asynchronous shocks and 2 joule/kg for synchronised shock delivery (C). No diode is found in the defibrillator circuit but usually contain three switches (B, E).

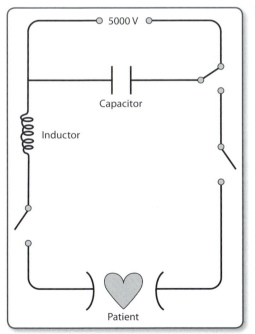

Figure 3.10 Defibrillator circuit.

Answers: SBAs

61. D Advancing the endotracheal tube to 24 cm at the lips

Dead space is defined as the volume of inspired air that does not partake in gas exchange and can be divided into:

- Anatomical dead space – the volume of the conducting airways, normally 150 mL, that may be measured by Fowler's method using nitrogen washout
- Alveolar dead space – the volume of gas from ventilated areas of lung that do not eliminate CO_2, i.e. not perfused. Normally 0 mL
- Physiological dead space – anatomical + alveolar dead space, i.e. total dead space. Normally, approximately 30% of tidal volume or 2–3 mL/kg and is measured with the Bohr equation

$$\text{Expired } CO_2 \text{ \% } (F_{ECO_2}) = \text{Inspired \% } CO_2 \text{ } (F_{ICO_2}) + \text{Alveolar \% } CO_2 \text{ } (F_{ACO_2})$$

As inspired CO_2 is negligible, therefore:

$$\text{Tidal volume } (V_T) \times F_{ECO_2} = \text{Alveolar volume } (V_A) \times \text{Alveolar } CO_2 \text{ } (F_{ACO_2})$$

Because $V_A = V_T$ – Dead space volume (V_D), therefore:

$$V_T \times F_{ECO_2} = (V_T - V_D) \times F_{ACO_2}$$

By expanding:

$$V_T \times F_{ECO_2} = (V_T \times F_{ACO_2}) - (V_D \times F_{ACO_2})$$

Dividing by V_T:

$$F_{ECO_2} = F_{ACO_2} - (V_D/V_T) \times F_{ACO_2}$$

Rearranging this:

$$V_D/V_T = F_{ACO_2} - F_{ECO_2}/F_{ACO_2}$$

Because concentration (F, %) is proportional to partial pressure (P), and alveolar P_{ACO_2} approximately equates to arterial P_{aCO_2}, therefore:

$$V_D/V_T = P_{aCO_2} - P_{ECO_2}/P_{aCO_2}$$

By reducing the conducting volumes, including reducing apparatus dead space such as shortening the circuit removing the heat and moisture exchanger (HME) filter, this will reduce anatomic dead space. Advancing the endotracheal tube by 2 cm will not affect the volume of either conducting airways or apparatus and thus will not have any effect on dead space. Increasing tidal volumes will increase traction exerted on bronchi by the lung parenchyma and therefore increase the dead space, hence reducing the tidal volumes will also reduce the dead space. Bronchodilation will increase the volume of conducting airways and therefore will increase the anatomical dead space. This can be achieved pharmacologically by bronchodilators such as β_2-agonists or anticholinergics such as atropine sulphate.

The causes altered dead space is summarised in Table 1.1.

JB West. Respiratory physiology: the essentials, 8th edn. Baltimore: Lippincott Williams & Wilkins; 2006.

62. D Give a fluid challenge

The patient is hypotensive and tachycardic with a suggestion that she might be bleeding. The most appropriate steps would be to fully assess the patient and treat any hypotension immediately with a fluid challenge. Although an arterial blood gas sample might be indicated, it is not an immediate priority. In addition, it is not yet clear if there is an indication for a blood transfusion although this may become necessary later. If there are any bleeding concerns, the surgeons must be allowed to meticulously control any bleeding points.

Dutton RP. Fluid management for trauma: Where are we now? Contin Educ Anaesth Crit Care Pain 2006; 6:144–147.

63. C Diabetic ketoacidosis

Diabetic ketoacidosis (DKA) is an endocrine emergency presenting with the triad of hyperglycaemia, ketosis and metabolic acidosis. It most commonly occurs in type I diabetics but may also present less commonly in type II diabetics. The underlying pathogenesis is due to an actual or effective insulin deficiency leading to excess ketone body production, including β-hydroxybutyrate and acetoacetate, from acetyl-CoA as a source of energy for the brain and muscle. The ketone bodies are proton donors, thereby generating a metabolic acidosis. The lack of insulin also increases gluconeogenesis and glycogenolysis leading to hyperglycaemia. High-glucose concentrations lead to an osmotic diuresis with urinary loss of water, K^+ and Na^+. This explains the features of polydipsia, polyuria, dehydration and weight loss. An attempt to compensate for the metabolic acidosis is made by hyperventilating to eliminate CO_2, the pattern known as Kussmaul breathing with characteristically deep, rapid efforts. Management includes treating the underlying cause of the DKA, usually infection, inadequate insulin therapy or trauma and cautious correction of dehydration and electrolyte imbalance.

Hyperosmolar non-ketotic coma (also known as hyperglycaemic hyperosmolar non-ketotic syndrome) is a clinical entity occurring in type II diabetics in response to infection, trauma or myocardial infarction. It is characterised by slower onset deterioration with dehydration, focal neurological signs and confusion. Very high concentrations of glucose are possible but ketoacidosis does not occur because small amounts of effective insulin prevent lipolysis and ketone production.

Diabetes insipidus (DI) is due to a deficiency of antidiuretic hormone (ADH), in cranial DI, or a renal insensitivity to ADH when nephrogenic DI presents. Patients present with polyuria, polydipsia but no hyperglycaemia would be expected.

Salicylate toxicity usually presents with a mixture of metabolic acidosis and respiratory alkalosis; however, significant changes to glucose concentrations would be unlikely.

Decompensated liver failure may present with significant metabolic acidosis; however, hypoglycaemia is more common.

Chaithongdi N, Subauste JS, Koch CA, Geraci SA. Diagnosis and management of hyperglycemic emergencies. Hormones 2011; 10:250–260.

64. E 2000 mL 0.9% NaCl in 24 hours

Assessment of paediatric dehydration and water deficit may be estimated using clinical assessment and physiological parameters, see **Table 3.10**.

Table 3.10 Clinical signs with extent of dehydration in paediatric patients			
Sign	**<5% dehydration**	**5–10% dehydration**	**>10% dehydration**
Skin	Unchanged	Reduced turgor	Mottled
Eyes	Unchanged	Sunken	Deeply sunken
Heart rate	Unchanged	Increased	Markedly increased
Respiratory rate	Unchanged	Increased	Markedly increased
Urine output	Unchanged	Reduced	Markedly reduced

The fluid deficit volume is calculated by the equation:

Fluid deficit volume = Weight (kg) × % dehydration × 10

This volume is replaced over 24 hours in addition to any fluid boluses or maintenance fluids.

Maintenance fluids, as opposed to deficit replacement as is the case here, should be prescribed according to the '4-2-1' rule:

- 4 mL/kg/hour for the first 10 kg
- 2 mL/kg/hour for the second 10 kg
- 1 mL/kg/hour for each kilogram thereafter

The choice of fluid used includes 0.9% NaCl, 0.9% NaCl/5% dextrose solution or Hartmann's solution. The National Patient Safety Agency recommended the discontinuation of routine use of 0.18% NaCl/4% glucose due to the risk of hyponatraemia.

Cunliffe M. Fluid and electrolyte management in children. BJA CEPD Reviews 2003; 3:1–4. doi:10.1093/bjacepd/mkg001.

65. B Right ventricle

The pulmonary artery catheter was the main method used to measure cardiac output for many years, but it has recently been superseded by less invasive techniques of cardiac output measurement.

A catheter is passed from the internal jugular vein into the right atrium. It is then passed into the right ventricle and out into the pulmonary artery, while the pressure waveforms are visualised, which confirms the position of the catheter tip.

A balloon at the tip of the catheter aids the positioning of the catheter and helps to wedge it in the pulmonary artery. Once wedged, the pulsatile waveform is lost and the tip of the catheter is looking ahead down the pulmonary tree towards the left atrium (see Figure 2.15).

Allsager CM, Swanevelder J. Measuring cardiac output. BJA CEPD Reviews 2003; 3:15–19.

66. E Type CF

Equipment which is connected to the patient's heart must be type CF. Type CF equipments are class 1 or 2 mains powered with an internal electrical power source. This type of equipment provides the most stringent protection against shock. Type BF and CF both have an F-type isolated floating applied part, which means that part of the equipment which is applied to the patient is isolated from all other parts of the equipment. Type B equipment maybe class 1, 2 or 3 mains powered equipment and is not suitable for direct connection to the heart.

These stringent leakage levels must be applied to all equipment making contact with the patient's heart to prevent microshock, and they must conform to a leakage specification of less than 10 mA. This equipment should be battery operated and fully isolated from earth whenever possible.

Boumphrey S, Langton JA. Electrical safety in the operating theater. BJA CEPD Reviews 2003; 3:10–14.

67. B Commence facemask ventilation

This scenario is an unanticipated difficult tracheal intubation during a rapid sequence induction in an adult patient. There are specific Difficult Airway Society guidelines for managing this situation. Here, the initial intubation plan (plan A) has resulted in a failed intubation; no more than three attempts to intubate the trachea should be made. Now you must concentrate on maintaining oxygenation and ventilation, postponing surgery and awakening the patient. Plan B, or the secondary intubation plan is not appropriate in this situation; therefore, an intubating laryngeal mask airway should not be inserted. If ventilation using a facemask is not successful, then relaxation of cricoid pressure and the insertion of a supraglottic airway would be the appropriate next step.

Henderson JJ, Popat MT, Latto IP, Pearce AC. Difficult Airway Society guidelines for management of the unanticipated difficult intubation. Anaesthesia 2004 Jul; 59(7):675–694. http://www.das.uk.com/files/rsi-Jul04-A4.pdf (Last accessed 01/10/2012).

68. C Insertion of an intra-aortic balloon pump

Intra-aortic balloon pumps are inserted to assist cardiac function in patients with severe cardiac failure. They increase myocardial oxygen supply and decrease myocardial oxygen demand by the inflation and deflation of a balloon placed in the descending aorta. They are usually inserted by cardiac surgeons or cardiologists using a percutaneous femoral artery approach. Indications for use include refractory ventricular failure, cardiogenic shock, unstable refractory angina and weaning from cardiopulmonary bypass.

In this case, insertion of an intra-aortic balloon pump would be the most appropriate next step as the patient is in a district hospital under the care of the cardiologists and is in severe left ventricular failure requiring cardiovascular support.

The patient may require urgent coronary artery bypass grafting, if occlusion of coronary arteries is the cause of his failure, but this will need to be done at a cardiac centre and will take time to arrange and the patient will need to be transferred. Therefore, this would not be the next step in his management. This would also apply to a heart transplant.

Adrenaline is a sympathomimetic drug which acts on α- and β-receptors. In this case, there is a risk that an adrenaline infusion may cause arrhythmias, further ischaemia and increase the heart rate and work of the heart, so it would not be an appropriate choice.

Milrinone is a phosphodiesterase III inhibitor and this increases cyclic adenosine monophosphate by decreasing its breakdown. It enhances right ventricular contractility, reduces pre-load and reduces pulmonary artery vasoconstriction. It is particularly useful in right ventricular failure and pulmonary hypertension.

Krishna M, Zacharowski K. Principles of intra-aortic balloon pump counterpulsation. Contin Educ Anaesth Crit Care Pain 2009; 9:24–28.

69. B Increased analgesia requirements

A number of prospective randomised trials have shown that mild peri-operative hypothermia results in a number of adverse outcomes:

- Myocardial ischaemia
- Arrhythmias
- Increased intraoperative blood loss
- Increased allogeneic transfusion requirement
- Increased risk of surgical wound infection
- Longer duration of action of neuromuscular blockade
- Longer duration of post-anaesthetic recovery
- Longer duration of hospital stay

All of these adverse outcomes resulted from a core hypothermia of 35–35.7°C. Increased analgesic requirement has not been directly associated with peri-operative hypothermia.

There are three basic strategies used to prevent mild peri-operative hypothermia, and these are minimising the redistribution of heat, cutaneous warming and internal warming.

Kirkbride D, Buggy DJ. Thermoregulation and mild peri-operative hypothermia. Br J Anaesth CEPD Reviews 2003; 3:24–28.

70. A Sciatic nerve

The nerves of the lumbar plexus (nerve roots L1–L5) are the subcostal, iliohypogastric, ilioinguinal, lateral cutaneous nerve of the thigh, femoral, genitofemoral and obturator nerves.

The sciatic nerve is part of the lumbosacral plexus (L4–S3) and is not blocked during a lumbar plexus block.

The first nerve of the lumbar plexus is the subcostal nerve followed by the iliohypogastric nerve. The ilioinguinal nerve penetrates the iliacus muscle at the anterior superior iliac spine and is the next nerve of the plexus. On the lateral border of the psoas muscle is the femoral nerve, immediately anterior to the psoas muscle is the genitofemoral nerve and medial to the psoas muscle is the obturator nerve which penetrates the obturator internus muscle.

All of these nerves can be blocked when a high volume of local anaesthetic is used during a lumbar plexus block.

Grant CRK, Checketts MR. Analgesia for primary hip and knee arthroplasty: The role of regional anaesthesia. Contin Educ Anaesth Crit Care Pain 2008; 8:56–61.
Mannion S. Psoas compartment block. Contin Educ Anaesth Crit Care Pain 2007; 7:162–166.

71. D Cochlear implant

Absolute contraindications to MRI scans include implanted surgical devices such as cochlear implants, cardiac pacemakers, implanted defibrillators, intra-ocular metallic foreign bodies and ferromagnetic neurovascular surgical clips. Many other implanted prosthetic devices are not ferromagnetic and are therefore safe. These include joint prosthesis, general surgical clips, artificial heart valves and sternal wires. These are all generally safe as they are fixed in fibrous tissue and the forces induced by the magnetic field are insignificant and will be unable to dislodge them.

Breast implants are generally safe but some breast tissue expanders have a metal port which allows for more accurate detection of the injection sites, these are contraindicated as they are attracted to the magnetic field and so maybe uncomfortable or cause injury.

All contraindications should be identified using a pre-scan checklist.

Penden CJ, Twigg SJ. Anaesthesia for magnetic resonance imaging. BJA CEPD Reviews 2003; 3:97–101.

72. C Remifentanil

The volume of distribution, clearance and protein binding can change for some drugs in morbidly obese patients. Highly lipophilic substances such as barbiturates and benzodiazepines all have significant increases in the volume of distribution in this group of patients. It is the less lipophilic compounds that have little effect on the volume of distribution with obesity.

Remifentanil is a highly lipophilic drug, but despite this shows no significant change in the volume of distribution in obese patients. Therefore, the absolute volume of distribution remains largely unchanged so the dosage should be calculated using the patient's ideal body weight.

De Baerdemaeker LEC, Mortier EP, Struys MMRF. Pharmacokinetics in obese patients. Contin Educ Anaesth Crit Care Pain 2004; 4:152–155.
Lotia S, Bellamy MC. Anaesthesia and morbid obesity. Contin Educ Anaesth Crit Care Pain 2008; 8:151–156.

73. A Mapleson A

Mapleson first described five semi-closed breathing systems (A–E), to which a sixth (F) was later added. In order to achieve adequate pre-oxygenation, a circuit that is efficient when a patient is spontaneously ventilating is required, which is best suited to the Mapleson A breathing system, or the co-axial version called the Lack breathing system. The most efficient for controlled ventilation is the Mapleson D or its co-axial modification the Bain system (see **Table 3.11**).

Mapleson WW. Anaesthetic breathing systems – Semi-closed systems. BJA CEPD Reviews 2001; 1:3–7.

Table 3.11 Gas flow rates for Mapleson breathing systems		
	Gas flow rates required	
Mapleson system	**Spontaneous ventilation**	**Controlled ventilation**
A	70 mL/kg/minute	2–3 × minute volume
B & C	2–3 × minute volume	2–3 × minute volume
D	2–3 × minute volume	70 mL/kg/minute
E & F	2–3 × minute volume	2–3 × minute volume

74. B Left-sided double-lumen tube

All of the above are potential options for unilateral lung isolation; however, double-lumen tubes provide the most secure and versatile approach as it allows not only lung isolation but also suctioning and application of continuous positive airway pressure (CPAP) to non-ventilated lungs, see **Table 3.12**. This patient needs to have their left lung isolated, therefore only ventilating the right lung.

Table 3.12 Tubes allowing single-lung ventilation	
Single lumen	**Double lumen**
Gordon-Green	Robertshaw (right or left)
Macintosh-Leatherdale	Bryce-Smith
Brompton-Pallister	Bryce-Smith-Salt

Double-lumen tubes can be right-sided or left-sided, each having an endobronchial lumen and a tracheal lumen with a cuff on each. Left-sided tubes are generally preferred because they avoid the risk of right upper lobe bronchial occlusion that could be caused by a right-sided double-lumen tube.

Carlens tubes are rubber left-sided tubes with a carinal hook that allow one-lung ventilation, but are less frequently used in modern practice. The carinal hook may increase difficulty in intubation, and its main use was for bronchospirometry.

White tubes are right-sided modifications of the Carlens tube.

Endobronchial blockers can be used in a patient with endotracheal tubes in situ, and act by occluding a single bronchus to prevent ventilation of that lung. They do not allow reinflation of that lung, application of CPAP, or suctioning of the occluded lung.

Other tubes that may allow single lung ventilation include:

Eastwood J, Mahajan R. One-lung anaesthesia. BJA CEPD Reviews 2002; 2:83–87.

75. A Defective CYP2D6 isoenzyme

Codeine phosphate undergoes O-demethylation to morphine, which is the only metabolite with significant μ-receptor activity. This process is dependent on cytochrome P450 isoenzyme CYP2D6 which demonstrates significant genetic variability. Those with defective or 'slow' CYP2D6 activity do not gain significant therapeutic effect of codeine phosphate, accounting for 10% of the UK population, but up to 30% of the Chinese population. The other isoenzyme demonstrating genetic polymorphism is CYP2C9.

The CYP3A5 isoenzyme is not involved in analgesic drug metabolism, but predominantly in benzodiazepine metabolism. Hepatic enzyme inducers such as phenytoin may reduce the clinical effect of certain drugs; however, this is not the case for codeine phosphate, diclofenac or paracetamol. Hepatic enzyme inhibitors may increase the plasma concentration of drugs metabolised by similar hepatic isoenzymes, but again this does not apply to codeine phosphate.

The dosing of the above drugs is at or approaching the maximal recommended regimes; thus, it is unlikely that her ongoing pain is due to suboptimal dosing.

Park GR. Drug metabolism. BJA CEPD Reviews 2001; 1:185–188. doi:10.1093/bjacepd/1.6.185

76. D Reduced phase II metabolism

Morphine is metabolised in the liver via phase II metabolism to morphine-3-glucuronide, morphine-6-glucuronide and normorphine. There is evidence that morphine-6-glucuronide has significant analgesic properties. In states of hepatic dysfunction, there will be a reduction in the metabolism of morphine, giving it a prolonged half-life and reduced clearance.

Although liver failure will also reduce phase I metabolism and plasma protein levels while increasing volume of distribution, these factors are unlikely to contribute to the pronounced effects of morphine. Of note, oral bioavailability of morphine is increased due to reduced first-pass metabolism.

Sasada M, Smith S. Drugs in anaesthesia and intensive care, 3rd edn. New York: Oxford University Press; 2003.

77. E Lidocaine is more ionised in infected tissue

Activity of local anaesthetic agents is dependent on them being present in the unionised state in order to cross the phospholipid bilayer and reach the intracellular component of sodium channels. The degree of ionisation of local anaesthetics is dependant on local pH and drug pKa. The pKa is the pH at which there is equilibrium between ionised and unionised forms of the agent and is 7.9 for lidocaine. As lidocaine is a weak base, it is more ionised below its pKa, leaving only 25% unionised at pH of 7.4. At the site of infections, such as abscesses, the pH is more acidic; therefore, the agent becomes ionised even further making it less active.

Another potential reason for a reduction in activity of local anaesthetics at the site of infected tissue is that there is increased blood flow that can remove the drug from the target tissue. This is less likely to be the cause here because of the use of adrenaline in the mixture.

Covino BG. Pharmacology of local anaesthetic agents. Br J Anaesth 1986; 58:701–716.

78. C Serum potassium of 3.3 mmol/L

This patient has suxamethonium apnoea caused by a reduced activity of plasma cholinesterase producing the characteristically prolonged neuromuscular blockade. Causes can be congenital or acquired.

In congenital cases, amino acid substitutions on chromosome three produce four potential allels: Eu (usual/normal), Ea (atypical), Es (silent) and Ef (Fluoride-resistant). The Eu:Eu genotype accounts for 96% of the population with a normal duration of block, with the remaining 4% being a combination of homozygous or heterozygous genotypes with a mildly prolonged block of minutes to a significantly prolonged block of hours. The Ea:Ea, Es:Es and Es:Ea demonstrate the most significantly prolonged blocks.

The dibucaine number signifies the degree of inhibition of plasma cholinesterase, with the higher numbers (80 in normal individuals with Eu:Eu genotype) providing normal duration of block and the lower numbers (20 in Ea:Ea and Es:Ea genotype) demonstrating a prolonged block.

Acquired causes include:

- Renal failure
- Hepatic failure
- Cardiac failure
- Thyrotoxicosis
- Malignancy
- Drugs
- Ketamine, lithium, local anaesthetics, the oral contraceptive pill, magnesium, neostigmine, cytotoxic agents and metoclopramide.

Appiah-Ankam J, Hunter JM. Pharmacology of neuromuscular blocking drugs. Contin Educ Anaesth Crit Care Pain 2004; 4:2–7.

79. A Nicotinic

Chlorpromazine (Largactil) is a phenothiazine drug that is used to treat schizophrenia, nausea and vomiting and intractable hiccups. It antagonises dopaminergic D_2 receptors, muscarinic, α-adrenergic, histaminergic H_1, and serotonergic receptors.

Chlorpromazine is a negative inotrope, causing reduced systemic vascular resistance, postural hypotension and tachycardia. It is an antisialagogue and a respiratory depressant, also causing reduced gastric motility and secretion with weight gain and increased appetite. The central effect of neurolepsis, sedation and anxiolysis occur, but neuroleptic malignant syndrome, extrapyramidal side effects and thermoregulatory disturbance may also be present.

Because of extensive first-pass metabolism, chlorpromazine only has an oral bioavailability of 30%, is 95% protein bound and undergoes extensive hepatic metabolism. It has more than 160 metabolites, many that are active, and most are excreted in the urine and faeces.

Peck T, Wong A, Norman E. Anaesthetic implications of psychoactive drugs. Contin Educ Anaesth Crit Care Pain 2010; 10:177–181.

80. A Autonomic neuropathy

Autonomic neuropathy may be central or peripheral due to conditions such as diabetes mellitus, causing impaired baroreceptor reflexes, conduction defects, delayed gastric emptying and bladder dysfunction. With spinal anaesthesia, there is a reduction in systemic vascular resistance leading to a reduced venous return and cardiac output. In normal patients, this leads to a compensatory tachycardia and increase in myocardial contractility due to the baroreceptor reflex. This, however, is lost in the elderly and diabetics, which would account for the profound hypotension without tachycardia.

A high spinal blockade would be one that rises to a level above T4. In this patient, the sensation on her chest wall precludes this diagnosis.

Hypovolaemia may be present in this patient; however, following a spinal anaesthetic a reflex tachycardia would be expected. Again the absence of tachycardia means that the underlying pathology is likely to be autonomic dysfunction.

Myocardial ischaemia may present with chest pain and electrocardiograph changes. Hypotension is not a common presentation of ischaemia; however, this may be present in massive myocardial infarction, which is not the case in this scenario.

Reduced ventricular compliance is common in the elderly and is usually due to an increased afterload. It will not cause an acute deterioration in blood pressure.

Murray D, Dodds C. Perioperative care of the elderly. Cont Educ Anaesth Crit Care Pain 2004; 4:193–196.

81. C A$^+$ crossmatched blood

This patient has symptomatic massive haemorrhage and needs to receive a blood transfusion. The most appropriate blood to transfuse would be A$^+$ crossmatched blood as this is the same as her blood group. Although the administration of O$^-$ blood would be acceptable practice, it is not crossmatched and would be inferior to fully crossmatched blood. Neither crystalloids such as Hartmann's solution nor colloids such as Gelofusine would replace the deficient haemoglobin, but would be measures to buy time until blood could be transfused. AB$^-$ would be inappropriate in this case as the patient would have antibodies to the B antigen, and therefore generate an immune response to the transfusion.

Al-Khafaji A, Webb AR. Fluid resuscitation. Contin Educ Anaesth Crit Care Pain 2004; 4:127–131.

82.　E The Haldane effect

The mechanisms in place to maximise oxygen supply to the fetus include:

- Fetal haemoglobin: this has a higher affinity for oxygen than maternal haemoglobin because of a reduced 2,3-diphosphoglycerate (2,3-DPG) causing a leftward shift of the oxyhaemoglobin dissociation curve
- Higher fetal haemoglobin concentration: the fetus has a haemoglobin concentration of 16–17 g/dL
- High uterine blood flow: this can be up to 750 mL/minute at term, of which 85% goes to the placenta
- The double Bohr effect: CO_2 diffuses across the placenta from the fetus to the maternal circulation causing an increase in maternal CO_2 and a reduced fetal CO_2. This causes a right shift of the oxyhaemoglobin dissociation curve in the mother and a left shift of the curve in the fetus, thereby favouring offloading of oxygen from the mother to the fetus

The Haldane effect refers to the increased ability of deoxygenated haemoglobin to carry CO_2 as carbamino compounds when compared with oxygenated haemoglobin. It does not directly contribute to improved fetal oxygen delivery, but contributes to CO_2 clearance.

Murphy PJ. The fetal circulation. Cont Educ Anaesth Crit Care Pain 2005; 5:107–112.

83.　D Aspiration pneumonitis

Obesity and laparoscopic surgery leave patients at a greater risk of aspiration pneumonitis. In addition, a laparoscopic salpingectomy requires patients to be in the head down position leaving her at an even greater risk of aspiration. The clinical features of aspiration include dyspnoea, tachypnoea, hypoxia, bronchospasm, airway obstruction and distal atelectasis.

Pneumonia is unlikely to occur acutely in the intraoperative period, while pulmonary oedema would present with evidence of reduced bilateral basal airway entry and bilateral basal crackles. Pneumothorax is a risk of laparoscopic surgery; however, there would be no added sounds on the affected side. Venous thromboembolism may occur in obese patients undergoing pelvic surgery; however, crackles are not a typical clinical feature of pulmonary embolism.

Levy DM. Pre-operative fasting—60 years on from Mendelson. Contin Educ Anaesth Crit Care Pain 2006; 6:215–218.

84.　B Metabolic acidosis with a large anion gap

The cardinal feature on the arterial blood gas sample would be a lactic acidosis. Elevated lactate (>2 mmol/L) occurs when there is cellular hypoxia leading to a failure of conversion of pyruvate to carbon dioxide and water; thus, it is converted to lactate in order to generate adenosine triphosphate. This is the case in acute mesenteric ischaemia, with a lactate of >5 mmol/L giving a 96% sensitivity and 60% specificity.

The anion gap is the difference between measured cations and anions.

$$\text{Anion gap} = (Na^+ + K^+) - (Cl^- + HCO_3^-)$$

A large anion gap, usually above 18 mmol/L, may indicate the underlying diagnosis and can be caused by:

- Lactic acidosis
- Ketoacidosis
- Uraemia
- Toxins – methanol, salicylates, biguanides

This patient is likely to have a metabolic acidosis with a large anion gap due to the lactate. There is no evidence in the history of ketoacidosis, and due to the tachypnoea this patient is unlikely to have a respiratory acidosis. Although a respiratory alkalosis may be present, it would not support the diagnosis of acute mesenteric ischaemia.

Badr A, Nightingale P. An alternative approach to acid–base abnormalities in critically ill patients. Contin Educ Anaesth Crit Care Pain 2007; 7:107–111.
Chawla G, Drummond G. Water, strong ions, and weak ions. Contin Educ Anaesth Crit Care Pain 2008; 8:108–112.

85. D Fibreoptic examination

Unilateral lung isolation has absolute indications (bronchopleural fistula, unilateral lung lavage, massive haemorrhage) and relative indications (improving surgical access). A double-lumen tube has a tracheal lumen and an endobronchial lumen. The definitive method confirming endobronchial intubation is using fibreoptic bronchoscopic examination of both the endotracheal lumen, looking for the carina and the endobronchial cuff in the correct lumen, and the endobronchial lumen confirming presence of bronchial branches. The risk with a right-sided double-lumen endotracheal tube is obstruction of the right upper lobe bronchus; thus, fibreoptic assessment is warranted.

Although auscultation and inspection of unilateral chest expansion may demonstrate endobronchial intubation, they are not definitive. Capnography would not demonstrate significant differences between endobronchial and endotracheal intubation, while direct laryngoscopy can only confirm endotracheal intubation.

Eastwood J, Mahajan R. One-lung anaesthesia. BJA CEPD Reviews 2002; 2(3):83–87.

86. A P_{50} of the oxyhaemoglobin dissociation curve is 2.8 kPa

The most likely diagnosis in this patient is CO poisoning. Inhalation of exhaust fumes, fires in enclosed spaces or smoking may lead to CO poisoning. Clinical features include headache, weakness, nausea and vomiting, confusion, ataxia, seizures and coma. The pathognomonic finding is a cherry-red complexion to the cheeks.

The underlying problem is that CO has 200–250 times greater affinity for haemoglobin than oxygen, thus forming the slowly dissociating carboxyhaemoglobin and reducing the available binding sites for oxygen. This causes a left shift of the oxyhaemoglobin dissociation curve whose P_{50} is normally 3.5 kPa. The cellular cytochrome oxidase system is inhibited leading to tissue hypoxia and metabolic acidosis. However, the arterial Po_2 is unaffected, although this is the primary determinant for the rate of CO dissociation from haemoglobin. Breathing room air, the half-life of carboxyhaemoglobin is 4 hours, 40 minutes with 100% oxygen and 20 minutes with hyperbaric oxygen therapy.

Pulse oximetry is unreliable in CO poisoning due to a similar absorption spectra to oxyhaemoglobin; thus, saturations tend towards 100%. Methaemoglobinaemia gives saturations approaching 85%.

Peripheral neuropathy is more likely to be a feature of chronic exposure or cyanide poisoning rather than acute CO poisoning.

CO poisoning leads to direct cardiovascular depression and low cardiac output states with arrhythmias ensuing.

Bishop S, Maguire S. Anaesthesia and intensive care for major burns. Cont Educ Anaesth Crit Care Pain 2012; 12:118–122.

87. D Perform a left lateral tilt

In any emergency, an ABCDE approach should be used, however this approach should be modified in pregnancy. High-flow oxygen should be administered immediately followed by a left lateral tilt of 15–30°. This is important beyond a gestational age of 20 weeks because the gravid uterus causes compression of the inferior vena cava and aorta leading to impaired venous return and cardiac output. Alternatively, manual lateral left displacement of the uterus may be attempted. Following this manoeuvre, intravenous access must be obtained with bloods being sent and fluid boluses administered. Early involvement of obstetricians is required and in the event of cardiac arrest, all advanced life support principles apply with some modifications.

Cardiopulmonary resuscitation should ensue with a left-sided tilt or manual displacement of the uterus. If initial resuscitation attempts fail, then a peri-mortem caesarean section within 5 minutes must be performed, particularly beyond 20 weeks gestation. Beyond a gestational age of 24–25 weeks the chances of both maternal and infant survival is the highest.

Resuscitation Council (UK). Advanced life support, 6th edn. London: Resuscitation Council (UK); 2011.

88. E Phenoxybenzamine

Phaeochromocytoma is a tumour of chromaffin cells secreting vasoactive amines such as noradrenaline, adrenaline or dopamine, but may also secrete other agents. Patients present with hypertension that can be difficult to control, along with palpitations, sweating, headache and potentially acute cardiovascular compromise. Hypertension is due to increased systemic vascular resistance.

The principles of pre-operative management is treatment of hypertension using firstly α-adrenoceptor blockers, followed by β-adrenoceptor blockers.

Unopposed β-blockade may lead to uncontrolled systemic vasoconstriction and hypertensive crises. The most common α-blockers used are prazosin, doxazosin and phenoxybenzamine. While phenoxybenzamine is predominantly an α_1-adrenoceptor blocker, it also has some α_2-effects. Prazosin and doxazosin are predominantly α_1-selective agents.

Pace N, Buttigieg M. Phaeochromocytoma. BJA CEPD Reviews 2003; 3:20–23.

89. D Dialysis may reduce plasma concentrations

Phenytoin is a hydantoin-derived anticonvulsant and antiarrhythmic agent with a high oral bioavailability (90%). It is highly plasma protein bound (>90%) to albumin and is metabolised in the liver by hydroxylation and glucuronidation. In sub-therapeutic doses, it undergoes first-order kinetics, but just above the therapeutic range it undergoes zero-order kinetics (saturation kinetics). This means that it has a narrow therapeutic window, above which plasma concentrations will rise linearly with administered dose (see **Figure 3.11**), increasing the potential for toxicity. It is excreted predominantly by the kidneys, although dose adjustment is only necessary in hepatic failure. As it is highly protein bound, it does not appear to be cleared by haemodialysis, peritoneal dialysis or haemofiltration.

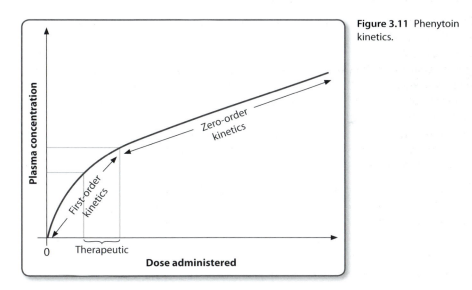

Figure 3.11 Phenytoin kinetics.

Phenytoin is a hepatic enzyme inducer, thus will reduce plasma concentrations of hepatically metabolised drugs such as lorazepam and warfarin leading to sub-therapeutic concentrations.

Sasada M, Smith S. Drugs in anaesthesia and intensive care, 3rd edn. New York: Oxford University Press; 2003.

90. A Flucloxacillin

There are a number of factors determining whether a drug will be cleared by haemofiltration or haemodialysis:

- Molecular size
- Protein binding
- Volume of distribution
- Lipophilicity
- Filter characteristics

It is important to consider drug dosing in renal impairment and while initiating haemodialysis or haemofiltration, although loading doses do not need readjustment as this is dependent on volume of distribution. In addition, only free drug is cleared; thus, highly protein bound drugs are less likely to be eliminated by the dialysis or filtration. The following antimicrobial agents may or may not need dosing adjustment during renal replacement therapy, see **Table 3.13**:

Paw H, Shulman R. Handbook of drugs in intensive care: An A–Z guide, 4th edn. Cambridge: Cambridge University Press; 2010.

Table 3.13 Dose adjustment of antibiotics for patients on renal replacement therapy

Dose adjustment not needed	Dose adjustment needed
Amphotericin	Aciclovir
Cefotaxime	Benzylpenicillin
Ciprofloxacin	Cefuroxime
Erythromycin	Co-amoxiclav
Flucloxacillin	Co-trimoxazole
Metronidazole	Fluconazole
	Gentamicin
	Meropenem
	Tazocin (piperacillin/tazobactam)
	Teicoplanin
	Vancomycin

Chapter 4

Mock paper 4

60 MTFs and 30 SBAs to be answered in three hours

Questions: MTFs

Answer each stem 'True' or 'False'.

1. **Regarding the pressure/volume loop of the left ventricle, which of the following is true:**
    A   It allows calculation of the stroke work
    B   It has a linear vertical line representing isovolumetric contraction even at increased volumes in the left ventricle
    C   The area inside the loop represents total volume of blood in the left ventricle
    D   It is the same as the right ventricle
    E   It represents preload as the left ventricular end-diastolic volume

2. **Regarding nervous control of the heart rate, which of the following is true:**
    A   At rest, both sympathetic and parasympathetic autonomic nerves have equal activity on the heart
    B   If both sets of autonomic nerves are blocked, the intrinsic heart rate would be approximately 60 beats per minute
    C   Sympathetic and parasympathetic fibres innervate both the sinoatrial and atrioventricular nodes
    D   The pacemaker rate is sensitive to temperature
    E   The parasympathetic nerve terminals release the neurotransmitter noradrenaline

3. **Regarding the Fick method for measuring cardiac output:**
    A   It involves the measurement of oxygen uptake rate as well as arterial and venous oxygen concentrations
    B   It can also be applied to other organs
    C   It is only accurate in the steady state
    D   Oxygen uptake rate cannot be calculated by spirometry
    E   Venous oxygen concentration can be calculated from a peripheral venous sample

4. **The following cranial nerves carry parasympathetic fibres:**
    A   Optic nerve
    B   Abducens nerve

    C   Trigeminal nerve

    D   Glossopharyngeal nerve

    E   Hypoglossal nerve

5. **Regarding nerve action potentials, which of the following is true:**

    A   The resting membrane potential is $-90\,mV$

    B   The nerve membrane is more permeable to K^+ than Na^+

    C   The absolute refractory period continues until repolarisation is complete

    D   During the relative refractory period, a supramaximal stimulus may cause excitation

    E   T-Type calcium channels are involved in the depolarisation phase

6. **The following are true regarding pain:**

    A   Allodynia is an exaggerated response to a painful stimulus

    B   Nociception is the same as pain

    C   Neuropathic pain is due to damage to the nervous system

    D   Hyperalgesia is a painful response to a normally painless stimulus

    E   Chronic pain is a pain that continues after normal recovery would be expected

7. **Regarding pain pathways:**

    A   The substantia gelatinosa is made up of laminae I and VI

    B   Primary afferents synapse in the dorsal horn

    C   Aδ fibres synapse in laminae II and III

    D   The spinothalamic tract decussates in the thalamus

    E   The main excitatory neurotransmitter at primary synapses is glutamate

8. **The following are true regarding the glomerular filtration rate (GFR):**

    A   GFR is volume divided by time that is filtered by all the glomeruli

    B   Approximately 50% of renal plasma flow is filtered by the glomeruli

    C   The ideal indicator for measuring GFR must enter the tubule by filtration only and not undergo resorption or metabolism

    D   A commonly used indicator for measuring GFR is para-aminohippurate

    E   Exogenous creatinine can also be used to calculate the GFR

9. **With respect to the renal handling of Na^+ and Cl^-:**

    A   The majority of NaCl is resorbed from the tubules

    B Na^+ and Cl^- ions are actively resorbed from the tubules

    C   As NaCl is resorbed in the proximal tubule, water moves in the opposite direction

    D   The proximal tubule resorbs about 70% of the filtered Na^+ and water

    E   The remaining 30% is resorbed at the distal convoluted tubules and collecting ducts

10. **The urinary excretion of potassium is increased by:**

    A   An increase in potassium absorption

    B   Alkalosis

    C   Acute acidosis

    D   Chronic acidosis

    E   Aldosterone

11. **Regarding respiratory disturbances in acid/base balance, which of the following is true:**

    A   They result in parallel changes in the concentration of bicarbonate and other buffer bases

    B   Acute respiratory acidosis is poorly compensated as compared with chronic respiratory acidosis

    C   High altitude can result in respiratory alkalosis

    D   Tuberculosis can cause a respiratory acidosis

    E   They cause minor changes in the pH of the cerebrospinal fluid

12. **The following factors increases functional residual capacity:**

    A   Supine position

    B   Male gender

    C   Asthma

    D   Exercise

    E   Intermittent positive pressure ventilation

13. **Regarding pulmonary shunt:**

    A   The $\dot{V}/\dot{Q}$ ratio is usually >1

    B   Venous admixture may be calculated from the shunt equation

    C   In an area of >50% shunt, as the FIO_2 is doubled the PaO_2 doubles

    D   End-capillary oxygen content can be measured directly

    E   The shunt equation requires knowledge of the haemoglobin

14. **Regarding responses modifying ventilation in healthy subjects:**

    A $PaCO_2$ is the most important factor controlling ventilation

    B   At a low PaO_2, ventilation is higher at any given $PaCO_2$

    C   Central chemoreceptors respond to a reduction in PO_2

    D   Response to an altered PaO_2 is minimal

    E   Ventilation increases up to 15 times the resting level during exercise

15. **Regarding carbon dioxide (CO_2) transport in the blood:**

    A   30% of CO_2 is carried as carbamino compounds in arterial blood

    B CO_2 is 50 times more soluble in blood than oxygen

    C   The chloride shift involves removal of chloride ions from erythrocytes to maintain electrical neutrality

    D   In arterial blood, the majority of CO_2 is dissolved

    E   The Haldane effect represents an increased capacity of deoxygenated haemoglobin to carry CO_2

16. **The pituitary gland:**

    A   Lies in the sella turcica

    B   Is connected to the hypothalamus via the pars intermedia

    C   Is mostly made up of the posterior lobe

    D The glandular part of the pituitary gland is in the anterior lobe

    E Only synthesises hormones in the anterior lobe

17. **The following hormone functions are correct:**

    A Luteinising hormone stimulates sperm production by the testes

    B Adrenocorticotrophic hormone stimulates the adrenal cortex to secrete mineralocorticoids

    C Human growth hormone stimulates general body growth and regulates metabolism

    D Prolactin initiates milk production in the mammary glands

    E Thyroid stimulating hormone stimulates the thyroid and parathyroid glands to secrete their hormones

18. **Regarding gastric function, which of the following is true:**

    A The stomach secretes about 1 L of juice per day

    B Chief cells are situated in the body of the stomach

    C Parietal cells secrete pepsins

    D Acid secretion is increased by gastrin

    E Acid secretion is decreased by secretin

19. **The following are synthesised by the liver:**

    A Albumin

    B Fibrinogen

    C Angiotensinogen

    D Transferrin

    E C-reactive protein

20. **Regarding platelets, which of the following is true:**

    A They have a lifespan of 3 days in the circulation

    B Aggregation is inhibited by adenosine diphosphate

    C They have nuclei

    D They contain α granules

    E Adhesion causes platelets to change shape

21. **The following antiarrhythmic drugs can be used to treat acute paroxysmal supraventricular tachycardia:**

    A Verapamil

    B Digoxin

    C Diltiazem

    D Flecainide

    E Adenosine

22. **Digoxin:**

    A Inhibits the Na^+ pump of myocardial cells

    B Has no inotropic effect

    C When taken orally only 25% is absorbed from the gastrointestinal tract

    D Sensitivity is increased in hyperkalaemia

    E Is contraindicated in hypertrophic obstructive cardiomyopathy

23. **When inducing systemic hypotension:**

    A   Sodium nitroprusside infusion could lead to cyanide toxicity
    B   Labetalol would be appropriate in hypertension with heart failure
    C   Isosorbide dinitrate infusion for hypertension plus ischaemia is appropriate
    D   Dopamine agonists can be used in severe hypertension with poor renal function
    E   Esmolol would be used for α- and β-blockade

24. **The following are true regarding β-adrenergic blocking drugs:**

    A   Atenolol is mainly excreted by the liver
    B   Propranolol is mainly excreted by the kidneys
    C   Esmolol has the shortest half-life of all the β-blockers
    D   They increase the risk of lidocaine toxicity
    E   Glucagon may be used to treat β-blocker overdose

25. **Diuretics have the following pharmacokinetic properties:**

    A   Bendroflumethiazide is mostly metabolised in the liver to inactive metabolites
    B   Amiloride is poorly absorbed from the gastrointestinal tract
    C   Furosemide is highly plasma protein bound
    D   Spironolactone can be administered intravenously and orally
    E   Mannitol is distributed throughout the extracellular fluid compartment

26. **The following drugs are contraindicated in patients suffering from porphyria:**

    A   Etomidate
    B   Enflurane
    C   Atropine
    D   Clonidine
    E   Cyclizine

27. **Propofol:**

    A   Is poorly water soluble
    B   Is a weak alkali
    C   Can elicit excitatory central nervous system effects on induction
    D   Causes severe complications following intra-arterial injection
    E   Has an increased context-sensitive half-time with prolonged infusion

28. **Regarding the commonly used benzodiazepines, which of the following is true:**

    A   They are all highly protein bound to albumin
    B   They all have active metabolites
    C   They are all well absorbed after administration
    D   They are all metabolised in the liver by oxidation
    E   They are all excreted in the urine as glucuronide conjugates

29. **Non-steroidal anti-inflammatory drugs:**

    A   Are more effective against somatic pain than opioids
    B   Have a large volume of distribution
    C   Are excreted in bile

D   Inhibit the production of prostaglandins and thromboxanes
E   All produce reversible enzyme inhibition

30. **The following are opioid partial agonists:**
  A   Nalbuphine
  B   Buprenorphine
  C   Codeine
  D   Pethidine
  E   Sufentanil

31. **The volume of distribution of the following drugs is greater than total body water:**
  A   Paracetamol
  B   Thiopentone
  C   Cocaine
  D   Vecuronium
  E   Amiodarone

32. **In a patient with chronic liver disease, dose reduction may be required for:**
  A   Thiopentone
  B   Morphine
  C   Midazolam
  D   Propofol
  E   Remifentanil

33. **Regarding log dose–response curves, which of the following is true:**
  A   In the presence of a reversible antagonist, an agonist may have full intrinsic activity
  B   A rightward shift indicates reduced potency
  C   A reduced ED_{50} is seen with a partial agonist
  D   Partial agonists act as competitive inhibitors
  E   Non-competitive inhibitors increase the ED_{50}

34. **Cocaine:**
  A   Undergoes hepatic metabolism
  B   Increases presynaptic uptake of noradrenaline
  C   Blocks fast ion channels
  D   Inhibits monoamine oxidase activity
  E   Is administered in a maximum dose of 5 mg/kg

35. **Non-depolarising neuromuscular blocking drugs:**
  A   Demonstrate a phase I block
  B   Need 30% receptor occupancy to be effective
  C   Include racemic mixtures
  D   Have a prolonged duration of action in the presence of plasma cholinesterase deficiency
  E   Cross the placenta

36. **Neostigmine:**

   A   Worsens paralytic ileus
   B   Causes sweating
   C   Increases heart rate
   D   Crosses the blood–brain barrier
   E   Prolongs the duration of action of suxamethonium

37. **Regarding anticonvulsants:**

   A   Sodium valproate acts via gamma-aminobutyric acid (GABA)-mediated transmission
   B   Gabapentin acts on GABA receptors
   C   Carbamazepine stabilises inactive Na^+ channels
   D   Phenytoin has a high oral bioavailability
   E   Sodium valproate is teratogenic

38. **Glycopyrrolate:**

   A   Crosses the blood–brain barrier
   B   Causes bronchoconstriction
   C   Increases respiratory dead space
   D   Has a tertiary amine structure
   E   Has a high oral bioavailability

39. **The following are bactericidal:**

   A   Vancomycin
   B   Teicoplanin
   C   Metronidazole
   D   Tetracycline
   E   Erythromycin

40. **The following are pro-drugs:**

   A   Clonidine
   B   Aspirin
   C   Enalapril
   D   Cortisone
   E   Lorazepam

41. **Amplifiers used for biological signals:**

   A   Require high common mode rejection ratio and low input impedance
   B   Have an attenuated signal when there is a high electrode impedance and a low amplifier input impedance
   C   Typically have a common mode rejection ratio in the region of 100:1
   D   Would require a bandwidth of 0.5–100 Hz frequency response for electrocardiogram
   E   Would require a bandwidth of about 1 kHz frequency response for electroencephalogram

42. **Modern defibrillators:**
    A   Are used to apply a large electric shock to the heart
    B   Use electric alternating current mains with a step-up transformer
    C   Discharge a monophasic current for maximum efficiency
    D   Typically require a voltage of 2500 V
    E   Typically discharge the current over 0.5 second

43. **Regarding different types of lasers:**
    A   The laser medium can be solid
    B   Class I lasers emit hazardous levels of laser radiation
    C   Class IV lasers are a skin hazard
    D   Infrared and visible are the only types of radiant energy available
    E   Neodymium (Nd) type laser is an example of a solid state laser

44. **Concerning MRI:**
    A   Fat produces high signals due to its high proton density
    B   The patient re-emits radio waves which are detected and used to construct an image
    C   The largest magnetic resonance signals are produced by nuclei of carbon atoms
    D   The magnetic field causes protons in the body to line up and spin
    E   Air produces no signal

45. **The following are not derived SI units:**
    A   Calorie
    B   Kilogram weight
    C   Pascal
    D cmH_2O
    E   Electron-volt

46. **Regarding temperature measurement, which of the following is true:**
    A   A thermistor's electrical resistance varies with temperature
    B   A thermocouple requires 2 different metals joined together
    C   Thermistors rely on the Seebeck effect to function
    D   The electrical resistance of a platinum wire varies linearly with temperature
    E   A thermistor, thermocouple or infrared thermometer can be used to measure the temperature at the tympanic membrane

47. **Regarding heat capacity, which of the following is true:**
    A   Heat capacity is the amount of heat required to raise the temperature of a 1 kg substance by 1 K
    B   The quantity of heat required to produce a change in temperature of an object depends on the specific heat capacity
    C   The SI units for heat capacity are J/kg/K
    D   Water has a high specific heat capacity
    E   Only small amounts of heat are usually required to warm up gases

48. **The following methods are employed to keep patients warm during anaesthesia:**
   A   Blowing warmed air directly onto the patient
   B   Lying the patient on a conductive surface
   C   Attaching a conductive heat exchanger to the infused fluids
   D   Using high anaesthetic gas flows
   E   Covering the patient with a metallic reflective blanket

49. **Regarding osmosis and osmotic pressure, which of the following is true:**
   A   Osmosis refers to the movement of water and molecules across a semipermeable membrane
   B   Osmotic pressure is the hydrostatic pressure that develops as a result of water diffusion into the space
   C   Osmotic pressure is dependent on the number and size of particles in solution
   D   Osmolarity is the potential of a fluid to exert osmotic pressure
   E   Osmolality is the millimolar solute per kilogram of solvent

50. **Regarding direct blood pressure measurement, which of the following is true:**
   A   Only systolic, diastolic and mean arterial pressures can be assessed using this method
   B   The transducers tend to be resistive strain gauge type
   C   Resonance tends to increase the amplitude of the reading
   D   Damping is a measure of the frictional forces acting on the measurement system
   E   Optimal damping of 0.9 is ideal

51. **Regarding electrical circuits, which of the following is true:**
   A   Resistance wires may contain a Wheatstone bridge
   B   Photoelectric cells are a form of transducer
   C   Transducers may convert sound into electrical energy
   D   Pressure transducers often contain four-strain gauges
   E   A transistor converts mechanical energy into electrical energy

52. **Cylinder manifolds:**
   A   Can be used to supply Entonox
   B   Should contain sufficient oxygen to last for 4 days
   C   Contain size J cylinders
   D   Have all cylinder valves open
   E   Have a change over of banks which is electronically controlled

53. **Vapourisers:**
   A   Are coded orange for halothane
   B   Are geometrically coded
   C   Must be removed prior to filling
   D   Are safe to tilt
   E   Can be used simultaneously in series

54. **1520 mmHg is approximately equal to:**

   A   2 bar
   B   1020 cmH$_2$O
   C   20.6 psi
   D   202.65 kPa
   E   2040 Torr

55. **Regarding the Mapleson E breathing system, which of the following is true:**

   A   It is suitable for a 45 kg child
   B   The Jackson-Rees modification has an open-ended bag
   C   It increases theatre pollution
   D   It allows application of continuous positive airway pressure
   E   The volume of tubing should be twice the patients tidal volume

56. **Regarding the Clark electrode, which of the following is true:**

   A   Electrons are liberated at the cathode
   B   It has a voltage of 6 V between the electrodes
   C   It is thermoregulated
   D   It measures oxygen tension in both gas and solution
   E   It is inaccurate when used with nitrous oxide

57. **Sidestream end-tidal carbon dioxide analysers:**

   A   Increase dead space significantly
   B   Are more rapid than mainstream analysers
   C   Only analyse carbon dioxide in the sample
   D   Require fresh gas flow rates greater than 450 mL/minute
   E   Cannot be used in patients who are not intubated

58. **Regarding pH measurement, which of the following is true:**

   A   A change of 1 pH unit causes a change in output of 60 mV
   B   There is a linear relation with H$^+$ ion concentration
   C   A pH of 7.4 is equal to a hydrogen ion concentration of 40 mmol/L
   D   It uses a calomel measuring electrode
   E   It is temperature controlled

59. **Cardiac output monitoring:**

   A   Uses the Stewart–Hamilton equation in thermodilution techniques
   B   Is accurate even when right heart methods are used
   C   May be measured using echocardiography
   D   May be measured using thermistors
   E   Is accurate when using bioimpedance

60. **The following are true regarding the bispectral index:**

   A   It eliminates the risk of awareness
   B   Five frontotemporal electrodes detect an electroencephalogram trace
   C   A value of 60–80 indicates adequate levels of anaesthesia
   D   It is affected by nitrous oxide use
   E   It is inaccurate when used with ketamine

Questions: SBAs

For each question, select the single best answer from the five options listed.

61. A 32-year-old woman with inflammatory bowel disease presents for an elective laparoscopic hemicolectomy. She has been taking 20 mg of prednisolone daily for the last 4 months.

What is the most appropriate perioperative steroid regimen?

A   125 mg methylprednisolone
B   4 mg dexamethasone
C   50 mg hydrocortisone
D   20 mg cortisone
E   200 µg fludrocortisone

62. You are called to assess a 74-year-old man with a 90-pack year history of smoking who presented with suspected bowel obstruction and difficulty in breathing. Arterial blood gas analysis shows a pH of 7.38, $Paco_2$ of 9.5 kPa, Pao_2 of 6.4 kPa and standard bicarbonate of 40.1 mmol/L.

Which is the most appropriate initial action?

A   Rapid sequence induction and ventilation
B   Administer high flow oxygen via a non-rebreath mask
C   Request a chest X-ray
D   Contact intensive treatment unit and arrange a bed
E   Administer 28% oxygen via a Venturi mask

63. A 65-year-old man is scheduled for laryngectomy and free flap surgery, which will take 6–8 hours.

Which of the following methods used to warm the patient is the most efficient?

A   Gel heat pad
B   Forced warm air blankets
C   Infusion of warmed fluids
D   Heat and moisture exchanger filter (HME filter)
E   Low flow anaesthetic gases

64. A 48-year-old man, who is otherwise fit and healthy, is having an elective laparoscopic cholecystectomy. Intubation has been unsuccessful despite four attempts at direct laryngoscopy and two attempts through an intubating laryngeal mask airway (ILMA).

What should be the next step?

A   Try a third attempt to intubate through the ILMA
B   Apply external laryngeal manipulation to aid direct laryngoscopy
C   Postpone surgery and wake the patient up
D   Pass a bougie and feel for 'clicks' under direct laryngoscopy
E   Give a further dose of muscle relaxant

65. An 18-year-old fit and healthy man is having a tonsillectomy as a day-case procedure. General anaesthesia is being induced with propofol and remifentanil infusion as part of his total intravenous anaesthesia regimen.

Which of the following would be the most likely immediate complication requiring treatment at induction of anaesthesia?

A   Chest wall rigidity
B   Awareness
C   Laryngospasm
D   Bradycardia
E   Histamine-induced bronchospasm

66. You have been asked to place an epidural for labour analgesia in a 28-year-old woman.

Which one of the following structures does *not* form a boundary of the epidural space?

A   Sacrococcygeal membrane
B   Pedicles and intervertebral foramina
C   Capsules of the facet joints and laminae
D   Posterior longitudinal ligament
E   Supraspinous ligament

67. A patient is having intracranial surgery for excision of a tumour. The consultant anaesthetist routinely uses nitrous oxide as part of his anaesthetic technique.

Which of the following is *not* a cerebral effect of nitrous oxide?

A   Increased intracranial pressure
B   Impaired cerebral sensitivity to carbon dioxide
C   Increased cerebral blood flow
D   Increased cerebral metabolic rate for oxygen consumption
E   Impaired autoregulation

68. A 50 kg, 23-year-old woman is in recovery having had a straightforward bilateral breast reduction and abdominoplasty, she was in theatre for 5 hours. She is otherwise fit and healthy. In recovery, she has a heart rate of 110 beats per minute, blood pressure of 140/85, respiratory rate of 25 breaths per minute and appears pale. She had 20 mg morphine in theatre and has not required any further analgesia in recovery.

Which of the following is the most likely cause of her clinical condition?

A   Angina
B   Pain
C   Hypothermia
D   Anaphylaxis
E   Hypovolaemia

69. A patient is due for a surgical procedure on the afternoon list which is scheduled to start at 1 pm and you are assessing him for anaesthesia. He says he ate breakfast at 7 am, which consisted of a large bowl of porridge.

Which one of the following causes the most rapid rate of emptying of food from the stomach?

A   Gastrin
B   Sympathetic stimulation
C   Cholecystokinin
D   Largely carbohydrate meal
E   Largely fatty meal

70. A 73-year-old man on warfarin for atrial fibrillation presents with an international normalised ratio (INR) of 5.2, having been previously well controlled. He has recently been commenced on a new drug by his general practitioner for a chest infection.

What is the most likely drug?

A   Cefalexin
B   Amoxicillin
C   Rifampicin
D   Ketoconazole
E   Clarithromycin

71. A 29-year-old woman presents following an aspirin overdose. She has oxygen saturations of 98% on air, respiratory rate of 34 breaths per minute, heart rate of 108 bpm, blood pressure of 84/56 mmHg and a Glasgow coma score (GCS) of 13/15. Her arterial blood gas result shows pH 7.24, $Paco_2$ 3.6 kPa, Pao_2 11.4 kPa and HCO_3^- 18.0 mmol/L.

Which best describes the therapeutic effect of sodium bicarbonate in this patient?

A   Increases tubular secretion of salicylates
B   Increases tubular ionisation of salicylates
C   Reduced urine pH will reduce reabsorption
D   Treats the metabolic acidosis
E   Binds to salicylates in renal tubules

72. A 42-year-old woman with a past medical history of hypertension, schizophrenia and post-operative nausea and vomiting presents for an open reduction and internal fixation of her ankle.

In this patient, why would an enantiopure preparation of S-ketamine be advantageous compared with a racemic mixture?

A   Less intense emergence phenomena
B   Reduced ischaemic preconditioning
C   More potency than R-ketamine
D   Is more cardiostable
E   Produces less frequent emergence phenomena

73. A 24-year-old man has a rapid sequence induction for a laparoscopic appendicectomy. He is given 5 mg morphine, 1 g of paracetamol, 1.2 g of co-amoxiclav, with anaesthesia maintained on sevoflurane with a minimum alveolar concentration of 1.1. Over the last 15 minutes, his end-tidal CO_2 increased from 4.6 to 8.4 kPa, his FIO_2 up to 80% with a SpO_2 of 93%, his heart rate has risen from 76 to 114 bpm, and his temperature increased from 36.5°C to 37.1°C.

What is the most likely underlying mechanism?

A   Reduced adenosine triphosphate consumption
B   Uncontrolled Ca^{2+} release into the sarcoplasmic reticulum
C   Abnormality of the Ryanodine-1 receptor
D   Autosomal recessive condition
E CO_2 absorption from pneumoperitoneum

74. At the end of a total abdominal hysterectomy performed on a 54-year-old woman, she has no twitches on a train-of-four nerve stimulation as she has been given 20 mg of rocuronium 5 minutes previously. You administer 400 mg of sugammadex to reverse the neuromuscular blockade.

Which best explains the mode of action of sugammadex?

A   Directly hydrolyses rocuronium
B   Forms complexes that are rapidly metabolised in the liver
C   Inhibits acetylcholinesterase
D   Creates a concentration gradient for rocuronium to diffuse away from the neuromuscular junction
E   Forms a lipid-soluble complex

75. An electroencephalogram trace shows a signal frequency of 9 Hz.

Which rhythm is this most likely to be?

A   α-rhythm
B   β-rhythm
C   γ-rhythm
D   δ-rhythm
E   θ-rhythm

76. A 28-year-old woman had an epidural inserted for labour analgesia. During injection of 15 mL 0.1% bupivacaine with 2 µg/mL of fentanyl, the patient complains of an abnormal sensation around her lips and becomes agitated.

What is the immediate management of this patient?

A   Give 100% oxygen
B   Call for help
C   Insert an intravenous cannula
D   Stop injecting the local anaesthetic
E   Send a full set of blood tests

77. A 21-year-old woman has had a laparoscopic salpingectomy for an ectopic pregnancy. She received a total of 50 mg of atracurium during the procedure. At the end of the operation, a nerve stimulator is used to assess depth of neuromuscular blockade.

Which of the following nerves best reflects the extent of neuromuscular blockade of the diaphragm?

A   Common peroneal nerve
B   Ulnar nerve
C   Accessory nerve
D   Tibial nerve
E   Facial nerve

78. A 22-year-old asthmatic woman with appendicitis is given 1 g paracetamol, 400 mg ibuprofen and 30 mg codeine. After 20 minutes, she finds it difficult to breath, is wheezy and hypoxic.

What is the most likely cause of her clinical features?

A   Histamine
B   Leukotrienes
C   Mast cell activation
D   Prostacyclin
E   Prostaglandins

79. A 61-year-old man with no past medical history of note presents with a 24-hour history of palpitations. A 12-lead electrocardiogram (ECG) is performed showing an irregularly irregular rhythm at a rate of between 100 and 112 beats per minute with no discernable P waves. His blood pressure is 138/80 mmHg, Glasgow coma score (GCS) is 15/15, has no chest pain and is not dyspnoeic.

What is the next course of action for this patient?

A   Heparin
B   Direct current cardioversion
C   Transoesophageal echocardiogram
D   Amiodarone
E   Bisoprolol

80. A 44-year-old non-insulin dependant diabetic woman with a background history of asthma and chronic back pain presents with anxiety and irritability. Her blood glucose is 2.9 mmol/L.

Which drug is most likely to have caused her hypoglycaemia?

A   Metformin
B   Salbutamol
C   Acarbose
D   Codeine
E   Glibenclamide

81. A 32-year-old woman, who is 24 weeks pregnant, presents with acute appendicitis. She is consented for a rapid sequence induction as well as a transversus abdominis plane block. She is worried about the effects of anaesthesia on the developing baby.

Which drug crosses the placenta the least?

A   Thiopentone
B   Suxamethonium
C   Morphine
D   Atracurium
E   Lidocaine

82. A 49-year-old woman with hypertension has been started on a diuretic by her general practitioner. She presents 2 months later with dysmenorrhoea and serum biochemistry revealing:

Na$^+$	129 mmo/L
K$^+$	5.6 mmol/L
Urea	5.3 mmol/L
Creatinine	72 µmol/L

Which drug is most likely to have been started?

A   Metolazone
B   Bumetanide
C   Acetazolamide
D   Amiloride
E   Spironolactone

83. A 59-year-old man presents with central crushing chest pain and shortness of breath. A 12-lead electrocardiogram shows ST segment elevation in leads II, III and aVF.

Which coronary artery is most likely to be affected?

A   Circumflex artery
B   Left anterior descending
C   Marginal artery
D   Right coronary artery
E   Posterior interventricular artery

84. Gas exchange occurs at the placenta, rather than the lungs, in the fetus.

What is most important factor in optimising fetal haemoglobin oxygenation?

A   Maternal blood alkalosis
B   Elevated fetal P_{CO_2}
C   Fetal blood has a pH of 7.28

D   Fetal haemoglobin has a P_{50} of 3.6 kPa
E   Fetal haemoglobin has a concentration of 16 g/dL

85. A 19-year-old man is undergoing a laparoscopic appendicectomy. His end-tidal carbon dioxide ($ETco_2$) increases to 8.3 kPa.

What is the most likely effect of an elevated arterial Pco_2?

A   Reduced pulmonary vascular resistance
B   Arrhythmias
C   Increased renal bicarbonate loss
D   Reduced intracranial pressure
E   Reduced plasma H^+ concentration

86. A 47-year-old woman presents with a subarachnoid haemorrhage. After 3 days, her urine output decreases and she is noted to be hyponatraemic.

Which of the following features is *least* likely to be attributed to excessive anti-diuretic hormone secretion?

A   Reduced pulmonary vascular resistance
B   Clotting factor production
C   Aquaporin-2 activity
D   Splanchnic vasoconstriction
E   Plasma osmolality of 265 mOsmol/kg

87. A 27-year-old man requires a manipulation under anaesthetic for a dislocated shoulder. He is given 200 mg of propofol and 75 µg of fentanyl. He wakes up 4 minutes after administration of propofol.

Which of the following best explains the short duration of action of propofol?

A   Hepatic conjugation
B   Extra-hepatic sulphation
C   Urinary excretion
D   High protein binding
E   Redistribution

88. A 74-year-old man had an open supra-renal abdominal aortic aneurysm repair 24 hours ago. He developed neurological deficits post-operatively.

Which of the following clinical features are most likely in anterior spinal artery syndrome?

A   Arm weakness more than leg weakness, bladder dysfunction, variable sensory loss
B   Preserved proprioception, touch and vibration sense with paralysis below the lesion
C   Loss of proprioception, touch and vibration and paralysis below the lesion
D   Ipsilateral paralysis, loss of vibration touch and proprioception
E   Loss of touch and temperature sensation below the lesion

89. When checking the anaesthetic circle breathing circuit, it appears to be incorrectly arranged.

    What is the ideal arrangement of a circle breathing system?

    A   Reservoir bag on the inspiratory limb; soda lime on the expiratory limb
    B   Vapouriser and soda lime on the expiratory limb; reservoir on the inspiratory limb
    C   Vapouriser on inspiratory limb; soda lime and reservoir bag on expiratory limb
    D   Soda lime and reservoir bag on the expiratory limb
    E   Soda lime, reservoir bag and vapouriser on the inspiratory limb

90. During routine theatre pollution testing, it was found that the concentration of nitrous oxide was 500 particles per million (ppm).

    What is the most likely cause for this finding?

    A   It is a paediatric theatre
    B   Excessive use of nitrous oxide
    C   Air changes are set at 15 times per hour
    D   Regular spillage during vapouriser filling may occur
    E   Passive scavenging systems are in use

Answers: MTFs

1. **A** True

   B False

   C False

   D False

   E True

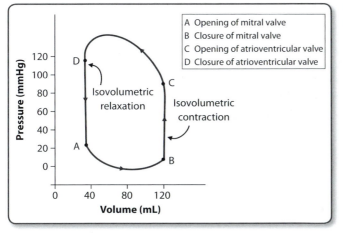

Figure 4.1 Left ventricular pressure–volume loop.

Ventricular blood pressure varies throughout the ejection phase, and in order to evaluate stroke work it is necessary to construct a graph of ventricular pressure plotted against volume (A), see **Figure 4.1**. During ventricular filling, there is an initial rapid filling phase, where pressure is falling because elastic recoil of the relaxing ventricle exerts a suction effect. During the later, slow filling phase, there is a rise in pressure which drives an increase in volume. During isovolumetric contraction, there is a steep rise in pressure, but no change in volume. The aortic valve then opens, at a pressure set by the diastolic arterial pressure and ejection occurs. The aortic valve closes at end-diastolic pressure, and isovolumetric relaxation begins. Here, there is a rapid drop in pressure and the mitral valve then opens to start ventricular filling once again.

$$SV = LVEDV - LVESV \approx \text{normally 70 mL.}$$

where SV is stroke volume, LVEDV is left ventricular end-diastolic volume and LVESV is left ventricular end-systolic volume. Isovolumetric contraction has rapid pressure changes which are seen as a straight upward vertical line on the pressure/volume loop at normal physiological volumes, but as the ventricles continue to fill it becomes increasingly more difficult to fill, so the left ventricle filling curve changes from linear to a gradually increasing gradient (B).

The area inside the loop represents the work done (pressure × volume) (C).

The pressure/volume loop of the right ventricle is the same shape as the left ventricle, but will have a smaller area, due to the lower pressures and volumes (D).

Preload is the end-diastolic stretch or tension of the ventricular wall and this is best shown as the LVEDV on the X-axis (E).

2. A False

   B False

   C True

   D True

   E False

The normal resting heart rate in the adult human is between 50 and 100 beats per minute. The pacemaker is innervated by autonomic nerves, and its intrinsic rate is continuously modified by activity in these nerves. Both sets of autonomic nerves are continually active at rest, but vagal inhibition predominates (A).

The intrinsic heart rate is 100 beats per minute if both sympathetic and parasympathetic innervations are blocked (B).

Sympathetic stimulation at the sinoatrial node results in increased heart rate, while parasympathetic stimulation causes a decrease in heart rate. They both also innervate the atrioventricular node, sympathetic stimulation resulting in shortening of the transmission delay and parasympathetic stimulation lengthening it (C).

Increased temperature, e.g. during pyrexia, causes an increase in the heart rate, and cooling of the heart, e.g. during cardiac surgery or hypothermia, slows the heart rate (D).

The parasympathetic nerve terminals release the neurotransmitter acetylcholine, which binds to the receptors in the cell membrane (E). The sympathetic nerve terminals release adrenaline and noradrenaline.

3. A True

   B True

   C True

   D False

   E False

Blood flow to an organ can be calculated using the Fick principle if the following details are known:

• The amount of marker substance taken up by an organ per unit time
• The concentration of marker substance in the arterial blood supply to the organ
• The concentration of marker substance in the venous blood leaving the organ

The Fick principle states that the rate at which the circulation takes up oxygen from the lungs must equal the change in oxygen concentration in the pulmonary blood multiplied by the pulmonary blood flow. Since the pulmonary blood flow represents output from the right ventricle, this allows us to calculate cardiac output.

Cardiac output is the oxygen uptake rate divided by the difference between the arterial and venous oxygen concentrations (A).

The Fick principle is quite general and applies to any organ in which there is exchange of products at a steady state (B).

Fick method is the gold standard for measuring cardiac output, but is slow and beat-to-beat changes in stroke volume cannot be followed. It is only valid in the resting state (C).

The resting oxygen consumption is measured over 5–10 minutes by spirometry or expired gases can be collected in a Douglas bag (D).

Peripheral venous blood is unsuitable as mixed venous blood is required to calculate cardiac output (E). The mixed venous blood is usually sampled from the pulmonary artery or right ventricle via a cardiac catheter.

4. **A** False

    B False

    C False

    D True

    E False

Parasympathetic nerve fibres are carried in the occulomotor, facial, glossopharyngeal and vagus nerves (cranial nerves III, VII, IX and X) (see **Table 4.1**).

Table 4.1 Parasympathetic cranial nerves

Number	Name	Target organ	Ganglion
III	Oculomotor	Eye	Ciliary
VII	Facial	Submandibular, sublingual, lacrimal glands	Pterygopalatine and submandibular
IX	Glossopharyngeal	Lungs, larynx, tracheobronchial tree	Otic
X	Vagus	Heart, parotid gland, proximal GIT	Superior and inferior (nodose)

5. **A** False

    B True

    C False

    D True

    E False

The resting membrane potential of a nerve depends predominantly on the balance between Na^+ and K^+ ions, achieving a potential of −70 mV (A). The membrane is more permeable to K⁺ ions that leak out of the neurones than Na⁺ that enters (B). An action potential arises when a stimulus exceeds the threshold potential which then causes membrane depolarisation. The absolute refractory period is the time between a threshold potential and one-third completion of repolarisation and is the time when no further stimulus can cause an action potential (see **Figure 4.2**) (C). The relative refractory period immediately follows the absolute refractory period until hyperpolarisation begins. A supramaximal stimulus may cause an action potential during this phase (D). Calcium channels are not involved in nerve action potentials, but in cardiac action potentials (E).

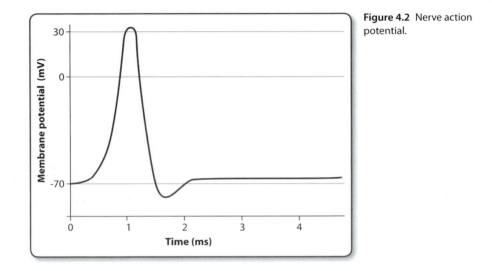

Figure 4.2 Nerve action potential.

6. **A** False

    B False

    C True

    D False

    E True

The International Association for the Study of Pain defines pain as 'an unpleasant sensory and emotional experience associated with actual or potential tissue damage or described in terms of such damage'. It serves predominantly as a protective function to body tissue.

- Nociception: the sensation of noxious stimuli in the central nervous system. This is different from pain, but is a component of pain symptoms (B)
- Allodynia: painful responses to normally painless stimuli (A)
- Hyperpathia: increased sensation from a sensory stimulus with a raised sensation threshold
- Hyperalgesia: exaggerated pain response to normally painful stimuli (D)

- Neuropathic pain: Pain initiated or caused by a primary lesion or dysfunction of the nervous system (C)
- Chronic pain: pain persisting beyond removal of stimulus and beyond the period of time expected for healing and recovery (E)

7. A False

    B True

    C False

    D False

    E True

Noxious stimuli are sensed by either unmyelinated, slow C-fibres in the case of heat, mechanical or chemical stimuli, or by myelinated, quick Aδ fibres. The cell bodies of these fibres are in the dorsal root ganglion, and they terminate in the dorsal horn (B). Aδ fibres terminate onto second-order neurones in Rexed laminae I and V, while C-fibres terminate in the substantia gelatinosa which is laminae II and III (A, C). Glutamate acts as the main excitatory neurotransmitter at these synapses, whereas gamma-amino butyric acid and glycine are the main inhibitory neurotransmitters here (E). The majority of these second-order neurones then decussate and travel in the lateral spinothalamic tract, whereas a small proportion pass posterolaterally on the ipsilateral side (D). These fibres then terminate on the ventral posterior and medial nuclei of the thalamus that then feed onto cortical areas such as the somatosensory cortex and cingulate gyrus.

8. A True

    B False

    C True

    D False

    E False

Glomerular filtration rate (GFR) is measured in mL/minute and is the total volume of renal plasma flow that is filtered over time by the glomeruli (A). To measure GFR, an indicator substance which has specific properties must be used. It must only enter the tubule by filtration and must not undergo absorption, tubular excretion or metabolism. It must also be inert and not have any influence on renal function (C). Examples of such indicators are inulin (which is injected into the blood) and endogenous creatinine (already present in the blood) (E).

An average of 20% of the total renal plasma flow is filtered by the glomeruli (B). The ratio of GFR to renal plasma flow is the filtration fraction.

Para-aminohippurate is used to calculate renal plasma flow as about 90% of it is removed from the kidney in just one pass, due to its secretion by the tubular cells, making it unsuitable for measuring GFR (D). Any solute which is used to calculate the GFR should be freely filtered and should be neither reabsorbed nor secreted by the kidneys.

9. A True

    B False

    C False

    D True

    E False

    NaCl (99%) is absorbed from the tubules, so only 1% is normally excreted in the urine (A). The amount of Na^+ excreted varies according to the intake in order to keep the extracellular volume as constant as possible.

    Na^+ tubular transport requires metabolic energy, but Cl^- is resorbed passively or by secondary active transport (B).

    The resorbed NaCl in the proximal tubule is followed passively by water, so both are moving in the same direction across the tubular membrane (C).

    By the end of the proximal tubule about 70% of the filtered Na^+ and water is resorbed back to the blood (D).

    The thick ascending limb of the loop of Henle resorbs about 15% of the NaCl as do the distal convoluted tubules and the collecting ducts (E).

10. A True

    B True

    C False

    D True

    E True

    An increase in the uptake of potassium ions (K^+) causes a rise in the plasma and intracellular concentration of K^+, this then increases the chemical driving force for K^+ secretion, hence an increase in K^+ excretion (A).

    Alkalosis causes an increase the intracellular concentration of K^+, which increases the excretion of K^+ by increasing distal urinary flow and the release of aldosterone (B).

    Acute acidosis lowers the intracellular K^+ concentration and so causes a reduction in K^+ excretion (C).

    Chronic acidosis also causes an increase in the intracellular K^+ concentration, as with alkalosis; hence, it results in increased K^+ excretion (D).

    Aldosterone increases the activity of Na^+-K^+-ATPase at the luminal membrane, therefore increasing the K^+ excretion by Na^+ and K^+ channels (E).

11. A False

    B True

    C True

    D True

    E False

In metabolic disturbances, there are parallel changes in the concentrations of bicarbonate (HCO_3^-) and non-bicarbonate buffer bases, but in respiratory disturbance these concentrations are independent of each other (A). The HCO_3^- and CO_2 buffer is no longer effective as the change in $Paco_2$ is the cause of the disturbance and not the result as is the case in metabolic disturbances. The non-bicarbonate buffer bases work to compensate for the changes in pH.

Respiratory acidosis is due to elevated $Paco_2$ and this lowers the pH. This is buffered by the non-bicarbonate bases, which results in a small increase in HCO_3^-, resulting in only a small compensation of the high $Paco_2$. If the $Paco_2$ remains high, as in chronic respiratory acidosis, the kidneys will increase the H^+ ion secretion after 1–2 days (B). This renal compensation aims to normalise the pH.

At high altitude, there is an acute deficiency in oxygen and this results in hyperventilation which reduces $Paco_2$ in the blood, producing a respiratory alkalosis (C).

Respiratory acidosis occurs due to the inability of the lungs to eliminate CO_2, as seen in tuberculosis and pneumonia, where there is a reduction in pulmonary tissue (D). Reduced ventilation and rib cage abnormalities have a similar effect.

Acute respiratory acidosis and alkalosis cause large fluctuations in the pH of the cerebrospinal fluid (CSF) (E). This is because CO_2 rapidly enters the CSF from the blood as compared with bicarbonate and H^+ ions, and the low protein concentration in the CSF means that there is less buffering capability.

12. **A** False

   B True

   C True

   D True

   E False

Supine position and general anaesthesia with intermittent positive pressure ventilation reduce the functional residual capacity. In addition, there is a 10% reduction in FRC in females when compared with males. Conditions that increase airway resistance including asthma as well as exercise increase the FRC (see Table 3.1).

13. **A** False

   B True

   C False

   D False

   E True

Shunt causes hypoxaemia because it is an extreme form of $\dot{V}/\dot{Q}$ mismatch with a ratio of zero as it is perfused but not ventilated blood (A). A high $\dot{V}/\dot{Q}$ ratio is associated with dead space. Venous admixture refers to the amount of mixed venous blood that would have to be added to pulmonary end-capillary blood to produce the observed drop in arterial Pao_2 (Pao_2) from the Po_2 in the end-capillary blood (Pco_2) (B). It may be calculated using the shunt equation:

$$\frac{\dot{Q}s}{\dot{Q}t} = \frac{(CcO_2 - Cao_2)}{(CcO_2 - C\bar{v}o_2)}$$

where $\dot{Q}s$ is blood flow to unventilated alveoli, $\dot{Q}t$ is total pulmonary blood flow, CcO_2 is end-capillary O_2 content, Cao_2 is arterial O_2 content, $C\bar{v}o_2$ is mixed venous O_2 content.

To calculate O_2 content, knowledge of the volume of haemoglobin, saturation and the partial pressure of O_2 in the mixed venous and arterial blood is needed (E).

In regions of the lung where there is a large amount of shunt, the Pao_2 will only increase minimally as the blood there is under ventilated (C), this region is essentially perfused but not ventilated. The end-capillary cannot be measured directly, but can be calculated using the alveolar gas equation (D).

14. **A** True

   B True

   C False

   D True

   E True

The main factors modifying ventilation normally include Pco_2, Po_2, pH and exercise.

- Pco_2: this is the most important factor controlling ventilation normally and has a very high sensitivity, being maintained to within 0.3–0.4 kPa (A). At a Pco_2 between 5 and 11 kPa, there is a linear increase in minute ventilation, above which there is respiratory depression and a reduction in minute ventilation (see **Figure 4.3**). The response to Pco_2 is reduced in increased age, sleep, genetic factors, trained

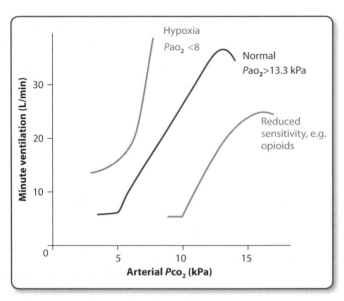

Figure 4.3 Relationship of minute ventilation and Pco_2.

athletes, divers, opiate and barbiturate use. The response to P_{CO_2} is augmented in response to hypoxic conditions

- P_{O_2}: under normal conditions, there is minimal response to a reduced P_{O_2} unless it falls below 8 kPa when there is a steep increase in minute ventilation. Ventilatory response to hypoxia is therefore only relevant in chronic lung conditions and at

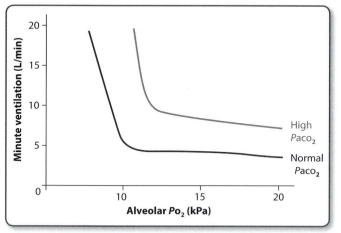

Figure 4.4 Relationship of minute ventilation and Pa_{O_2}.

high altitude. In conditions of hypercarbia, the response to hypoxia is augmented (see **Figure 4.4**). A reduction in P_{O_2} is sensed by peripheral chemoreceptors only

- pH: a reduced pH will act predominantly on the peripheral chemoreceptors to increase minute ventilation
- Exercise: this increases minute ventilation significantly, while P_{CO_2} is maintained or reduces slightly, P_{O_2} increases slightly and pH is maintained. Therefore, the mechanisms are thought to be multifactorial including cortical stimulation and afferent impulses from proprioceptors, but are poorly understood. Minute ventilation can increase more than 15 times, oxygen uptake increasing to 4 L/min and carbon dioxide excretion increasing to 8 L/min

15. A False

  B False

  C False

  D False

  E True

CO_2 is carried in the blood either dissolved, as bicarbonate or as carbamino compounds (see **Figure 4.5**). In arterial blood 90% is carried as bicarbonate, 5% as carbamino compounds and 5% dissolved (A, D).

- Dissolved CO_2 is 20 times more soluble than O_2 (B)
- Bicarbonate is formed in a two-stage reaction, the first stage being catalysed by carbonic anhydrase to form carbonic acid (H_2CO_3). Carbonic acid is then

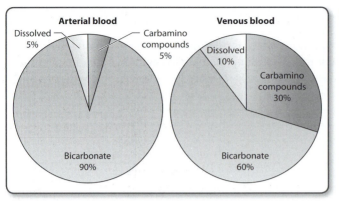

Figure 4.5 Distribution of CO_2 in arterial and venous blood.

converted to H$^+$ and HCO$_3^-$. The subsequent reaction results in H$^+$ intracellularly while HCO$_3^-$ diffuses out of the cell. To maintain electrical neutrality, chloride diffuses into erythrocytes: the chloride shift (C)

$$CO_2 + H_2O \rightleftharpoons H_2CO_3 \rightleftharpoons H^+ + HCO_3^-$$

- Carbamino compounds: CO_2 binds to the amine terminal of haemoglobin forming carbamino haemoglobin, an enzyme independent reaction

The Haldane effect is the increased capacity of deoxygenated haemoglobin to carry CO_2 and hydrogen ions in compared to oxygenate haemoglobin (E).

16. **A** True

    B False

    C False

    D True

    E True

The pituitary gland is a pea-sized structure which lies in the sella turcica of the sphenoid bone, and it is attached to the hypothalamus by the infundibulum (A, B).

It is made up of two anatomically and functionally separate parts: the anterior and posterior pituitary glands. The anterior pituitary gland (in the anterior lobe) makes up about 75% of the gland (C). It mostly contains glandular epithelial cells and forms the glandular part of the pituitary (D). It secretes hormones that regulate many bodily activities, such as growth and reproduction.

The posterior pituitary gland, which is in the posterior lobe, does not synthesise hormones, but it does store and release two hormones: oxytocin and anti-diuretic hormone (E).

17. **A** False

    B False

    C True

D True

E False

Luteinising hormone (LH) stimulates secretion of testosterone by the testes and together with follicle-stimulating hormone (FSH) stimulates secretion of oestrogen by the ovaries and ovulation. It also stimulates the formation of the corpus luteum and its secretion of progesterone. FSH stimulates sperm production by the testes and stimulates ova production and secretion of oestrogens by the ovaries (A). Both LH and FSH are secreted from gonadotrophin cells in the anterior pituitary.

Adrenocorticotrophic hormone is secreted from the corticotrophin cells and stimulates the adrenal cortex to secrete glucocorticoids from the zona fasciculata. Mineralocorticoids are secreted from the zona glomerulosa of the adrenal cortex, and their secretion is not controlled by the pituitary gland hormones (B).

Human growth hormone is the most abundant of the anterior pituitary hormones and is secreted from the somatotrophin cells of the anterior pituitary gland. It stimulates body growth and regulates metabolism by stimulating protein synthesis, inhibiting protein breakdown and stimulating lipolysis (C).

Prolactin is secreted from lactotrophin cells and initiates and maintains milk secretion by the mammary glands (D). The ejection of milk depends on the hormone oxytocin, released from the posterior pituitary gland.

Thyroid-stimulating hormone is secreted from the thyrotrophin cells and stimulates the thyroid gland to secrete thyroxine and triiodothyronine, not the parathyroid glands (which exhibits a negative feedback control system that does not involve the pituitary gland) (E).

18. A False

B False

C False

D True

E True

The stomach secretes up to 3 L of gastric juice daily (A). The main content is pepsinogens, mucus, hydrochloric acid, intrinsic factor and gastroferrin. Secretion is from the tubular glands of the gastric mucosa.

Mucus is secreted from specialised mucus cells and protects the inner surface of the stomach; hydrochloric acid is formed in the parietal cells of the fundus, while pepsinogens which form pepsins (once the pH is below 6) are made in the chief cells situated in the fundus of the stomach (B, C).

Gastrin is released as a result of mechanical and chemical stimulation and it increases the secretion of gastric acid. Release of gastrin is inhibited by a low luminal pH (D).

A low pH and fat content in the duodenal chyme causes inhibition of the secretion of gastric acid by the release of hormones such as secretin and gastric inhibitory peptide (E).

19. A True

   B True

   C True

   D True

   E True

Albumin is a binding and carrier protein present in the plasma. It binds to hormones, amino acids, steroids, vitamins and fatty acids to aid in their transport. It is also an osmotic regulator, as it exerts an osmotic force across the capillary wall that pulls water into the blood. It also plays a role in the buffering capacity of blood. Normal plasma levels of albumin are about 3.5–5 g/dL. The synthesis of albumin by the liver is closely regulated and is decreased during fasting and increased in conditions where there are large losses of albumin (e.g. nephritic syndrome) (A).

Fibrinogen is a plasma protein synthesised by the liver and is the precursor to fibrin (B). The soluble fibrinogen is converted to insoluble fibrin; this process is catalysed by thrombin to form a stable clot.

Angiotensinogen is the precursor of the vasopressor peptide angiotensin II. It is present in the plasma and synthesised in the liver (C). Renin acts on angiotensinogen to convert it to angiotensin I, which is then converted to angiotensin II by the actions of angiotensin II-converting enzyme. The circulating levels of angiotensinogen are increased by glucocorticoids, thyroid hormones and angiotensin II.

Transferrin is a hepatically synthesised glycoprotein whose main function is to transport iron and regulate free iron concentrations (D). It is also produced in other organs such as the brain. In the plasma iron is converted from the ferrous state (Fe^{2+}) to the ferric (Fe^{3+}) form and then binds to transferrin. Transferring that is not bound to iron is called apotransferrin.

C-reactive protein is an acute phase protein synthesised in the liver in response to macrophage and adipocyte activity (E). It is released in response to inflammation and injury, and when its levels increase it activates monocytes and causes the further production of cytokines.

20. A False

   B False

   C False

   D True

   E True

Platelets are non-nuclear megakaryocyte derivatives with a circulating lifespan of between 8 and 14 days (A, C). They are involved in coagulation via a number of mechanisms. Vessel wall damage exposes microfibrils and collagen that activates von Willebrand's factor and thus platelets. The platelets become spherical and corrugated upon adhesion and release contents of cytoplasmic α-granules including adenosine triphosphate, fibrinogen, fibronectin, calcium, adrenaline and 5-HT (D, E). These factors encourage more platelet recruitment as well as further coagulation, vasoconstriction and vessel repair. In addition, at the site of tissue injury damaged cells release adenosine diphosphate (ADP) that binds to glycoprotein IIb/IIIa complex along with fibrinogen (B). Production of thromboxane A_2 further increases ADP levels.

21. A True

B False

C True

D False

E True

Paroxysmal supraventricular tachycardias (SVTs) can be treated by vagal manoeuvres such as the Valsalva or carotid sinus massage, but these can become less effective if the arrhythmia persists because the sympathetic tone increases. The drugs of choice for acute therapy are intravenous adenosine, verapamil or diltiazem (A, C, E).

Verapamil and diltiazem are alternates to adenosine. They affect the calcium-dependent atrioventricular (AV) nodal block. They are vasodilators so may produce hypotension if the paroxysmal SVT does not terminate. They should not, however, be used to treat pre-existing arrhythmias such as Wolff–Parkinson–White syndrome or broad-complex tachycardias.

The administration of intravenous boluses of adenosine result in transient AV nodal block, but it is very rapidly cleared from the circulation by cellular uptake and metabolism. Transient dyspnoea or chest pain may occur after administration. Adenosine is preferred in patients with severe hypotension, history of heart failure and poor left ventricular function. The calcium channel blockers would be preferred in patients with acute bronchospasm and if only small bore intravenous access is available.

Digoxin and flecainide are used for atrial fibrillation (B, D).

22. A True

B False

C False

D False

E True

Digoxin inhibits the sodium pump ($Na^+/K^+/ATPase$) and as a result there is a transient increase in the intracellular sodium close to the sarcolemma (A). This promotes calcium influx by the sodium–calcium exchange mechanism to enhance myocardial contractility, with arrhythmogenic risk (B).

Important therapeutic benefits of digoxin are the slowing of the heart rate and inhibition of the atrioventricular node by vagal stimulation and decreased sympathetic nerve discharge.

Seventy-five per cent of the oral dose of digoxin is rapidly absorbed, while the rest is inactivated in the lower gut (C). It circulates in the blood unbound to plasma proteins and binds to tissue receptors in the heart and skeletal muscle. It is lipid soluble and is excreted unchanged in the urine.

There are many factors affecting the sensitivity to digoxin; hypokalaemia is the most common and sensitises to the toxic effects of digoxin. Hyperkalaemia protects against digitalis-induced arrhythmias (D). Hypercalcaemia increases sensitivity to digitalis and hypocalcaemia decreases sensitivity.

Hypertrophic obstructive cardiomyopathy is a contraindication because the inotropic effect can worsen outflow obstruction (E). Other contraindications include AV nodal heart block, the possibility of digitalis toxicity and some cases of Wolff–Parkinson–White syndrome.

23. **A** True

   B False

   C True

   D True

   E False

Sodium nitroprusside relaxes smooth muscle. This is non-selective for arterioles and veins. It is the result of intracellular release of nitric oxide, which activates guanylate cyclase, resulting in accumulation of cyclic guanosine monophosphate. Two metabolites of nitroprusside are cyanide and thiocyanate, both of which may cause toxicity (A). The toxicity of thiocyanate is significantly increased in the presence of renal failure. Cyanide rapidly enters the blood cell and can affect oxygen transport. Toxicity is associated with prolonged infusion and warning signs include tachycardia, metabolic acidosis and elevation of venous oxygen saturation.

The drugs of choice in patients with hypertension plus heart failure would be angiotensin-converting enzyme inhibitors, such as enalapril. Negative inotropic drugs, such as α- and β-blockers, should be avoided (B).

Nitric oxide donors such as isosorbide dinitrate or nitroglycerin infusions are the drugs of choice for reducing hypertension in patients with ischaemia (C).

Fenoldopam is a dopamine receptor (DA_1) agonist and is used to induce hypotension in patients with severe or malignant hypertension combined with poor renal function (D).

Esmolol is an ultrashort-acting $β_1$-blocker, which is rapidly converted to inactive metabolites by blood esterases (E). Labetalol is a combined α- and β-blocking antihypertensive agent.

24. **A** False

   B False

   C True

D True

E True

β-Blockers that are most hydrophilic and least lipid soluble are excreted unchanged by the kidneys. Those most lipophilic and least water soluble are largely metabolised by the liver. Atenolol is mostly lipophilic so is excreted by the kidney and propranolol is mostly hydrophilic so is excreted by the liver (A, B).

Esmolol is an ultra-short acting β-blocker with a half-life of about 9 minutes (C). It is rapidly converted to inactive metabolites by blood esterases. Full recovery from β-blockade is about 30 minutes. Indications of use include the perioperative management of supraventricular tachycardia and hypertension.

β-Blockers depress hepatic blood flow so that the blood levels of lignocaine can increase resulting in a greater risk of toxicity (D).

Glucagon can theoretically be used as an infusion to treat β-blocker overdose because it stimulates the formation of cyclic adenosine monophosphate (AMP) by bypassing the occupied β-adrenoceptors (E). An infusion of a phosphodiesterase inhibitor such as milrinone could also be used as it helps cyclic AMP to accumulate.

25. A False

   B True

   C True

   D False

   E True

Bendroflumethiazide is well absorbed when administered orally and produces its effects within 90 minutes. It is approximately 70% metabolised in the liver to active metabolites and the rest is eliminated in the urine unchanged (A).

Amiloride is poorly absorbed from the gut, has a very low plasma protein binding and is not metabolised (B).

Furosemide is well absorbed from the gut and is highly plasma protein bound (approximately 95%) (C). Excretion is in the urine with the drug largely unchanged.

Spironolactone is only available as an oral preparation; it is incompletely absorbed from the gut and is highly protein bound (D).

Mannitol is distributed throughout the extracellular fluid compartment following intravenous administration (E). At the glomerulus, it is freely filtered and none is reabsorbed.

26. A True

   B True

   C False

   D True

   E False

The following drugs can precipitate an acute porphyric crisis:

- Barbiturates
- Cocaine
- Clonidine
- Diclofenac
- Etomidate
- Enflurane
- Halothane
- Hyoscine
- Lidocaine
- Metoclopramide
- Prilocaine
- Ranitidine

Therefore, these drugs should be avoided in patients suffering from porphyria.

27. **A** True

    B False

    C True

    D False

    E True

Propofol is a phenolic derivative, 2,6-diisopropylphenol. It is highly lipid soluble and is presented as a lipid water emulsion due to its poor water solubility (A). The solution contains soya bean oil and purified egg phosphatide.

Propofol is a weak acid and has a pKa of 11, and at physiological pH it is almost completely unionised, which explains its rapid onset of action (B).

In about 10% of patients excitatory effects can be seen; these are not true cortical seizure activity, but are probably a result of an imbalance between subcortical excitatory and inhibitory mechanisms (C). The movements produced are dystonic. Propofol also has antiemetic properties.

Upon intra-arterial injection, propofol is relatively safe as it does not crystallise in the same manner as thiopentone (D).

With prolonged infusion, the context-sensitive half-life is prolonged (E). It is 98% protein bound to albumin and has a large volume of distribution. Immediately after intravenous administration, it is rapidly redistributed to well-perfused tissues and so has a short duration of action.

28. **A** True

    B False

    C False

    D False

    E True

All the commonly used benzodiazepines (midazolam, diazepam and lorazepam) are highly protein bound (approximately 95%) to albumin (A).

Midazolam and diazepam are metabolised to active metabolites, although lorazepam does not have any active metabolites (B). Less than 5% of the metabolised midazolam is to oxazepam which is active. Diazepam is metabolised in the liver to desmethyldiazepam, oxazepam and temazepam.

Diazepam and lorazepam are well adsorbed after oral administration due to their high lipid solubility. Midazolam only has 40% bioavailablilty following oral administration (C).

Midazolam is metabolised in the liver by hydroxylation and conjugation with glucuronic acid. Diazepam undergoes oxidation in the liver and lorazepam is conjugated with glucuronic acid to inactive metabolites and then excreted in the urine (D).

All the benzodiazepines are ultimately conjugated with glucuronic acid, thus producing inactive metabolites and then excreted in the urine (E).

29. **A** True

  B False

  C True

  D True

  E False

Non-steroidal anti-inflammatory drugs (NSAIDs) are generally used to treat mild-to-moderate pain and reduce opioid consumption in the perioperative period. They are known to be more effective against somatic pain than opioids (A).

They can be administered orally, rectally, intravenously or intramuscularly, although not every NSAID can be administered by all of these routes. They are well absorbed from the gastrointestinal tract and are generally highly protein bound (except paracetamol). They have a low volume of distribution and are metabolised in the liver to inactive metabolites that are excreted in the urine and bile (B, C).

They work by inhibiting the enzyme cyclo-oxygenase that converts arachidonic acid to the cyclic endoperoxides (prostaglandins and thromboxanes), thereby inhibiting their production (see **Figure 4.11**) (D).

Apart from aspirin, all of the NSAIDs produce reversible inhibition of the enzyme cyclo-oxygenase, so that as the plasma levels of the NSAIDs fall, the activity of cyclo-oxygenase resumes (E). Aspirin causes irreversible inhibition of the enzyme, so that the production of new cyclic endoperoxides can only occur when new cyclo-oxygenase is produced.

30. **A** True

  B True

  C False

  D False

  E False

A partial agonist is a drug with receptor affinity but limited efficacy or intrinsic activity compared full agonists. They may also have antagonistic effects at that receptor. The following are opioid receptor partial agonists (**Table 4.2**).

Table 4.2 Opioid partial agonist activity

Drug	Agonist at	Antagonist at
Nalbuphine	σ, κ	μ
Buprenorphine	μ (partial agonist)	
Nalorphine	σ, κ	μ
Pentazocine	σ, κ	μ

31. A True

  B True

  C True

  D False

  E True

Total body water is normally approximately 0.6 L/kg in the average adult; thus, a volume of distribution (Vd) greater than this accounts for greater than total body water. The Vd is affected by protein binding, ionisation and lipid solubility. Paracetamol is unionised and lipid soluble, despite having a low protein binding of only 10%, thus has a high Vd of 1 L/kg (A).

With a pKa of 7.6, 60% of thiopentone is unionised at plasma pH of 7.4, but the high protein binding (to albumin) of 70–80% means that only 12% is free in the plasma. With high lipophilicity, the Vd is 2–2.5 L/kg (B).

Both cocaine (95%) and amiodarone (98%) are highly protein bound, thus have large Vds (C, E).

All neuromuscular blocking drugs are highly polar, leading to small Vds of less than 0.3 L/kg, including vecuronium (D).

32. A True

  B True

  C True

  D True

  E False

Liver disease has a number of effects relevant to drug administration:

- Drug clearance: reduced phase I and II metabolism, increasing plasma levels of drug; and reduced first-pass metabolism due to presence of portacaval shunts, thus increasing bioavailability

- Plasma proteins: reduce protein synthesis, protein concentrations and plasma protein binding, thereby increasing free drug
- Volume of distribution: ascites increases volume of distribution

Dose reduction is required for thiopentone because there is an increase in the free fraction and a prolonged distribution half-life (A). Propofol and benzodiazepine dosing should be carefully titrated as patients may have an increased sensitivity to their depressant effects (C, D). A reduction in hepatic blood flow and extraction ratio, as well as a sensitivity to opioid effects means morphine dosing would need to be reduced (B). However, because of its rapid metabolism by esterases, remifentanil dosing does not need modification (E).

33. A True

   B True

   C False

   D True

   E True

Log dose–response curves are useful to compare the effect of drugs on desired response. The ED_{50} is the dose needed to achieve 50% of the maximal effect, or the dose required to achieve a given response in 50% of the population. Any rightward shift to the sigmoid-shaped curves (see **Figure 4.6**) indicates a reduction in potency or presence of a competitive antagonist, thereby increasing the ED_{50} (B). Partial agonists may shift the curve right, and reduce the maximal effect; thus, the ED_{50} might be increased rather than reduced (C). This is similar to the effect of non-competitive inhibitors (E). In the presence of a full agonist, partial agonists may act as competitive inhibitors (D). An agonist will have full intrinsic activity, therefore

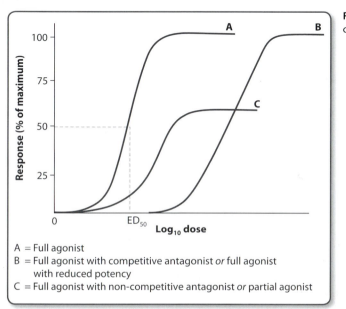

Figure 4.6 Dose–response curves.

A = Full agonist
B = Full agonist with competitive antagonist *or* full agonist with reduced potency
C = Full agonist with non-competitive antagonist *or* partial agonist

achieving maximal response, in the presence of a reversible antagonist, but will have a rightward shift, i.e. an increase in the ED_{50} (A).

34. A True

  B False

  C True

  D True

  E False

Cocaine is an ester local anaesthetic agent predominantly used for topical anaesthesia, presented as a paste or spray. Its local anaesthetic effects include blocking fast sodium channels, but it also inhibits uptake 1 of noradrenaline from the presynaptic nerve endings while inhibiting monoamine oxidase activity (B, C, D). This causes an increased activity of active amines leading to central nervous system toxicity, sympathetic stimulation and hyperthermia. It can cause confusion, hallucinations, convulsions, apnoea as well as arrhythmias, tachycardias, hypertension and myocardial ischaemia. It is associated with addiction in chronic use. Cocaine is 95% plasma protein bound, with a pKa of 8.6 having a short duration of action and a maximum safe dose of 1.5–3 mg/kg (E). Cocaine is metabolised primarily in the liver, undergoing ester hydrolysis (A).

35. A False

  B False

  C True

  D False

  E False

Non-depolarising neuromuscular blocking drugs act by competitively binding to the α-subunit of nicotinic acetylcholine receptors on post-junctional neuromuscular membranes. They demonstrate characteristics of a phase II block, including a train-of-four ratio of <0.7, fade to a 1 Hz stimulus, post-tetanic facilitation and reduced block in response to the use of anticholinesterases (A). Seventy per cent receptor occupancy is required before detection of neuromuscular blockade can be seen with a peripheral nerve stimulator (B). They undergo variable metabolism, but only mivacurium is metabolised by plasma cholinesterases; thus, it is the only agent that may demonstrate prolonged block to plasma cholinesterase deficiency (D). Mivacurium and atracurium are racemic mixtures of stereoisomers (C). Non-depolarising muscle relaxants are large charged molecules, therefore generally do not cross the placenta (E).

36. A False

  B True

  C False

  D False

  E True

Neostigmine is an anticholinesterase with a quaternary amine structure that increases the availability of acetylcholine. It reverses the effect of non-depolarising neuromuscular blocking drugs but is also used to treat myasthenia gravis, paralytic ileus and urinary retention. Because of its cholinergic effects, it may cause bradycardia, reduced cardiac output and hypotension (C). Bronchospasm and increased airway secretions can occur, and miosis, increased salivation, increased gastrointestinal motility, nausea and vomiting, sweating and lacrimation may be precipitated by its use (A, B). It may also prolong the duration of action of suxamethonium (E). Neostigmine is poorly absorbed orally, is less than 10% protein-bound and is highly ionised due to its quaternary amine structure, therefore does not cross the blood–brain barrier (D). It is predominantly excreted unchanged in the urine, and clearance is reduced in renal impairment.

37. A True

B False

C True

D True

E True

Anticonvulsants can act either via enhancing gamma-aminobutyric acid-mediated pathways or stabilisation of sodium channels (**Table 4.3**).

Phenytoin, carbamazepine and sodium valproate all have teratogenic properties , and the pharmacokinetic differences can be seen below (**Table 4.4**).

Table 4.3 Mechanism of action of anticonvulsants

Enhancing GABA-mediated pathways	Stabilising sodium channels
Sodium valproate	Phenytoin
Benzodiazepines	Carbamazepine
Barbiturates	Lamotrigine
Vigabatrin	

Table 4.4 Pharmacokinetics of common anticonvulsants

Drug	Bioavailability (%)	Volume of distribution (L/kg)	Protein binding (%)	Metabolism	Elimination
Carbamazepine	100	1.0	75	Hepatic, active metabolites	Urine
Phenytoin	90	0.7	90	Hepatic, zero-order	Urine
Sodium valproate	100	0.4	90	Hepatic, active metabolites	Urine

38. A False

   B False

   C True

   D False

   E False

Glycopyrrolate is an antimuscarinic agent with a charged quaternary amine structure, thus does not cross the blood–brain barrier or the placenta (A, D). It therefore has no central effects such as sedation, mydriasis or antiemetic effects. However, it is a potent antisialagogue, and causes tachycardias. It has a long-lasting bronchodilatory effect, increasing physiological dead space (B, C).

It has an oral bioavailability of less than 5%, is minimally metabolised and is excreted predominantly unchanged in the urine (E).

39. A True

   B True

   C True

   D False

   E False

Bactericidal agents are those that kill bacteria and can be either disinfectants or antibiotics. In contrast, bacteriostatic antibiotics prevent bacterial reproduction without causing direct bacterial damage or death (**Table 4.5**).

Table 4.5 Classes of antibiotics	
Bactericidal	**Bacteriostatic**
β-lactams – penicillins, cephalosporins	Macrolides
Aminoglycosides	Tetracyclines
Ciprofloxacin	Sulphonamides
Glycopeptides	Trimethoprim
Metronidazole	Chloramphenicol
Rifampicin	Clindamycin

40. A False

   B True

   C True

   D True

   E False

Pro-drugs are substances whereby the parent compound is inactive, and must be converted to an active compound in the body.

Clonidine and lorazepam have direct actions at target sites, while aspirin is metabolised to salicylic acid, enalapril is converted to the active form enalaprilat and cortisone is converted to hydrocortisone.

41. A False

   B True

   C False

   D False

   E True

In order to detect and interpret biological signals, they must be amplified and any unwanted noise and interference must be minimised. For best results, the biological signals require a high common mode rejection ratio and high input impedance (A). If there is a high electrode impedance and a low amplifier input impedance, then this will attenuate the signal across the amplifier because the input and electrode impedances act as a potential divider (B). Common mode rejection is the attenuation of electrical signals that are common to two input signals. This is why having differential amplification helps reduce unwanted noise, the potential difference between the two signals is amplified, but the common signals are attenuated. In modern devices, the common mode rejection ratio is usually greater than 100,000:1, but can go up to 1,000,000:1 in modern electrocardiogram (ECG) amplifiers (C).

The amplifier bandwidths must cover these ranges of frequency in order to produce the best signals: for ECG; 0.15–50 Hz, for electroencephalogram; 0.5–100 Hz, for electromyography; 20 Hz–2kHz (D, E).

42. A True

   B False

   C False

   D True

   E False

Defibrillators are devices that apply large electric shocks to the heart to try and restore sinus rhythm (A). They have three main uses: elective cardioversion to correct dysrhythmias such as atrial fibrillation and atrial flutter, emergency cardioversion for ventricular fibrillation and direct defibrillation during heart surgery.

The earlier defibrillators used domestic alternating current mains with a step-up transformer to achieve the high voltage needed, but these were not very efficient or accurate as the maximum power achievable from the mains socket was much lower than the required value of about 125 kW. Modern defibrillators use capacitors that store the required charge (B). The defibrillator circuit can be seen in Figure 3.9.

Monophasic defibrillators typically have a critically damped sine wave waveform and the current flows from one electrode to the other in one direction. Modern defibrillators now use a biphasic waveform where the current first flows in one direction and then reverses to flow in the opposite direction (C). These types of waveforms are more efficient, require less energy and have a higher success rate for first shock as compared with monophasic.

The voltage required for defibrillation is typically about 2500 V, producing a current of 50 A with a resistance of 50 Ω (D). The duration of the discharge is usually about 4 ms for each waveform, so for biphasic defibrillators this would be about 8 ms (E).

43. **A** True

   B False

   C True

   D False

   E True

There are many different types of laser medium that can either be solid, liquid, gas or semiconductor (A). Examples of a solid-state laser are ruby or neodymium (Nd):yttrium–aluminium garnet (E). Examples of a gas laser medium are CO_2, while organic dyes can be used as mediums for dye lasers. A classification for lasers has been developed which has four classes:

- **Class I:** lasers which cannot emit laser radiation at known hazard levels (B)
- **Class II:** low-power visible lasers
- **Class III:** intermediate- and moderate-power lasers, hazardous only when the beam is viewed directly
- **Class IV:** high-power lasers, hazardous to view and are hazardous to the skin (C)

There are three types of radiant energy available, each producing different tissue responses (D):

- Infrared causes molecules to vibrate and then heat up
- Visible light produces photochemical effects
- Ultraviolet radiation causes dissociation of the molecular bond.

44. **A** True

   B True

   C False

   D True

   E True

MRI is an imaging technique that takes advantage of the behaviour of atomic nuclei in strong magnetic fields to produce high-quality images of the human body, especially the soft tissues. They work by placing the patient in a strong magnetic field and applying radio-wave energy to the patient. This electromagnetic field causes atoms with unpaired protons to align in axis, spin and generate their own magnetic field (D). The most abundant unpaired proton substance is hydrogen that produces the highest signal density (C). Exposure to a second magnetic field at right angles to the first causes displacement of the aligned nuclei. This leads to change of the axis of nuclei in a process called precession. After stopping the transmission of the electromagnetic energy of the scanner, nuclei return to their original state and the patient then re-emits radio waves as a result of the magnetic resonance that occurs within the atomic nuclei (C). These signals are detected where the time taken for nuclei within tissue to return to their normal position varies according to the properties of that tissue. Tissue with high proton (or hydrogen) density, such as soft tissue, fats and water, produces the highest signals (A). Tissue with low proton content such as air produces the lowest signal densities (E).

45. A True

   B False

   C False

   D True

   E False

The following units are not used in the SI system:

- mmHg
- cmH_2O
- atmosphere
- calorie

Despite the international recognition of this system, there are a few units that are still used in medicine, despite not being in this system. The measurement of blood pressure is still given the units of mmHg and the measurement of central venous pressure is still given the units of cmH_2O.

46. A True

   B True

   C False

   D True

   E True

The electrical resistance of a thermistor varies with temperature and it requires a source of current and a method of measuring the current so that the resistance can be converted to temperature (A).

A thermocouple consists of an electrical circuit with two wires made of different metals attached together at their ends (B). One end is in the temperature probe and the other is kept at a standard reference temperature. A current will flow in the circuit and this will be proportional to the temperature difference between the two ends. Thermocouples, not thermistors, rely on the Seebeck effect (C). This is where a potential difference is generated when two metal conductors are joined together to form a circuit; the potential difference produced is proportional to the temperature difference at the two junctions.

The electrical resistance of a platinum wire varies linearly with temperature, so this property can be used in a similar way to thermistors (D).

The temperature at the tympanic membrane is an attractive site for temperature measurement because of its anatomical position deep within the skull and in close proximity to the internal carotid artery. The temperature can be measured by a thermistor, thermocouple or infrared thermometer (E).

47. A False

B True

C False

D True

E True

Specific heat capacity is defined as the amount of heat required to raise the temperature of 1 kg of a substance by 1 K and the SI units are J/kg/K. Heat capacity is the amount of heat required to raise the temperature of a given object by 1 K and the SI units are J/K (A, C).

To change the temperature of an object, the amount of heat required to achieve this depends on the specific heat capacity of the object (B). Water has a high specific heat capacity, more than most other substances (D). This property is used in the design of vapourisers, where water is used as a heat sink, a reservoir of heat, in order to maintain a constant temperature.

Gases have low specific heat capacities, so only a small amount of heat is required to increase their temperature (E).

48. A False

B False

C True

D False

E False

During anaesthesia and surgery, patients can lose heat as a result of exposure, vasodilatation, infusion of cold fluids and breathing cold dry gases. Warm air is blown over the patient into warm thin-walled air blankets which cover the patient. Hot air should not be blown directly onto the patient as this may cause heat damage (A).

A conductive heating pad could be placed under the patient, but this is not as efficient as the warm air blankets. The patients should not be placed on a conductive surface as this can cause heat loss by conduction (B).

Warming of intravenous fluids by passing them through a conductive heat exchanger is an effective way of administering warmed fluids and maintaining thermostasis of patients (C).

Low-flow anaesthesia should be used as this will help to warm the inspired gases, which occur as a result of the exothermic reaction when soda lime absorbs carbon dioxide (D).

Metallic reflective blankets should not be used in the theatre setting as they are a fire hazard and may cause electric shocks (E).

49. A False

B True

C False

D True

E True

If two solutions of different concentrations are separated by a semipermeable membrane, then water will diffuse across the membrane from the lower concentration solution to the greater one. This process of water diffusion is called osmosis and does not apply to other molecules (A). As the water diffuses it dilutes the solution it is moving to, creating a hydrostatic pressure on that side called the osmotic pressure (B). The osmotic pressure depends on the number of particles in the solution; the size of the particles does not matter (C). Thus, a solution containing twice as many small molecules as a solution containing much larger particles will exert double the osmotic pressure.

Osmolarity is the potential of fluid to exert an osmotic pressure because of the different types of molecules present in the fluid compartment (D). The plasma osmolarity is about 300 mmol/L.

Osmolality is the millimole solute per kilogram of solvent, which is the amount of osmotically active particles present per kilogram of solvent, usually 290 mOsmol/kg in the plasma (E). It is more useful than osmolarity as it does not need to consider the volume changes that occur in solutions as a result of temperature changes.

50. A False

B True

C True

D True

E False

When the waveform of a direct blood pressure measurement is obtained, in addition to systolic, diastolic and mean arterial pressures, additional indices can be obtained. Heart rate, myocardial contractility, stroke volume and the resistance and compliance of the vascular bed can be estimated (A).

The most common type of transducers used for direct pressure measurement consists of a diaphragm with a resistive strain gauge (B). Other types used can be resistive, capacitive or inductive.

Resonance can be defined as the state when a system is subjected to an oscillating force with a frequency close to that systems natural frequency. Damping is that which opposes the amplitude of oscillations due to energy loss in the form of resistive or frictional forces (D). The more resonant the system, the higher the possibility for increased amplitude of readings, while the reverse is true for more damp systems (C).

The damping coefficient is a dimensionless number indicating the level of damping within a system. A damping coefficient of 0 indicates no damping and that of 1 indicates critical damping. Optimal damping has a damping coefficient of 0.64 and at this value the best compromise between response time and overshoot is achieved (E).

51. A True

   B True

   C True

   D True

   E False

A resistance wire operates on the principle that electrical resistance of a metal increases linearly with temperature. In order to increase sensitivity of such a system, a Wheatstone bridge circuit (see **Figure 4.7**) may be used (A). This is composed of four resistors, a battery and a galvanometer. In order to ensure the galvanometer reads zero, the variable resistor (R_3) is adjusted according to the unknown resistor (R_4), which can be a resistance wire or a strain gauge. Most pressure transducers contain four strain gauges forming the four resistors of the Wheatstone bridge circuit (D).

A transducer is a device that converts one form of energy into another (C). This includes devices such as microphones, strain gauges, photoelectric cells and

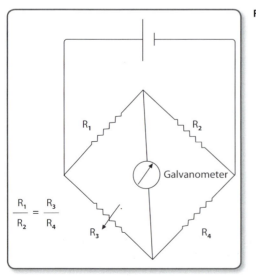

Figure 4.7 Wheatstone bridge circuit.

$$\frac{R_1}{R_2} = \frac{R_3}{R_4}$$

thermocouples (**B**). A transistor is a semiconductor device with three electrical contacts that may act as an amplifier, detector or a switch (**E**).

52. **A** True

 B False

 C True

 D True

 E False

Cylinder manifolds are used to supply oxygen, nitrous oxide and Entonox to gas piping, although a vacuum-insulated evaporator (VIE) supplies most oxygen (**A**). VIEs should have sufficient oxygen to last 6 days' use, while the manifolds supply a reserve to last a further 2 days (**B**). Cylinders used in manifolds are size J, containing 6800 L of oxygen at a pressure of 137 bar, with two banks of three cylinders, all of which have fully open valves, each connected by a pneumatically controlled change-over valve (see **Figure 4.8**) (**C**, **D**). Magnets hold the shuttle mechanism in position until the pressure of one of the banks decreases below the other at which point the valve pneumatically shuttles allowing the cylinder bank with higher pressure to supply the oxygen. This is not electronically controlled, but electrical signaling systems alarm when this occurs to prompt changing the empty cylinders (**E**).

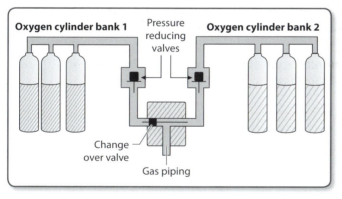

Figure 4.8 Oxygen cylinder manifold.

53. **A** False

 B True

 C False

 D False

 E False

Vapourisers are filled with agent-specific geometric and colour-coded bottles to reduce the risk of incorrect vapouriser filling (**B**) (**Table 4.6**).

Table 4.6 Vapouriser colour codes	
Volatile agent	**Colour code**
Desflurane	Blue
Enflurane	Orange
Halothane	Red (A)
Isoflurane	Purple
Sevoflurane	Yellow

The keyed filling devices reduce the risk of vapouriser overflow, spillage and ensure complete emptying of filling bottles.

Tilting a vapouriser may lead to administration of unsafe concentrations of volatile agent as volatile agent may enter the bypass chamber, although vapourisers may be filled without removing them from the anaesthetic machine (C, D). Modern anaesthetic machines only allow single vapouriser use by the Selectatec mechanism ensuring only one vapouriser is in use at any given time (E).

54. **A** True

    B False

    C False

    D True

    E False

Pressure is defined as the force per unit area. The SI unit of pressure is the Pascal, while that of force is the Newton.

$$Pressure = Force \, / Area$$

$$Force = Mass \times Acceleration$$

$$Pa = 1 \, N/m^2$$

$$N = kg \times m/s^2$$

1520 mmHg is equivalent to 2 atmospheres, while 1 atmosphere is equivalent to:

- 1 bar
- 760 mmHg
- 760 torr
- 101.325 kPa
- 1020 cmH$_2$O
- 14.5 psi (lb/in^2)
- 30 inches of Hg

55. **A** False

    B True

C True

D False

E False

The Mapleson E breathing system is also known as the Ayres T-piece system, while the Jackson-Rees modification is the Mapleson F, containing an open-ended bag allowing continuous positive airway pressure administration (B, D). It is suitable for use in paediatric patients under 30 kg of weight, and is inefficient during spontaneous ventilation (A). Because of its open-ended nature, it provides minimal resistance but also is responsible for a significant amount of theatre pollution by ventilatory gases as scavenging is difficult (C). The volume of the tubing should be equal to the patients' tidal volume (E). If the volume is too large, rebreathing may occur, if it is too small then atmospheric air may be entrained.

56. **A** False

B False

C True

D True

E False

The Clark polarographic electrode is the device utilised in arterial blood gas analysers, operating with a platinum cathode and silver/silver chloride anode within a potassium chloride electrolyte solution (see **Figure 4.9**). A voltage of 0.6 V is applied across the electrodes, where electrons are liberated at the silver/silver chloride anode and utilised at the cathode (A, B):

$$O_2 + 4 \cdot (electrons) + 2 \cdot H_2O \rightarrow 4 \cdot OH^-$$

As oxygen tension in either gas or solution samples increases, more electrons are utilised at the cathode generating a current flow.

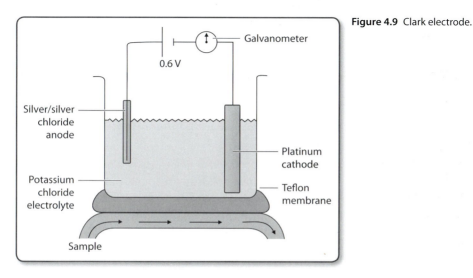

Figure 4.9 Clark electrode.

The analyser must maintain a solution temperature of 37°C, and readings are affected by the presence of halothane (C). It is the fuel cell device that is affected by nitrous oxide (E). Oxygen tension can be measured in either gas or solution (D).

57. **A** False

    B False

    C False

    D True

    E False

End-tidal carbon dioxide ($ETco_2$) can be measured using the principles of either photoacoustic spectroscopy or, more commonly, infrared absorption spectroscopy. There are two modes of analysis: side stream analysis or mainstream analysis.

Side-stream analysis involves connecting a 1.2 mm tube via a Luer connector to a breathing system in either an intubated or a non-intubated patient that samples gas at rates of up to 200 mL/minute (D, E). As the minimal oxygen flows required for a patient are 250 mL/min, this must be accounted for with the gas sampling, thus a minimum fresh gas flow rate of 450 mL/minute is required. In addition, as gas is sampled, there is minimal increase in dead space (A). Because gas samples have to be removed, there is a delay on up to 4 seconds in analysing the sample, in contrast to mainstream analysers which are more rapid (B). Side-stream $ETco_2$ analysers can also interpret other gas concentrations including volatile anaesthetic agents, while mainstream analysers can only analyse CO_2 concentrations (C).

58. **A** True

    B True

    C False

    D False

    E True

The pH is defined as:

$$pH = - \log [H^+]$$

Thus, the relationship between pH and $[H^+]$ is a logarithmic one. At a pH of 7 the $[H^+]$ is 100 nmol/L, and at pH of 7.4 it is 40 nmol/L and at pH 10 it is 10 nmol/L (C). However, the measuring system using the pH electrode demonstrates a linear change in electrical output rather than a logarithmic one, with a change of approximately 60 mV per unit pH (A, B).

The pH electrode consists of a calomel reference electrode of a mercury/mercury chloride electrode in a potassium chloride solution and a measuring silver/silver chloride electrode within pH-sensitive glass (see **Figure 4.10**) (D). The whole device is maintained at a temperature of 37°C (E). Upon contact with the measuring electrode an electrical potential is generated between this and the calomel reference electrode and displayed as an output.

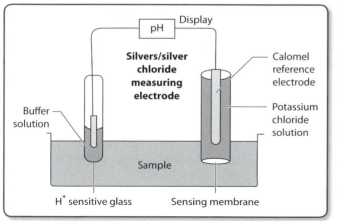

Figure 4.10 pH electrode.

A similar principle is used for the Severinghaus carbon dioxide electrode using pH-sensitive glass.

59. A True

B True

C True

D True

E False

The cardiac output (CO) is the volume of blood ejected by the heart per minute and is equal between right and left sides of the heart (B). It is normally approximately 70 mL/kg/minute and may be measured by non-invasive or invasive methods.

Non-invasive methods include:

- Transthoracic echocardiography (C)
- Transcutaneous Doppler: a probe placed on the suprasternal notch determines the velocity of blood flow in the pulmonary arteries and across valves
- Transthoracic electrical bioimpedance: electrodes on the neck and thorax will change bioimpedance depending on aortic blood flow. This method is only accurate in healthy individuals, and is mainly useful for monitoring trends (E)
- Non-invasive cardiac output monitor: this uses the Fick principle and continuous end-tidal carbon dioxide (ET_{CO_2}) values to calculate cardiac output:

$$CO = \frac{\dot{V}_{CO_2}}{Ca_{CO_2} - C\bar{v}_{CO_2}}$$

Because Ca_{CO_2} is negligible, $C\bar{v}_{CO_2}$ and ET_{CO_2} grossly equates to , thus

$$CO = \frac{\dot{V}_{CO_2}}{ET_{CO_2}}$$

Invasive methods include:

- Transoesophageal Doppler: a probe placed in the distal third of the oesophagus measures velocity of flow in the descending aorta; CO is calculated using estimated aortic diameter
- Dye dilution techniques: indocyanine green or lithium is injected into a central vein; an arterial sensing electrode is used to plot concentration-over-time curves. The area under the curve is used to calculate cardiac output
- Transthoracic thermodilution (PiCCO): cold saline is injected into a central vein (for example the internal jugular vein), and the change in temperature, as detected by an arterial cannula thermistor, is plotted over time and the Stewart–Hamilton equation is used to calculate the cardiac output (A, D)
- Transpulmonary thermodilution: in this technique a pulmonary artery catheter is inserted and then cold saline is injected into a proximal lumen which is sensed by a distal thermistor. Once again, the Stewart–Hamilton equation is used to calculate the cardiac output

60. A False

B False

C False

D False

E True

Bispectral index (BIS) analysis uses a device with four frontotemporal electrodes detecting electroencephalogram signals that are analysed to give a continuous value indicating level of sedation or anaesthesia (B). The value produces is a dimensionless number between 0 and 100 (C):

- 80–100: awake, alert
- 60–80: sedation
- 40–60: anaesthesia
- <40: cortical suppression

As well as increasing depth of anaesthesia, the BIS value is lower in hypothermia, cerebral ischaemia and the use of neuromuscular blocking drugs. It is not affected by nitrous oxide or opioids but cannot be used in conjunction with ketamine because of the dissociative qualities ketamine has (D, E). Interference from electrical muscular activity and surgical diathermy may occur.

The evidence base for use of BIS is equivocal with two large-powered studies carried out with similar methodology showing that BIS may or may not reduce the risk of awareness. It certainly does not eliminate the risk of awareness, and due to the high risk of inter-patient variability, clinical judgement is still vital (A).

Answers: SBAs

---

61. C 50 mg hydrocortisone

This patient is on long-term steroids for inflammatory bowel disease. Use of greater than 10 mg of prednisolone is thought to increase the risk of hypothalamic–pituitary–adrenal insufficiency in the perioperative period; thus, steroid replacement therapy is indicated. Patients taking less than 10 mg of prednisolone daily or having stopped steroids more than 3 months preoperatively do not require additional steroid replacement. However, patients who have stopped steroids less than 3 months preoperatively or are taking more than 10 mg of prednisolone daily require supplementation:

Minor surgery: routine preoperative steroid or 25–50 mg hydrocortisone at induction

Intermediate surgery: routine preoperative steroid, 25–50 mg hydrocortisone at induction, 100 mg hydrocortisone daily in divided doses for 24 hours

Major surgery: routine preoperative steroid, 25–50 mg hydrocortisone at induction, 100 mg hydrocortisone daily in divided doses for 48–72 hours

Conversion factors for steroids can be calculated, as prednisolone 5 mg is equivalent to

- Methylprednisolone: 4 mg
- Hydrocortisone: 20 mg
- Cortisone acetate: 25 mg
- Betamethasone: 750 mg
- Dexamethasone: 750 mg

Nicholson G, Burrin JM, Hall GM. Peri-operative steroid supplementation. Anaesthesia 1998; 53:1091–1104.

---

62. E Administer 28% oxygen via a Venturi mask

This patient has type 2 respiratory failure with a suspected bowel obstruction. The most likely cause is chronic obstructive pulmonary disease given his smoking history. His arterial blood gas results suggest that he is a chronic retainer and is compensating with elevated bicarbonate. Although he is hypoxic, there is still no indication for intubation on the information provided and the patient's hypoxia is best managed carefully initially with an F_{IO_2} of 28% via a Venturi mask. A chest X-ray and intensive treatment unit admission may be necessary later. Administering high flow oxygen via a non-rebreathing mask may eliminate his hypoxic drive and cause hypoventilation.

Ely J, Clapham M. Delivering oxygen to patients. BJA CEPD Reviews 2003; 3:43–45.

---

63. B Forced warm air blankets

The most effective way to warm a patient having a laryngectomy would be using a forced warm air blanket. Most of the patient's body surface can be covered. The temperature of the warm air blanket is maintained between 32°C and 38°C, which reduces heat loss as a result of convection. It also acts as a radiative reflective surface, thereby reducing heat loss by radiation. A conductive heat pad could also be used, but this is not as efficient as the forced warm air blankets. There are various ways of warming intravenous fluids before they are infused; they can be passed through a heat exchanger, by wrapping coils of the giving set around a heater or passing them inside a heating device. The use of low-flow anaesthetic gases and HME filters all help reduce heat loss, but are not very efficient in heating the patient.

Sullivan G, Edmondson C. Heat and temperature. Contin Educ Anaesth Crit Care Pain 2008; 8:104–107.

64. C Postpone surgery and wake the patient up

This scenario is of an adult male who has an unanticipated difficult tracheal intubation. The initial intubation plan (plan A) has been unsuccessful, so the secondary tracheal intubation plan was attempted (plan B). This too has proved to be unsuccessful; the next appropriate step should be to move onto plan C, which is to maintain oxygenation and ventilation and then postpone surgery and awaken the patient.

No more than two insertions of the intubating laryngeal mask airway should be attempted. Optimising manoeuvres for direct laryngoscopy such as head and neck positioning and applying external laryngeal manipulation should have been attempted during the initial intubation plan (plan A), before moving onto the secondary intubation plan (plan B). Use of the bougie and ensuring full muscle relaxation are also part of the initial intubation plan.

Difficult Airway Society Guidelines Default Strategy for Intubation Including Failed Direct Laryngoscopy, 2004. http://www.das.uk.com/files/ddl-Jul04-A4.pdf (Last accessed 01/10/2012)

65. D Bradycardia

Remifentanil is a pure μ-receptor agonist and is a synthetic phenylpiperidine derivative of fentanyl. In combination with propofol, it is commonly used to induce and maintain anaesthesia. For induction, an initial bolus dose is usually administered, and it is at this point that some of the complications of remifentanil can occur.

It causes respiratory depression and chest wall rigidity and causes reduction in blood pressure and bradycardia. Bradycardia is more pronounced at induction of anaesthesia in young fit patients who already have a low heart rate, and when combining a large dose of remifentanil with laryngoscopy or airway manipulation, marked bradycardia can be elicited, often requiring atropine or glycopyrrolate and cessation of the vagal stimulus.

Remifentanil does not cause laryngospasm; in fact, it makes it less likely. There is no increase in histamine release.

Remifentanil is rapidly broken down by non-specific plasma and tissue esterases and as a result has an elimination half-life of 3–10 minutes. This is why it must be administered as a continuous infusion.

Komatsu R, Turan AM, Orhan-Sungur M, McGuire J, Radke OC, Apfel CC. Remifentanil for general anaesthesia: A systematic review. Anaesthesia 2007; 62:1266–1280.

66. E Supraspinous ligament

The boundaries of the epidural space are as follows:

- Superior: fusion of three spinal and periosteal layers of dura mater at the foramen magnum
- Inferior: sacrococcygeal membrane
- Anterior: posterior longitudinal ligament
- Lateral: pedicles and intervertebral foraminae
- Posterior: ligament flavum, capsule of facet joints and laminae

Despite the supraspinous ligament being posterior to the epidural space, it does not actually form the posterior boundary of the space.

Richardson J, Groen GJ. Applied epidural anatomy. Contin Educ Anaesth Crit Care Pain 2005; 5:98–100.

67. B Impaired cerebral sensitivity to carbon dioxide

The use of nitrous oxide during intracranial surgery is controversial. The effects of nitrous oxide are to raise intracranial pressure, cerebral blood flow and cerebral metabolic rate for oxygen consumption; it also impairs the brain's ability to autoregulate its blood supply. These effects are mostly antagonised by opioids, benzodiazepines, barbiturates and propofol.

Nitrous oxide has no effect on the sensitivity to carbon dioxide.

It is important to avoid the use of nitrous oxide in the presence of air in the ventricles, when there is increased risk of venous air embolism and pneumocephalus.

Banks A, Hardman JG. Nitrous oxide. Contin Educ Anaesth Crit Care Pain 2005; 5:145–148.

68. C Hypothermia

Hypothermia causes sympathetic nervous system excitation resulting in shivering, hypertension, tachycardia, tachypnoea and vasoconstriction. She has been in theatre for a number of hours and had a large surface area exposed to the cold theatre environment; this would all contribute to her hypothermia. With a large surface area being exposed for such a long duration of time, active warming measures such as infusion of warm fluids and use of a warm air blanket may still result in the patient becoming hypothermic.

She is young, fit and healthy with no previous cardiac history, so angina is an unlikely explanation. Anaphylaxis would cause a profound hypotension and maybe a rash, so this could not be the diagnosis either.

Hypovolaemia would cause a tachycardia, but this would normally be associated with a drop in the blood pressure which is not the case here, so this too is unlikely.

Pain could also cause excitation of the sympathetic nervous system, but this woman has had a large dose of morphine and has not required any further analgesia in recovery, which suggests that she is not in any pain.

Luscombe M, Andrzejowski JC. Clinical applications of induced hypothermia. Contin Educ Anaesth Crit Care Pain 2006; 6:23–27.

69. D Largely carbohydrate meal

Emptying of the stomach during digestion is primarily dependent on the tone of the proximal stomach and the pylorus. These are both under reflex and hormonal control.

Cholinergic fibres of the vagus nerve increase the tone of the proximal stomach, thereby increasing emptying and adrenergic sympathetic fibres inhibit the tone, decreasing the emptying.

Motilin is a hormone that promotes gastric emptying, whereas gastrin and cholecystokinin both inhibit emptying.

The emptying rate for carbohydrates is faster than that for proteins, which in turn is faster than that for fats.

Jolliffe DM. Practical gastric physiology. Contin Educ Anaesth Crit Care Pain 2009; 9:173–177.

70. E Clarithromycin

First-line treatment for a community-acquired pneumonia is amoxicillin; however, clarithromycin is an appropriate alternative, particularly in those with penicillin allergies. Amoxicillin has no interaction with the anticoagulant effect of warfarin, while clarithromycin is a hepatic enzyme inhibitor, enhancing the anticoagulant effect of warfarin. Although ketoconazole is an hepatic enzyme inhibitor, it is unlikely to be prescribed for a bacterial chest infection.

Lim WS et al. Guidelines for the management of community-acquired pneumonia in adults: Update 2009. Thorax 2009; 64(suppl iii):1–55.
Joint Formulary Committee. British National Formulary. London: Pharmaceutical Press; 2013.

71. B Increases tubular ionisation of salicylates

Salicylates are weakly acidic drugs, thus are unionised in acidic environments and ionised in alkaline environments. Administration of sodium bicarbonate has the effect of alkalinising the urine in the distal tubules. Thus as the salicylate diffuses across the tubules, it becomes ionised and therefore trapped in the tubules thereby increasing excretion. Sodium bicarbonate should be considered in patients with plasma levels of 300 mg/L, whereas renal replacement therapy should be considered in plasma levels greater than 700 mg/L.

Ward C, Sair M. Oral poisoning: An update. Contin Educ Anaesth Crit Care Pain 2010; 10:6–11.

72. A Less intense emergence phenomena

Ketamine is a phencyclidine derivative that contains a chiral centre giving either S- or R-forms. It can be presented as a racemic mixture or as an enantiopure S-ketamine, which has a number of advantages. The S-ketamine enantiomer is more potent, more cardiostable and does not demonstrate ischaemic myocardial preconditioning. Therefore, it is thought to have advantages in patients with known ischaemic heart disease over the racemic mixture. Ketamine is associated with emergence phenomena, including delirium, hallucinations and altered behaviour. The S-ketamine preparation has significantly less intense emergence phenomena, but occurring with the same frequency as the racemic mixture. They appear to be less common in younger and older patients, but may occur with increased frequency or intensity in those with psychiatric conditions.

Pai A, Heining M. Ketamine. Contin Educ Anaesth Crit Care Pain 2007; 7:59–63.

73. C Abnormality of the Ryanodine-1 receptor

The clinical picture described fits with a diagnosis of malignant hyperthermia (MH). This is an autosomal dominant disorder of chromosome 19 affecting the Ryanodine-1 receptor (RYR1). Triggering agents including suxamethonium and volatile anaesthetics cause uncontrolled release of Ca^{2+} through the RYR1 channel from the sarcoplasmic reticulum into the cytoplasm. This causes uncontrolled, sustained muscle contraction and activation leading to increased adenosine triphosphate consumption, increasing CO_2 production and O_2 consumption. The speed of increase in end-tidal CO_2 along with the rise in temperature and O_2 consumption make MH more likely than CO_2 absorption from pneumoperitoneum.

Halsall PJ, Hopkins PM. Malignant hyperthermia. BJA CEPD Reviews 2003; 3:5–9.

74. D Creates a concentration gradient for rocuronium to diffuse away from the neuromuscular junction

Sugammadex (Bridion) is a modified γ-cyclodextrin and is classified as a selective relaxant-binding agent. It allows very rapid reversal of neuromuscular blockade from any depth of block due to rocuronium and to a lesser extent vecuronium. It acts by forming a complex with rocuronium in a 1:1 ratio, thereby reducing the potential for rocuronium binding to nicotinic acetylcholine receptors. The water-soluble complex generates a concentration gradient for the neuromuscular blocking drug to diffuse away from the neuromuscular junction into the plasma.

Sugammadex is not significantly bound to plasma proteins and undergoes minimal metabolism having no active metabolites, before excretion in the urine, either isolated or bound to rocuronium.

Makri I, Papadima A, Lafioniati A, et al. Sugammadex, a promising reversal drug. A review of clinical trials. Rev Recent Clin Trials 2011; 6:250–255.

75. A α-rhythm

The electroencephalogram is a compiled recording of electrical activity from a number of scalp electrodes that can suggest the state of brain activity. The amplitude of signal is between 1 and 500 μV with a signal frequency range of 0 and 60 Hz. There are a number of different rhythms depending on the signal frequency (**Table 4.7**):

Whyte SD, Booker PD. Monitoring depth of anaesthesia by EEG. BJA CEPD Reviews 2003; 3:106–110.

Table 4.7 EEG rhythms

Rhythm	Frequency	Occurrence
α	8–10 Hz	Closed eyes; in coma
β	13–30 Hz	Alert or active
δ	4 Hz	During sleep; in children
θ	4–8 Hz	Drowsiness; in children

76. D Stop injecting the local anaesthetic

Local anaesthetic toxicity presents with neurological and cardiovascular disturbance. Neurological changes include peri-oral paraesthesia, agitation, tremor, confusion, seizures and coma. Cardiovascular changes include hypotension, arrhythmias, myocardial depression and cardiac arrest.

Immediate management of severe local anaesthetic toxicity includes

- Immediate cessation of injection of local anaesthetic
- Call for help
- Maintain and secure the airway
- Administer 100% oxygen
- Confirm intravenous access
- Control seizures
- Consider sending a full set of bloods without delaying treatment

Treatment of local anaesthetic toxicity depends on whether circulatory arrest is present or not. In circulatory arrest, cardiopulmonary resuscitation, as outlined in advanced life support guidelines, must proceed. 20% intravenous lipid emulsion solution must be used as soon as possible as a bolus of 1.5 mL/kg over 1 minute followed by an infusion of 15 mL/kg/hour. Two further bolus doses may be administered and the rate of the infusion may be increased to 30 mL/kg/hour if there is no return of cardiovascular stability within 5 minutes.

In the absence of circulatory arrest, treatment of hypotension, bradycardia and tachyarrhythmias with standard therapy is indicated and lipid emulsion may be considered.

In this clinical scenario, the most prudent action is to stop injecting the local anaesthetic solution because it is likely that the epidural catheter is intravenous in location.

The Association of Anaesthetists of Great Britain & Ireland. AAGBI Safety Guideline: Management of Severe Local Anaesthetic Toxicity. London: The Association of Anaesthetists of Great Britain & Ireland, 2010.

77. E Facial nerve

Stimulation of the facial nerve causes contraction of the orbicularis oculi muscle, which is more similar to the extent of diaphragmatic neuromuscular blockade than adductor pollicis muscle stimulation via the ulnar nerve. The ulnar nerve is, however, more sensitive to neuromuscular blockade than the diaphragm.

The accessory nerve may be used to assess depth of neuromuscular blockade because it is easily visible, however may lead to indirect vagal stimulation and asystole. The tibial nerve may also be used but is less commonly used than the common peroneal nerve looking for foot dorsiflexion.

Gill SS, Donati F, Bevan DR. Clinical evaluation of double-burst stimulation. Its relationship to train-of-four stimulation. Anaesthesia 1990; 45:543.

78. B Leukotrienes

This asthmatic patient is most likely to have non-steroidal anti-inflammatory drug (NSAID)-sensitive asthma that affects 10–23% of asthmatics. The underlying mechanism is due to inhibition of conversion of arachidonic acid to the cyclic endoperoxides of thromboxane A_2 (TXA_2), prostacyclin (PGI_2) and prostaglandins (PGE_2, $PGF_{2\alpha}$, PGD_2) via cyclo-oxygenase (COX). Therefore, there is an excess of arachidonic acid that is converted to leukotrienes (LT) by lipoxygenase (see **Figure 4.11**). LTs can directly induce bronchospasm, particularly in asthmatics.

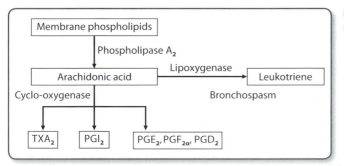

Figure 4.11 Leukotriene synthesis.

Although anaphylaxis-producing histamine via mast cell activation is also possible, NSAID-sensitive asthma is a more likely diagnosis in this patient.

Peck TE, Hill, SA, Williams M. Pharmacology for anaesthesia and intensive care, 3rd edn. Cambridge: Cambridge University Press; 2008.

79. A Heparin

This patient has evidence of new onset atrial fibrillation (AF) with no evidence of haemodynamic compromise. As the onset is likely less than 48 hours, full anticoagulation with intravenous heparin is indicated as this gives the opportunity for direct current cardioversion if the 48-hour onset time elapses. Once heparin has been initiated, either chemical (amiodarone, flecainide or sotalol) or electrical cardioversion may be attempted. A transoesophageal echocardiogram is only indicated if the onset time of AF is greater than 48 hours.

Bajpai A, Rowland E. Atrial fibrillation. Contin Educ Anaesth Crit Care Pain 2006; 6:219–224.

80. E Glibenclamide

Hypoglycaemia in diabetic patients is most commonly due to drug therapy. Although insulins most frequently cause hypoglycaemia in insulin-dependent diabetics, sulphonylureas (tolbutamide, glibenclamide) are the most common cause in non-insulin dependent diabetics. Sulphonylureas act by increasing insulin release from β-cells of the islets of Langerhans.

Metformin is a biguanide that acts to increase peripheral glucose uptake, delays glucose absorption from the gastrointestinal tract, as well as reduces gluconeogenesis. It is not significantly associated with causing hypoglycaemia.

Acarbose acts to inhibit intestinal α-glucosidases that delay digestion of starch and sucrose, therefore reducing post-prandial hyperglycaemia.

β-Blockers have been associated with hypoglycaemia, as have angiotensin-converting enzyme inhibitors. Salbutamol and codeine are not linked to hypoglycaemia.

Peck TE, Hill, SA, Williams M. Pharmacology for anaesthesia and intensive care, 3rd edn. Cambridge: Cambridge University Press; 2008.

81. D Atracurium

The factors governing placental transfer of drugs include degree of ionisation, which is dependent on pKa, protein binding, lipid solubility and molecular weight. Highly lipophilic, unionised molecules will cross more readily than ionised, large poorly lipophilic substances.

All induction agents cross the placenta, with propofol concentrations in the umbilical cord being 70% of maternal levels, and thiopentone being present in fetal blood within 1 minute of injection.

Suxamethonium does cross the placenta in small quantities, although in doses greater than 300 mg or with inherited or acquired maternal plasma cholinesterase deficiency significant transfer may occur. Non-depolarising neuromuscular blocking drugs, including atracurium, however, are large charged molecules that do not cross the placenta in significant quantities.

Morphine crosses the placenta significantly, with a fetomaternal transfer ratio of 0.92. Fentanyl, despite being significantly more lipid soluble than morphine, crosses to a lesser extent due to a higher protein binding. Pethidine is an opioid that is highly lipid soluble and only 60% protein bound with active metabolites that cross the placenta significantly.

Local anaesthetic agents cross the placenta depending on protein binding. Lidocaine is only 70% protein bound and crosses more freely than bupivacaine and ropivacaine that are 95% and 94% protein bound respectively. In addition, the relatively acidic fetal pH causes the local anaesthetic agents to become more ionised and therefore trapped in the fetal circulation.

Reynolds F, Knott C. Pharmacokinetics in pregnancy and placental drug transfer. Oxf Rev Reprod Biol 1989; 11:389–449.

82. E Spironolactone

Of the above options, spironolactone is most likely due to the biochemical effect (see **Table 4.8**) and the menstrual irregularities, which are recognised side effects.

Clarke P, Simpson KH. Diuretics and renal tubular function. BJA CEPD Reviews 2001; 1:99–103.

Table 4.8 Effects of diuretics

Drug	Target	Location	Biochemical effect
Acetazolamide	Carbonic anhydrase inhibition	Proximal convoluted tubule	$\downarrow pH$, $\uparrow Cl^-$
Bumetanide/furosemide	Inhibit Na^+/Cl^- reabsorption	Ascending loop of Henle	$\downarrow Na^+$, $\downarrow K^+$, $\downarrow Cl^-$, $\downarrow Mg^{2+}$, $\uparrow pH$
Bendroflumethiazide/metolazone	Inhibit Na^+/Cl^- reabsorption	Distal convoluted tubule	$\downarrow Na^+$, $\downarrow K^+$, $\downarrow Cl^-$, $\uparrow Ca^{2+}$, $\uparrow pH$
Amiloride	Inhibits Na^+/K^+ exchange	Distal convoluted tubule	$\uparrow K^+$
Spironolactone	Aldosterone antagonist	Distal convoluted tubule/collecting ducts	$\uparrow K^+$, $\downarrow Na^+$
Mannitol	Osmotic diuretic	Ascending loop of Henle	$\downarrow Na^+$, $\downarrow K^+$

83. D Right coronary artery

The patient has clinical features of acute myocardial infarction. The vessel affected may be derived based on the leads of the 12-lead electrocardiogram (ECG) demonstrating ischaemic changes (see **Table 4.9**).

Table 4.9 Distribution of ECG leads and blood vessels

Area affected	Leads affected	Blood vessels affected
Anterior	V2, V3, V4	Left anterior descending artery
Inferior	II, III, aVF	Right coronary artery
Lateral	I, aVL, V5, V6	Circumflex artery

If the left main stem is affected, the patient will likely have ischaemic ECG changes in both anterior and lateral distributions. This patient has ischaemic changes in the distribution of the right coronary artery. The marginal artery is a branch of the right coronary artery, is a smaller branch of the right coronary artery and is less likely to demonstrate features of a complete inferior myocardial infarction. The posterior interventricular artery is a branch of the right coronary artery and will demonstrate features of a posterior myocardial infarction.

Sheppard LP, Channer KS. Acute coronary syndromes. Contin Educ Anaesth Crit Care Pain 2004; 4:175–180.

84. D Fetal haemoglobin has a P_{50} of 3.6 kPa

Oxygen delivery to the fetus occurs at the placental unit where gas exchange takes place. To optimise oxygen transfer from mother to fetus, fetal haemoglobin must have a higher affinity for oxygen than maternal haemoglobin. A reduced 2,3-diphosphoglycerate (2,3-DPG) concentration causes leftward shift of the fetal oxyhaemoglobin dissociation curve to achieve this such that the fetal P_{50} is 3.6 kPa in comparison to maternal P_{50} of 4.8 kPa.

The fetal pH is normally 7.25–7.35, but this does not contribute to improved oxygen loading of fetal haemoglobin. However, fetal CO_2 does transfer across the placenta into maternal blood causing the double Bohr effect. This is when an elevated CO_2 in maternal blood causes a shift of the oxyhaemoglobin dissociation curve to the right, while a reduced CO_2 in fetal blood shifts the oxyhaemoglobin dissociation curve to the left, thereby favouring oxygen transfer to the fetus.

Maternal blood alkalosis does not improve oxygenation of fetal haemoglobin. A high haemoglobin concentration in the fetus improves oxygen delivery, but not oxygenation of haemoglobin.

Murphy PJ. The fetal circulation. Contin Educ Anaesth Crit Care Pain 2005; 5:107–112.

85. B Arrhythmias

An elevated arterial P_{CO_2} (Pa_{CO_2}) is when the Pa_{CO_2} is greater than 6 kPa. This has a number of effects on various body systems. Arrhythmias are the only likely effects resulting from an elevated arterial P_{CO_2} from the list provided.

The following are the effects of a raised arterial P_{CO_2}:

- Cardiovascular: sympathetic stimulation, myocardial depression, vasodilatation, arrhythmias
- Respiratory: increased central and peripheral chemoreceptor activation and respiratory drive, respiratory depression at high Pa_{CO_2} levels, increased sensitivity to hypoxia, increased pulmonary vascular resistance and respiratory acidosis, reduced haemoglobin affinity for oxygen
- Neurological: increased cerebral blood flow; increased intracranial pressure; increased intraocular pressure, pupillary dilatation, confusion, headache, coma
- Renal: increased bicarbonate retention and hydrogen ion excretion

Kregenow DA, Swenson ER. The lung and carbon dioxide: implications for permissive and therapeutic hypercapnia. Eur Respir J 2002; 20:6–11.

86. A Reduced pulmonary vascular resistance

This patient has a history consistent with syndrome of inappropriate anti-diuretic hormone release (SIADH). This can be caused by head injury; subarachnoid haemorrhage; infection such as meningitis or pneumonia, or paraneoplastic phenomena. The clinical features of this syndrome are due to the effects of ADH (vasopressin) that is normally released from the posterior pituitary gland.

ADH is released in response to an increased plasma osmolality, a reduced extracellular fluid volume and angiotensin II. It aims to retain water to restore fluid volume and plasma osmolality. This is done by increasing expression of aquaporin-2 receptors in the distal nephron to increase water reabsorption. The normal plasma osmolality is 280–295 mOsmol/kg, while in SIADH this may fall to below 270 mOsmol/kg.

It is also a potent vasoconstrictor, hence the name vasopressin, causing splanchnic, coronary and pulmonary vasoconstriction. ADH also increases the production of clotting factors, particularly factor VIII, while playing a role in thermoregulation, circadian rhythmic control and memory.

Davies M, Hardman J. Anaesthesia and adrenocortical disease. Contin Educ Anaesth Crit Care Pain 2005; 5:122–126.

87. E Redistribution

Propofol (2,6-diisopropylphenol) is an anaesthetic agent that is administered in doses of 1–2 mg/kg for intravenous induction of anaesthesia. It is 98% protein bound with a volume of distribution of 4 L/kg. Metabolism is predominantly hepatic conversion to quinol and conjugation to a glucuronide and sulphate derivatives, followed by hepatic excretion. The terminal elimination half-life is 5–12 hours; however, the short duration of action is mainly due to rapid redistribution, with a redistribution half-life of 1.3–4.1 minutes.

Hill SA. Pharmacokinetics of drug infusions. Contin Educ Anaesth Crit Care Pain 2004; 4:76–80.

88. B Preserved proprioception, touch and vibration sense with paralysis below the lesion

The arterial supply to the anterior two-thirds of the spinal cord is variable but commonly arises from a dominant radicular branch from low intercostal, high lumbar or iliac artery, known as the great anterior radicular artery of Adamkiewicz. During aortic cross-clamping, infarction of the spinal cord supplied by this artery may occur leading to anterior spinal artery syndrome. Because of the anatomical distribution of pathways, the posterior columns are spared thus preserving proprioception, touch and vibration sense. However, as the motor tracts carried in the anterior and lateral corticospinal tracts, as well as the pain and temperature sensation carried in the spinothalamic tracts are in the anterior two-thirds of the spinal cord, they are affected below the lesion. Thus, the overall picture is one of preserved proprioception, touch and vibration sense with paralysis below the level of the lesion. The other options represent variations in different forms of spinal injury.

Leslie RA, Johnson EK, Thomas G, Goodwin APL. Dr Podcast scripts for the final FRCA. Cambridge: Cambridge University Press; 2011.

89. D Soda lime and reservoir bag on the expiratory limb

The circle breathing system hasa highly efficient design allowing for minimal pollution and use of low gas flows. Unidirectional valves control direction of gas flow throughout the system, allowing for an inspiratory limb and an expiratory limb. The inspiratory limb contains a single unidirectional valve but no other adjuncts as this limits resistance in to inspiration. The expiratory limb contains a unidirectional valve, followed by a switch controlling the reservoir bag or ventilator with an adjustable pressure-limiting valve, followed by a soda lime canister (see **Figure 4.12**). The position of all the components is carefully selected to minimise rebreathing and maximise efficiency. For example, placing the reservoir bag on the inspiratory limb after the unidirectional valve could lead to rebreathing, as expired gases could enter the reservoir bag.

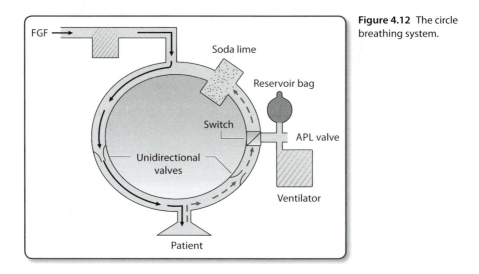

Figure 4.12 The circle breathing system.

Most commonly, vapourisers out of circuit are used, whereby the fresh gas flow passes through the vapouriser before entering the circle breathing system. This is because the most frequently used vapourisers are of the plenum design, which are highly efficient but have high internal resistance and are bulky. Therefore, they are placed outside the breathing system.

Sinclair CM, Thadsad MK, Barker I. Modern anaesthetic machines. Contin Educ Anaesth Crit Care Pain 2006; 6:75–78.
Nunn G. Low-flow anaesthesia. Contin Educ Anaesth Crit Care Pain 2008; 8:1–4.

90. A It is a paediatric theatre

The acceptable 8-hour time-weighted concentrations of nitrous oxide are 100 particles per million, and should be assessed annually. The reasons for increased theatre pollution include:

- Paediatric breathing systems: T-piece such as Mapleson E and F
- Failure of scavenging systems
- Theatre air changes of less than 15 times per hour
- Breathing system and connection leaks
- Spillage during vapouriser filling
- Use of uncuffed endotracheal tubes
- Use of cardiopulmonary bypass

In this scenario, a paediatric theatre is the most likely cause as it would involve increased use of nitrous oxide, use of uncuffed tubes and use of open breathing circuits such as T-piece circuits.

Thomas I, Carter JA. Occupational hazards of anaesthesia. Contin Educ Anaesth Crit Care Pain 2006; 6:182–187.
Banks A, Hardman JG. Nitrous oxide. Contin Educ Anaesth Crit Care Pain 2005; 5:145–148.

Chapter 5

Mock paper 5

60 MTFs and 30 SBAs to be answered in three hours

Questions: MTFs

Answer each stem 'True' or 'False'.

1. **Regarding lung volumes:**
   A   Vital capacity is the total lung capacity minus the residual volume
   B   Inspiratory reserve volume is approximately 2.5 L in adults
   C   Measurement of functional residual capacity utilises Boyle's law
   D   All volumes can be measured using spirometry except functional residual capacity
   E   Closing capacity always exceeds residual volume

2. **In an area of lung where the ventilation/perfusion ($\dot{V}/\dot{Q}$) ratio is greater than 1:**
   A   A pulmonary embolism may be present
   B   The alveolar oxygen value is low
   C   The alveolar carbon dioxide value will be normal
   D   This may represent shunt
   E   There will be compensatory hypoxic pulmonary vasoconstriction

3. **The following reduce pulmonary vascular resistance:**
   A   Alkalosis
   B   Increase in $P\text{a}_{CO_2}$
   C   Angiotensin
   D   Prostacyclin
   E   Sevoflurane

4. **In calculating oxygen flux, knowledge of the following variables is required:**
   A   Systemic vascular resistance
   B   Arterial oxygen saturation
   C   Hüfner's constant
   D   Stroke volume
   E   Haemoglobin concentration

5. **Regarding the conducting system of the heart:**
   A   The sinoatrial node is located on the anterior wall of the left atrium
   B   The sinoatrial node generates 60 action potentials per minute

C   The atrioventricular node is the only electrical connection between the atria
and ventricles

D   The bundle of His contains slow conducting muscle fibres

E   The Purkinje fibres distribute the electrical impulse to the endocardial cells

6.   **Regarding nervous control of the heart:**

A   Vagal stimulation results in the pacemaker cells becoming hyperpolarised

B   Hyperpolarisation is induced by an increase in permeability to potassium ions

C   Sympathetic stimulation causes an increase in the outward flow of sodium and
calcium ions

D   The inotropic effect of sympathetic stimulation is due to increased calcium ion
permeability

E   Sympathetic stimulation results in a more rapid effect on heart rate than
parasympathetic stimulation

7.   **Regarding exercise:**

A   At the onset, sympathetic activity increases and vagal activity remains
unchanged

B   Heart rate is increased whilst systolic and diastolic times are reduced

C   Ventricular contractility is increased mainly by secretion of catecholamines
from the adrenal medulla

D   The central venous pressure decreases

E   The systemic vascular resistance is reduced to minimise the rise in arterial
pressure

8.   **Cardiopulmonary receptors:**

A   Have an overall stimulatory effect on the heart

B   Are found in the venae cavae, atria and pulmonary vessels

C   Are mechanoreceptors

D   Are involved in the short-term regulation of blood pressure

E   Do not function in the transplanted heart

9.   **Regarding the kidney:**

A   The functional unit of the kidney is the nephron

B   The renal corpuscle is situated in the medulla

C   The glomerulus filters proteins from the blood

D   The proximal and distal tubules contain convoluted segments

E   The collecting ducts are mostly found in the cortex

10. **Regarding the renal handling of hydrogen ions, which of the following are true:**

A   Most of the hydrogen ions are secreted in the distal convoluted tubule

B   Hydrogen ion secretion occurs in exchange for potassium

C   The luminal pH in the collecting ducts may decrease to 4.5

D   Secretion of hydrogen ions allows the reabsorption of filtered bicarbonate

E   About 20% of the daily production of hydrogen ions is excreted in the urine in
its free form

11. **Regarding abnormalities in aldosterone secretion, which of the following are true:**

   A   Conn's syndrome results in hypokalaemic alkalosis
   B   Primary hyperaldosteronism is more common than secondary hyperaldosteronism
   C   Secondary hyperaldosteronism can be caused by adrenocortical tumours
   D   Adrenocortical insufficiency results in postural hypotension
   E   Adrenocortical insufficiency causes muscular weakness and paralysis

12. **The following are true regarding disturbances in salt and water homeostasis:**

   A   Isosmotic loss cannot be caused by diarrhoea and vomiting
   B   A salt deficit results in the shift of fluid from the extracellular to the intracellular fluid compartment
   C   Infusion of large volumes of glucose solution results in intracellular and extracellular oedema
   D   Excessive antidiuretic hormone (ADH) secretion has the same effect as infusion of large volumes of glucose solution
   E   Infusion of hypertonic saline results in fluid shifting from the intracellular to the extracellular space

13. **Regarding energy metabolism:**

   A   Fats are completely oxidised to CO_2 and H_2O
   B   Proteins are completely oxidised to CO_2 and H_2O
   C   Carbohydrates are completely oxidised to CO_2 and H_2O
   D   It can be calculated using the bomb calorimeter
   E   More energy is required to produce adenosine triphosphate (ATP) from proteins than from carbohydrates

14. **The following are true regarding the functional anatomy of the liver:**

   A   The portal space in the centre of each acinus contains the hepatic artery, hepatic vein and bile duct
   B   The central veins coalesce to form the portal vein
   C   Kupffer cells are present in the endothelium of the sinusoids
   D   Portal venous pressure is greater than hepatic venous pressure
   E   There is a small pressure drop across the hepatic arterioles

15. **Regarding nerve fibres:**

   A   Light touch is carried by sensory $A\gamma$ fibres
   B   B fibres transmit somatic motor impulses
   C $A\beta$ fibres conduct at a speed of 70–120 $m.s^{-1}$
   D   Sympathetic transmission can be via C fibres
   E $A\alpha$ fibres have the largest diameter

16. **The following tracts are correctly paired with the information transmitted within them:**

   A   Proprioception and dorsal columns
   B   Light touch and spinothalamic tracts

   C   Fibres from the legs and the fasciculus cuneatus
   D   Descending inhibition and the locus caeruleus
   E   Motor impulses and the lateral corticospinal tract

17. **Immediately following a spinal cord injury at the level of the 4th thoracic vertebra the following would be likely:**
   A   Bradycardia
   B   Hypotension
   C   Autonomic areflexia
   D   Arrhythmias
   E   Spastic paralysis

18. **The following are risk factors for postoperative nausea and vomiting:**
   A   Hypotension
   B   Cigarette smoking
   C   Neostigmine
   D   Trauma surgery
   E   Morphine

19. **Parathyroid hormone:**
   A   Has the same effect as calcitonin on osteoclasts
   B   Decreases serum levels of calcium and phosphates
   C   Increases magnesium reabsorption by the kidney
   D   Promotes the formation of calcitriol
   E   Secretion is ultimately controlled by the pituitary gland

20. **The following substances are routinely added to blood storage solutions:**
   A   Glucose
   B   Bicarbonate
   C   Adenosine
   D   Citrate
   E   Magnesium

21. **The following are caused by intravenous anaesthetics:**
   A   Thiopentone and pain on injection
   B   Etomidate and nausea and vomiting
   C   Etomidate and increased intraocular pressure
   D   Propofol and reduction in systemic vascular resistance
   E   Methohexitone and an increased heart rate

22. **Midazolam:**
   A   Is mainly in the ionised form in acidic conditions
   B   Has an oral bioavailability of approximately 40%
   C   Prolongs the effects of fentanyl
   D   Has no active metabolites
   E   Is metabolised in the liver

23. **Minimum alveolar concentration (MAC):**
    A   Is a measure of potency
    B   Is increased in pregnancy
    C   Is decreased in hypothermia
    D   Is increased in hyperthyroidism
    E   Is decreased in chronic alcohol intake

24. **Regarding prostaglandin synthesis and non-steroidal anti-inflammatory drugs (NSAIDs):**
    A   Phospholipase A2 is inhibited by NSAIDs
    B   Lipoxygenase is inhibited by NSAIDs
    C   Cyclo-oxygenase (COX) has three isoenzymes
    D   COX-2 produces prostaglandins which are responsible for the control of renal blood flow
    E   Inhibition of COX-1 is responsible for the side effects of NSAIDs

25. **Regarding opioids:**
    A   Diamorphine undergoes ester hydrolysis
    B   Fentanyl is a prodrug
    C   Pethidine has anticholinergic properties
    D   Codeine is a phenylpiperidine derivative
    E   Papaveretum contains morphine, codeine and papaverine

26. **Nitrates:**
    A   Reduce cardiac preload and afterload
    B   Increase venous return
    C   Increase local nitric oxide levels
    D   Produce tolerance with chronic use
    E   Preferentially dilate the smaller coronary arteries

27. **β-adrenergic blockers have the following effects on the heart:**
    A   Negative chronotropic action
    B   Positive dromotropic action
    C   Increased afterload
    D   Increased diastolic perfusion
    E   Increased contractility

28. **In the treatment of hypertension:**
    A   Angiotensin-converting enzyme (ACE) inhibitors inhibit aldosterone production
    B   Calcium channel blockers inhibit aldosterone release
    C   β-adrenergic blockers lower plasma triglyceride levels
    D   Calcium channel blockers should not be combined with β-adrenergic blockers
    E   ACE inhibitors should not be combined with thiazide diuretics

29. **The following drugs are cleared by haemodialysis:**

   A   Paracetamol
   B   Methanol
   C   Theophylline
   D   Digoxin
   E   Tramadol

30. **Context-sensitive half-time:**

   A   Is greater for fentanyl than thiopentone after an 8-hour infusion
   B   Is approximately constant for remifentanil
   C   For propofol is 15 minutes after a 2-hour infusion
   D   Is the time taken for the plasma concentration of a drug to fall by 50% after stopping an infusion
   E   Is dependent on drug metabolism

31. **Drugs containing a chiral centre include:**

   A   Propofol
   B   Morphine
   C   Ketamine
   D   Enflurane
   E   Prednisolone

32. **The following drugs undergo minimal (less than 15%) metabolism:**

   A   Rocuronium
   B   Diclofenac
   C   Fentanyl
   D   Mivacurium
   E   Ephedrine

33. **Rocuronium:**

   A   Is structurally related to vecuronium
   B   Is highly bound to plasma proteins
   C   Has a prolonged duration of action in hypocalcaemic patients
   D   Is more potent than vecuronium
   E   Has a shorter duration of action than pancuronium

34. **Flumazenil:**

   A   Is a non-competitive benzodiazepine antagonist
   B   Should be administered in an initial intravenous dose of 100 mg
   C   Is well absorbed orally
   D   Is metabolised in the liver
   E   Can cause convulsions

35. **The following drugs increase gastrointestinal motility:**

   A   Amitriptyline
   B   Hyoscine

C   Domperidone
D   Neostigmine
E   Alfentanil

36. **The following drugs readily cross the placenta:**

A   Atropine
B   Ephedrine
C   Heparin
D   Diclofenac
E   Edrophonium

37. **Unfractionated heparins:**

A   Cause non immune-mediated thrombocytopenia
B   Activate anti-thrombin III
C   Have a molecular weight of between 2000 and 8000 Daltons
D   Are synthetic
E   Are 10% plasma protein bound

38. **Aciclovir:**

A   Is an antimicrobial agent
B   Is a nucleoside reverse transcriptase inhibitor
C   May cause renal failure following rapid intravenous injection
D   Causes local thrombophlebitis
E   Causes anaemia and neutropenia

39. **Thiazide diuretics:**

A   Inhibit Na^+ and Cl^- reabsorption in the distal convoluted tubule
B   Cause hyponatraemic acidosis in 20% of users
C   Increase bicarbonate excretion
D   Increase plasma cholesterol and triglyceride levels
E   Decrease glycogenolysis and increase glycogenesis

40. **Which of the following drugs is considered safe to use in patients with malignant hyperthermia:**

A   Nitrous oxide
B   Ketamine
C   Desflurane
D   Alfentanil
E   Suxamethonium

41. **The following are electrical units:**

A   Farad
B   Watt
C   Joule
D   Ohm
E   Candela

42. **Concerning heat loss:**

    A   Significant amounts of heat are lost from the body via expired air, urine and faeces
    B   Radiation is the warming of air next to the skin
    C   Conduction is the transfer of heat between two substances that are in contact
    D   Radiation may contribute up to 50% of normal heat loss from the body
    E   Convection heat loss is due to the loss of latent heat of vaporisation of moisture on the skin's surface

43. **Concerning temperature:**

    A   Heat must be supplied when a substance changes from a vapour to a liquid
    B   The latent heat of crystallisation is released when a solid dissolves into a liquid
    C   At the critical temperature, a substance changes spontaneously from liquid to vapour
    D   Above its critical temperature, nitrous oxide is a liquid
    E   When a substance changes from a solid to a liquid, it is at a constant temperature

44. **Regarding the different modes of ultrasound scanning:**

    A   A-mode is the most basic mode
    B   A-mode is the most widely used mode in anaesthesia
    C   B-mode allows a two-dimensional view of the scanned tissue
    D   C-mode generates a three-dimensional view
    E   M-mode detects the movement of reflecting surfaces along a single scan line

45. **Regarding diffusion:**

    A   Fick's law applies to osmosis
    B   The rate of diffusion is directly proportional to the membrane surface area and thickness
    C   The rate of diffusion of a gas is inversely proportional to the square root of its molecular weight
    D   Diffusion cannot occur without the presence of a pressure gradient
    E   Carbon monoxide can be used to test the diffusion capacity of the lungs

46. **Modern automated blood pressure measurement devices:**

    A   Record systolic blood pressure as the point when the rate of increase in pulsation is maximal
    B   Record diastolic pressure as the point when pulsations disappear
    C   Calculate the mean arterial pressure from the systolic and diastolic values
    D   Are inaccurate if the patient has a bradycardia
    E   Are inaccurate when the blood pressure changes rapidly

47. **Oxygen concentrators:**

    A   Need solenoid valves to ensure uninterrupted oxygen supply
    B   Can deliver an oxygen concentration of up to 95%
    C   May be used to supply piped oxygen in hospitals
    D   Contain silica gel to absorb nitrogen
    E   May produce toxic concentrations of argon

48. **The pressure regulators on a standard anaesthetic machine:**
   - A   Reduce variable high inlet pressures to variable low inlet pressures
   - B   Have no effect on gas flow
   - C   Ensure downstream pressures do not exceed 400 kPa
   - D   Protect patients from barotrauma
   - E   Are upstream of the pressure relief valves

49. **Regarding soda lime:**
   - A   The granules are sized 4–8 mesh
   - B   It changes to a violet colour when exhausted
   - C   1 kg absorbs a maximum of 20 L of carbon dioxide
   - D   Higher gas flow rates result in quicker consumption of granules
   - E   It can be used in a Mapleson B breathing system

50. **The Humphrey ADE breathing system:**
   - A   Is driven by piped gas
   - B   Has a pressure relief valve which opens at $45 \, cmH_2O$
   - C   Has a reservoir bag
   - D   Can be used to pre-oxygenate patients
   - E   Is unsuitable for use in children weighing less than 30 kg

51. **Carbon dioxide can be measured with:**
   - A   Gas chromatography
   - B   Transcutaneous electrodes
   - C   Polarography
   - D   Haldane apparatus
   - E   Piezoelectric resonance

52. **Blood gas analysers directly measure the following:**
   - A   Oxygen saturation
   - B   Standard bicarbonate
   - C   Base excess
   - D $Paco_2$
   - E   Hydrogen ion concentration

53. **Regarding the oesophageal Doppler probe:**
   - A   The tip should be sited at the level of T5-6 vertebral bodies
   - B   Peak velocity is a marker of cardiac contractility
   - C   The corrected flow time is directly proportional to afterload
   - D   The aortic cross-sectional area may be measured
   - E   The cardiac index is the cardiac output multiplied by body surface area

54. **Regarding intravenous cannulae:**
   - A   20 G cannulae deliver flow rates of approximately 130 mL/min
   - B   24 G cannulae are yellow in colour
   - C   Peripheral cannulae may deliver faster flow rates than central venous catheters
   - D   Orange cannulae can achieve flow rates of 500 mL/min
   - E   Blood flows faster than Hartmann's solution

55. **Regarding chest drains:**
    A   They should be inserted in the 5th intercostal space, posterior axillary line
    B   The drain bottle should be 125 cm below the mid-axillary line of the patient
    C   Tubing should have a volume which is greater than 50% of the patients maximum inspiratory capacity
    D   The tubing within the drainage bottle should be at least 5 cm below the fluid surface
    E   Suction of 30 cmH$_2$O is usually applied

56. **Fuses:**
    A   Utilise the principles of heat production and current flow
    B   Melt to disconnect a circuit
    C   Vary the lengths of their wire element for different ratings
    D   Improve the safety of medical electrical equipment
    E   Are capacitors

57. **Safety features of surgical diathermy include:**
    A   The presence of a capacitor in the circuit
    B   A small passive electrode pad
    C   Ensuring the diathermy equipment is earthed
    D   Using as high a frequency as possible
    E   Alarms warning of high stray leakage currents

58. **The following safety measures are required when using lasers in the operating theatre:**
    A   Only appropriately trained staff should be present
    B   All staff must wear eye protection
    C   Dry swabs should be placed over the patient's face
    D   A maximum of 50% inspired oxygen concentration should be used
    E   The theatre doors should be locked

59. **The following have paramagnetic properties:**
    A   Nitrous oxide
    B   Nitrogen
    C   Oxygen
    D   Carbon dioxide
    E   Nitric oxide

60. **Parametric statistical tests:**
    A   Include the Mann–Whitney U test
    B   Assume mean, median and mode are the same
    C   Follow a Gaussian distribution
    D   May be used to analyse unpaired data
    E   Assess ordinal data

Questions: SBAs

For each question, select the single best answer from the five options listed.

61. A 31-year-old woman undergoing an emergency laparoscopic appendicectomy has an end-tidal CO_2 of 3.4 kPa with saturations of 97% on 35% O_2, heart rate of 114 beats per minute and a blood pressure of 74/42 mmHg. An arterial blood gas shows a pH of 7.28, $Paco_2$ of 6.8 kPa, Pao_2 of 18.3 kPa and standard bicarbonate of 20.1 mmol/L.

Which of the following is the most likely cause of the raised end-tidal carbon dioxide levels?

A   Basal atelectasis
B   Hypoventilation
C   Absorption of CO_2 from the pneumoperitoneum
D   Hypovolaemia
E   Increased pulmonary shunt

62. You have been called urgently to assess a patient with a tracheostomy in place who is struggling to breathe through the tracheostomy and is now becoming distressed and hypoxic.

Which of the following is the most appropriate next step in management?

A   Remove the inner tube
B   Apply high-flow oxygen to the face and tracheostomy
C   Remove the speaking valve
D   Pass a suction catheter through the tracheostomy tube
E   Deflate the cuff

63. You have been asked to see a patient on the ward who was anaesthetised 2 days previously for a mastectomy. She is complaining of numbness and tingling in the distribution of the ulnar nerve.

Which of the following is *least* likely to prevent ulnar nerve injury in a patient?

A   Padding of vulnerable areas
B   Ensuring no equipment is lying on the patient
C   Regional anaesthesia instead of general anaesthesia
D   Avoiding generalised ischaemia
E   Avoiding excessive abduction of the upper limb

64. A 20-year-old woman having gynaecology surgery has a history of post-operative nausea and vomiting following previous anaesthetics. You decide to give her a combination of anti-emetic drugs.

Which one of the following anti-emetic drugs acts on the chemoreceptor trigger zone?

A   Cyclizine
B   Metoclopramide
C   Ondansetron

    D Dexamethasone

    E Prochlorperazine

65. You perform a needle cricothyroidotomy for a 'can't intubate, can't ventilate' scenario.

Which one of the following is true regarding the cricothyroid membrane?

    A It is a vascular structure

    B It lies between the thyroid cartilage and hyoid bone

    C It is easier to locate in women then men

    D It is at the level of the 5th cervical vertebra

    E There are no vessels or nerves penetrating it

66. You have been called to the recovery area to assess a 75-year-old man who has had a total hip replacement. He has a temperature of 34.9°C.

Which of the following physiological processes is *least* likely to help maintain this patient's body temperature?

    A Vasoconstriction of skin blood vessels

    B Hyperglycaemia

    C Shivering

    D Increased heart rate

    E Increased metabolic rate

67. A 66-year-old patient has a glomerular filtration rate (GFR) of $20\,\text{mL/min}/1.73\,\text{m}^2$.

Which one of the following can be safely administered without dose adjustment?

    A Fentanyl

    B Digoxin

    C Rocuronium

    D Gentamicin

    E Lithium

68. A 33-year-old woman has been admitted with jaundice. She has a plasma bilirubin level of 83 μmol/L, brown discolouration of her urine and brown coloured stools.

What is the most likely diagnosis?

    A Haemolysis

    B Gallstones

    C Gilbert's syndrome

    D Steroid therapy

    E Hepatitis

69. A 58-year-old man is complaining of polyuria, polydipsia and weight loss. He undergoes a glucose tolerance test to establish a diagnosis.

Which of the following is the main stimulus for insulin release from the pancreas?

A   Elevated blood sugar level
B   Glucagon
C   Insulin releasing peptide
D   Adrenaline
E   Growth hormone

70. A 58-year-old man presents with a subarachnoid haemorrhage due to a ruptured cerebral aneurysm. After 3 days, his Glasgow coma score (GCS) begins to deteriorate and cerebral vasospasm is suspected. The neurosurgical team recommends administration of a calcium channel blocker.

Which calcium channel blocker would be the most appropriate in this patient?

A   Amlodipine
B   Diltiazem
C   Nifedipine
D   Nimodipine
E   Verapamil

71. A 32-year-old woman receives a spinal anaesthetic. Her blood pressure decreases from 132/84 mmHg to 96/48 mmHg within 5 minutes of administration of 2.5 mL 0.5% intrathecal heavy bupivacaine and her heart rate increases from 84 to 112 beats per minute.

Which is the most likely underlying pathogenesis?

A   Intravascular hypovolaemia
B   Reduced adrenaline transmission
C   Increased cardiac sodium channel activity
D   Reduced acetylcholine transmission
E   Increased smooth muscle intracellular calcium

72. A 36-year-old man has been kept nil by mouth for 18 hours whilst awaiting an open reduction and internal fixation of an ankle fracture.

Which of the following metabolic changes would be most likely to have occurred in this patient?

A   Increased ketone body production
B   Increased lipid breakdown
C   Increased glycogenolysis
D   Increased proteolysis
E   Reduced glucose production

73. A 56-year-old man presents with acute heart failure. He is started on a glyceryl trinitrate (GTN) infusion.

What best describes the mechanism of action of GTN?

A   Nitrous oxide production
B   Arteriolar vasodilatation

    C   Increased cytoplasmic calcium
    D   Increased intracellular phospholipase C
    E   Increased intracellular cyclic guanosine monophosphate

74. An 18-year-old woman presents with suspected meningitis. She is prescribed an antibiotic with good cerebral penetrance.

The single most important factor determining drug transport across the blood–brain barrier is?

    A   Barrier surface area
    B   Molecular weight
    C   Protein binding
    D   Plasma pH
    E   Drug concentration

75. A 34-year-old man breathing 21% humidified oxygen has a Pao_2 of 12.1 kPa and a $Paco_2$ of 5.3 kPa.

Which of the following is most likely to contribute to the difference between alveolar and arterial Po_2?

    A   Asthma
    B   Pulmonary embolism
    C   Pneumonia
    D   Atelectasis
    E   Bronchial veins

76. A 15-year-old boy presents with testicular torsion. He is known to have an isolated atrial septal defect (ASD) with left to right shunting of blood. Intraoperatively his saturations decrease suddenly from 97% to 80% on 100% oxygen.

Which of the following is most likely to cause reversal of flow through the ASD?

    A   Prostacyclin
    B   Acetylcholine
    C   Histamine
    D   Nitric oxide
    E   Hypocarbia

77. A 24-year-old man presents following a traumatic brain injury. He is induced with propofol and rocuronium for tracheal intubation prior to transfer to a regional centre for neurosurgical intervention.

Which of the following is most likely to be due to propofol?

    A   Reduced jugular bulb saturations
    B   Reduced cerebral blood flow
    C   Epileptic electroencephalogram activity
    D   Increased intracranial pressure
    E   Unchanged cerebral oxygen consumption

78. A size J oxygen cylinder reads a gauge pressure of 6850 kPa.

What is the volume of oxygen contained within it?

A   180 L
B   900 L
C   3400 L
D   1800 L
E   340 L

79. A patient with carbon monoxide poisoning is being anaesthetised at an atmospheric pressure of 200 kPa. 2.5% sevoflurane is dialed on a Tec Mark 5 vaporiser with an FIO_2 of 1.0 and a flow rate of 4 L/minute via a circle breathing system.

What single change should be made to maintain appropriate delivery of sevoflurane?

A   Double the fresh gas flow rates
B   Add nitrous oxide
C   Increase concentrations of sevoflurane to 5%
D   Reduce concentrations of sevoflurane to 1.25%
E   No changes are required

80. A 54-year-old, 80 kg woman is being pre-oxygenated with a Magill breathing system.

What is the minimum oxygen flow rate required to prevent re-breathing?

A   2.8 L/minute
B   4.2 L/minute
C   5.6 L/minute
D   10.5 L/minute
E   14 L/minute

81. A 42-year-old woman with a background of hypertension, schizophrenia and hyperthyroidism is anaesthetised for a laparotomy. She had a rapid sequence induction and anaesthesia is maintained with sevoflurane. Gradually, her end-tidal CO_2 starts to increase despite optimal ventilation.

What is the *least* likely cause for the capnograph abnormality?

A   Malignant hyperthermia
B   Myocardial infarction
C   Neuroleptic malignant syndrome
D   Thyrotoxicosis
E   Sepsis

82. An arterial blood gas sample is analysed with a galvanic fuel cell.

What is the reaction most likely to occur at the cathode?

$$\text{A}\quad K^+ + Cl^- \rightarrow AgCl + electron$$
$$\text{B}\quad CO_2 + H_2O \rightarrow H^+ + H_2O$$
$$\text{C}\quad Pb + 2OH^- \rightarrow PbO + H_2O + 2 \cdot (electrons)$$
$$\text{D}\quad Ag^+ + Cl^- \rightarrow AgCl + electron$$
$$\text{E}\quad O_2 + 4 \cdot (electrons) + 2 \cdot H_2O \rightarrow 4 \cdot OH^-$$

83. A 32-year-old woman has a working epidural during labour. The fetal cardiotocography shows a prolonged bradycardia and an emergency lower segment caesarean section is indicated. A top-up solution of levobupivacaine, bicarbonate and adrenaline is used.

   What is the principal purpose of using bicarbonate in this solution?

   A   It raises the height of the block
   B   It reduces the potential for toxicity
   C   It prolongs the duration of action
   D   It reduces the onset time of the block
   E   It increases the potency of levobupivacaine

84. A 38-year-old woman with an open distal radius fracture is given 100 mg intramuscular pethidine in the emergency department. She has a history of depression, for which she takes 15 mg of phenelzine daily. On induction of anaesthesia, her blood pressure decreases significantly and 6 mg of ephedrine is administered intravenously. Her blood pressure increases to 220/115 mmHg, persisting at this value for 20 minutes.

   What is the most likely underlying cause?

   A   Increased activity of vasoactive amines
   B   Reduced catechol-O-methyltransferase activity
   C   Altered activity of pethidine
   D   Reduced ephedrine metabolism
   E   Increased adrenoceptor sensitivity

85. A 63-year-old man presenting for an elective hip replacement has a history of hypertension, motion sickness and Parkinson's disease.

   Which drug is most prudent to avoid?

   A   Cyclizine
   B   Prochlorperazine
   C   Remifentanil
   D   Midazolam
   E   Glycopyrrolate

86. A 72-year-old man having a cataract procedure under local anaesthetic develops sudden bradycardia. Atropine 300 µg is given intravenously.

   Which effect is *least* likely to be due to atropine?

   A   Bradycardia
   B   Vomiting

C Bronchodilatation
D Anhidrosis
E Sedation

87. A 69-year-old, 50 kg woman on the intensive care unit has paralytic ileus, for which she has been treated with 2.5 mg of neostigmine intravenously.

Which other effect is likely to be caused by this dose of neostigmine?

A Bronchoconstriction
B Mydriasis
C Urinary retention
D Raised intraocular pressure
E Neuromuscular weakness

88. A 82-year-old woman presents with weight loss, weakness and reduced appetite. Her serum albumin is 21 g/L.

Which drug is most significantly bound to albumin?

A Warfarin
B Bupivacaine
C Thiopentone
D Alfentanil
E Pancuronium

89. A 47-year-old woman with a history of depression presents with an overdose of her medication. She is drowsy with dry mucous membranes, dilated pupils, has a heart rate of 115 bpm, a blood pressure of 94/56 mmHg and a temperature of 38.2°C. Her electrocardiogram shows sinus tachycardia with prolonged QT interval and a QRS complex of 220 ms.

What is the most likely drug to cause these clinical features?

A Moclobemide
B Lithium
C Phenelzine
D Fluoxetine
E Amitriptyline

90. A new drug is trialed assessing adequacy of suppressing the hypertensive response to tracheal intubation. Blood pressures are recorded pre- and post-intubation, with and without the drug being administered.

What statistical test best assesses whether a difference exists?

A Paired analysis of variance (ANOVA)
B Unpaired ANOVA
C Paired Student's t-test
D Unpaired Student's t-test
E Chi-squared (χ^2) test

Answers: MTFs

1. **A** True

    B True

    C True

    D False

    D True

    The vital capacity (VC) is the sum of the inspiratory reserve volume (IRV), tidal volume (TV) and expiratory reserve volume (ERV). This is also the same as total lung capacity (TLC) minus residual volume (RV) (A) (see **Figure 5.1**). The IRV is usually 2.5–3 L (B). Measurement of functional residual capacity (FRC) can be calculated using helium dilution methods, nitrogen washout or body plethysmography that utilises Boyle's law (C). The only volumes that cannot be measured using a spirometer are any volumes that include the RV, which are the FRC and TLC (D). Closing capacity is the lung volume when airway closure occurs and is the closing volume plus RV; therefore, it always exceeds RV (E).

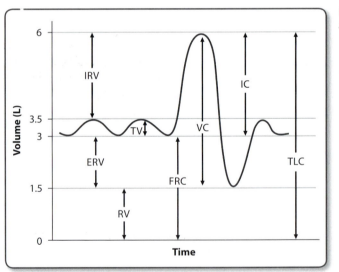

Figure 5.1 Lung volumes, as assessed by spirometry.

2. **A** True

    B False

    C False

    D False

    E False

    The ventilation/perfusion ($\dot{V}/\dot{Q}$) ratio varies in different areas of the lung. At the apex of the lungs, there is relatively better ventilation than perfusion; thus, $\dot{V}/\dot{Q}$ is greater than 1. At the bases of the lungs, there is a relatively greater perfusion than ventilation; therefore; $\dot{V}/\dot{Q}$ is less than 1.

Areas with a high $\dot{V}/\dot{Q}$ ratio (>0.8) are involved in dead space ventilation which could be caused by any cause of an increase in alveolar dead space (see Table 1.1), including pulmonary embolism (A). The alveolar gas in these areas tends to equilibrate with inspired air; therefore, Pao_2 will tend to increase and $Paco_2$ will decrease (B, C). As there is an increase in Pao_2, there will not be any hypoxic pulmonary vasoconstriction (E). However, a reduced Pao_2 in these areas causes regional vasoconstriction, thereby allowing ventilation to take part in better-perfused lung units.

Areas with a low $\dot{V}/\dot{Q}$ ratio (<0.8) contribute to physiological and pathological shunt (D). In these areas, alveolar gas equilibrates with mixed venous blood whereby Pao_2 decreases and $Paco_2$ increases. Hypoxic pulmonary vasoconstriction in these areas diverts blood to better-ventilated lung units.

3. A True

   B False

   C False

   D True

   D True

Pulmonary vascular resistance (PVR) decreases with an increased pH (A) and Pao_2, but increases with an increased $Paco_2$ (B). Angiotensin is a potent humoral vasoconstrictor, therefore will increase PVR (C). Prostacyclin is a humoral vasodilator, thus will reduce PVR (D). All volatile anaesthetic agents decrease PVR (E) (see Table 3.2).

4. A False

   B True

   C True

   D True

   E True

Oxygen flux (Do_2) is the oxygen delivered to tissues per unit time and it depends on both cardiac output (CO) and arterial O_2 content.

$Do_2 = CO \times$ arterial O_2 content

$= (SV \times HR) \times [(10 \times Hb \times Sao_2 \times 1.34) + (10 \times Pao_2 \times 0.0225)]$

where SV is stroke volume in mL (D), HR is heart rate in beats per minute, Hb is haemoglobin concentration in g/dL (E), Sao_2 is arterial O_2 saturation (B), 1.34 is Hüfner's constant which is the volume of O_2 carried by 1 g haemoglobin (C), Pao_2 is arterial partial pressure of O_2, 0.0225 is mL of O_2 dissolved per 100 mL of plasma per kPa. Knowledge of the SVR is not required (A)

The normal value is 850–1200 mL/min; if the cardiac output is indexed to body surface area the normal value is 500–700 mL/min/m². A knowledge of systemic vascular resistance is not required to calculate Do_2 (A).

5. **A** False

    B True

    C True

    D False

    E True

The sinoatrial node is a modified strip of cardiac muscle located in the posterior wall of the right atrium close to the superior vena cava (A) that initiates the heartbeat. It has an electrically unstable cell membrane and generates an action potential every second (B). This then excites the adjacent atrial cells and results in a wave of depolarisation across both atria.

The atrioventricular node is a small mass of cells and connective tissue situated in the lower posterior part of the atrial septum. It is the only electrical connection of the annulus fibrosus (C).

The bundle of His contains fast conducting muscle fibres (D) which conduct the electrical impulse from the atrioventricular node to the upper part of the interventricular septum. It then divides into the left and right bundle branches (see Figure 5.2). The fibres of the bundle of His terminate in an extensive network of large fibres in the subendocardium, the Purkinje fibres. The Purkinje cells have a large diameter so have a high conduction velocity, which allows them to distribute the electrical impulse rapidly to the endocardium work cells (E).

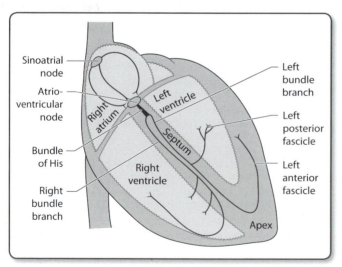

Figure 5.2 Conduction system of the heart.

6. **A** True

    B True

    C False

D True

E False

The parasympathetic nerve terminals act by releasing acetylcholine that then binds to muscarinic receptors in the cell membrane. Receptor activation causes immediate bradycardia. The pacemaker potential becomes more negative (hyperpolarisation) (A) and reduces the rate of the upward drift of the pacemaker potential. These changes cause an increased interval between beats because more time is required for the potential to reach threshold.

Hyperpolarisation is induced by an increase in membrane permeability to potassium (B) and is achieved by the opening of additional potassium channels which increases the outward background current and shifts the membrane potential closer towards the potassium equilibrium potential.

The chronotropic effect of sympathetic stimulation is due to an increase in the rate of rise of the pacemaker potential, which is able to reach threshold more rapidly. This is due to an increase in the inward background current produced by sodium and calcium ions (C).

The inotropic effect of sympathetic stimulation occurs as a result of an increase in the inward calcium current during the plateau phase, which increases intracellular calcium stores (D).

Vagal stimulation produces almost immediate bradycardia due to the rapid hyperpolarisation of the resting membrane potential. Sympathetic stimulation has a relatively slower onset, usually taking several heartbeats before there is an increase in firing rate (E).

7. **A** False

   B True

   C False

   D False

   E True

Vagal activity decreases and sympathetic nerve activity increases at the onset of exercise (A).

The increase in sympathetic activity increases the heart rate and shortens both systolic and diastolic times (B). Increased atrial contraction helps to offset the effect of reduced filling times by increasing the atrial contribution to ventricular filling.

Ventricular contractility is largely increased by cardiac sympathetic activity and to a lesser degree by catecholamine secretion from the adrenal medulla (C). This increases both the ejection fraction and the stroke volume.

Venoconstriction in the splanchnic circulation, induced by sympathetic stimulation and compression of the limb veins by the skeletal muscle pump, shifts blood into the central veins thus preventing the central venous pressure (CVP) from falling; in fact, the CVP may even increase (D).

Vasodilatation in the exercising skeletal muscle and skin causes a reduction in the systemic vascular resistance, which minimises any increase in arterial pressure (E). This helps maintain stroke volume during exercise.

8. A False

    B True

    C True

    D False

    E False

The cardiopulmonary receptors in the heart and pulmonary artery have an overall tonic inhibitory effect on heart rate and peripheral vascular resistance (A). The venoatrial receptors are branched, non-encapsulated nerve endings around the junctions of the great veins and atria (B). These receptors signal cardiac filling. They consist of three functional classes: mechanoreceptors (C) around the venoatrial junctions (myelinated fibres), mechanoreceptors scattered diffusely throughout the atria, ventricles and pulmonary arteries (non-myelinated fibres) and chemosensitive fibres travelling in the vagus and cardiac sympathetic nerves.

The cardiopulmonary receptors have an overall depressant effect on the heart and seem to be involved in the long-term regulation of blood pressure (D).

Patients who have had a heart transplant have good long-term blood pressure regulation, despite being denervated of the intrinsic cardiopulmonary receptors (E).

9. A True

    B False

    C True

    D True

    E False

Each kidney contains 1.2 million nephrons, its functional units (A). The renal corpuscle, which is made up of Bowman's capsule and the glomerulus, is situated in the renal cortex (B). The glomerulus, which is at the beginning of the nephron, filters protein (C), but allows water and small dissolved substances to pass into the proximal tubule.

The proximal tubules have a convoluted segment and a straight (pars recta) segment. The distal tubules begin with a straight segment (thick ascending loop of Henle) followed by a convoluted segment. Thus they both consist of convoluted segments (D) and are on either side of the loop of Henle.

The collecting ducts, which have several distal tubules draining into them, have cortical and medullary segments (known as outer and inner), so are present in both the cortex and medulla (E). These are anatomically and functionally distinct and make final modifications to the urine before excretion (see **Figure 5.3**).

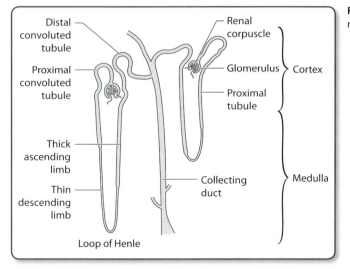

Figure 5.3 Structure of the nephron.

10. **A** False

B False

C True

D True

E False

The enzyme carbonic anhydrase plays a key role when a hydrogen ion gradient needs to be generated. It catalyses the reaction:

$$CO_2 + H_2O \rightleftharpoons H_2CO_3 \rightleftharpoons H^+ + HCO_3^-$$

The majority of the H^+ ions are secreted in the proximal convoluted tubule (A), not the distal convoluted tubules. There are two mechanisms for H^+ ion secretion:

- In the proximal tubule, H^+ ions are secreted in exchange for Na^+ ions (not K^+ ions, ATPase mediated) (B)
- In the collecting ducts, the H^+ ions are secreted primarily by the H^+ pumps in the intercalated cells; this allows the titration of phosphate and the pH may decrease to 4.5 (C)

One of the primary functions of H^+ ion secretion by the renal tubules is the resorption of filtered bicarbonate (D); the other is the excretion of fixed acid.

Less than 1% of the daily production of H^+ ions can be excreted in the free form (E). The majority of the H^+ ions are secreted as titratable acid, mostly (80%) phosphate.

11. **A** True

B False

C False

D True

E False

Conn's syndrome (primary hyperaldosteronism) is excess secretion of aldosterone from the adrenal gland and causes excessive K^+ loss (A).

Secondary hyperaldosteronism is much more common than primary hyperaldosteronism (B), occuring when there is a reduction in the effective plasma volume, such as in pregnancy, chronic diuretic therapy, nephrotic syndrome and heart failure (C). Activation of the renin–angiotensin mechanism results in the release of aldosterone.

Addison's disease causes reduced aldosterone release resulting in Na^+ loss and K^+ retention. Extracellular and plasma volume become depleted and contribute to the inability to maintain arterial blood pressure, which can result in postural hypotension (D).

Muscular weakness and paralysis are a result of hypokalaemia and, if severe, neurones and muscle fibres hyperpolarise which makes them less responsive to stimulation. This occurs with hypersecretion of aldosterone and not adrenocortical insufficiency (E).

12. **A** False

 B False

 C True

 D True

 E True

Diarrhoea and vomiting can result in isosmotic fluid loss (A). The osmolality remains unchanged and there is a decrease in extracellular fluid with no change in the intracellular space. Other examples of isosmotic loss are with diuretics, blood loss and burns.

- A water deficit results in a rise in the osmolality and fluid shifts from the intracellular to the extracellular compartment (B). This can occur in osmotic diuresis and sweating.

The intake of hypotonic fluid lowers the osmolality of the extracellular fluid compartment, excess water results in a decrease in the osmolality and fluid shifting to the intracellular space.

The infusion of large volumes of glucose solutions and excessive antidiuretic hormone (ADH) secretion both result in an excess of water and a decreased osmolality, resulting in fluid shifting to the intracellular compartment (C, D).

The infusion of hypertonic saline causes an excess of salt, which increases the osmolality and shifts fluid into the extracellular space (E). It can result in extracellular oedema. Steroid therapy and drinking seawater have the same effect.

13. A True

  B False

  C True

  D False

  E True

Fats and carbohydrates are completely oxidised to CO_2 and H_2O (A, C). Proteins are broken down to form urea (B).

The utilisable energy content of food, which is made available by its combustion, is called the physical caloric value and this can be determined with the bomb calorimeter. Here a known quantity of food is placed in a combustion chamber surrounded by water in an insulated chamber and is incinerated. The heat produced is taken up by the surrounding water, providing a measure of the caloric value. In humans, energy production is determined by indirect calorimetry (D). It is the oxygen utilisation that is measured, giving an indication of the energy liberation. About 90 kJ of energy is required to produce 1 mol of adenosine triphosphate from proteins but only 74 kJ is required from carbohydrates (E), so a protein diet can increase the metabolic rate by about 15%.

14. A False

  B False

  C True

  D True

  E False

The liver is made up of lobules and its functional unit is the acinus. Within the lobules, blood flows via sinusoids from branches of the portal vein to the central vein of each liver lobule (see **Figure 5.4**). The central veins eventually coalesce to form the hepatic veins (B), which then go on to drain into the inferior vena cava. Hepatic arterial blood also enters the sinusoids.

The portal space in the centre of each acinus contains a vascular stalk that consists of terminal branches of the portal vein, hepatic arteries and bile ducts (A). Blood flows from the vascular stalk to terminal hepatic venules that are located outside the acinus.

Kupffer cells, a form of macrophage, are anchored to the endothelium of the sinusoids and project into the lumen (C).

The portal venous pressure is normally about 10 mmHg, whereas the hepatic venous pressure is about 5 mmHg (D).

The mean arterial pressure in the hepatic artery branches that converge on the sinusoids is about 90 mmHg; then there is a marked pressure drop (E) along these arterioles, as the mean pressure in the sinusoids is less than the portal venous pressure.

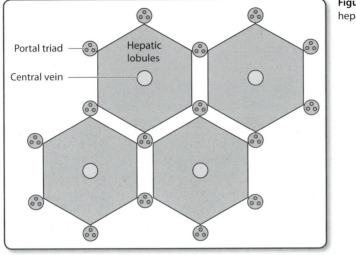

Figure 5.4 Microscopic hepatic anatomy.

15. **A** False

 B False

 C False

 D True

 E True

Transmission of nerve impulses may be sensory, motor or autonomic. The speed of transmission depends on the extent of myelination of neurones and fibre diameter, as shown in **Table 5.1**.

Table 5.1 Properties of nerve fibres				
Fibre	**Diameter (µm)**	**Myelination**	**Conduction velocity (m/s)**	**Function**
Aα	12–20	Yes	70–120	Motor, proprioception
Aβ	5–12	Yes	30–70	Touch, pressure
Aγ	3–6	Yes	15–30	Muscle spindle
Aδ	2–5	Thin	12–30	Pain, temperature, touch
B	3	Yes	3–15	Autonomic preganglionic
C dorsal root	0.4–1.2	No	0.5–2	Pain, temperature, mechanoreceptors, reflexes
C sympathetic	0.3–1.3	No	0.7–2.2	Postganglionic autonomic

16. **A** True

 B True

 C False

D True

E True

The spinal cord starts at the foramen magnum and terminates at L1–2 in adults. It is within the vertebral canal and gives off 31 paired spinal nerves. The central grey matter is surrounded by white matter that contains ascending and descending tracts (**Table 5.2**).

Table 5.2 Spinal tracts			
Ascending tracts		**Descending tracts**	
Lateral spinothalamic	Contralateral pain and temperature	Lateral corticospinal	Contralateral motor fibres (pyramidal)
Anterior spinothalamic	Contralateral touch and pressure	Anterior corticospinal	Ipsilateral motor fibres (extrapyramidal)
Dorsal columns	Ipsilateral touch and proprioception Fasciculus gracilis: lower body Fasciculus cuneatus: upper body	Rubrospinal	Extrapyramidal supply to lower motor neurones
Spinocerebellar	Proprioception	Vestibulospinal	
Spinotectal	Spinovisual reflexes	Tectospinal	

17. A False

B False

C False

D True

E False

Spinal cord injury is most prevalent in previously healthy young males in whom it is usually caused by motor vehicle accidents, sports injuries or assaults. It can be classified based on level of injury, stability and degree of neurological deficit. Clinical features include:

- Cardiac
  - Initial hypertension (B), vasoconstriction and arrhythmias (D). Subsequent effects are due to loss of sympathetic function and unopposed parasympathetic activity
  - *T1 and above:* hypotension and bradycardia
  - *T6 and above:* hypotension, no bradycardia (A)
- Respiratory
  - *C1–3:* complete paralysis of all respiratory muscles
  - *C3–5:* variable diaphragmatic involvement
  - *C6–8:* paralysis of intercostal and abdominal muscles

- Autonomic
  - *Above T5/6:* loss of descending inhibitory control causes autonomic hyperreflexia (C) up to 6 weeks after an injury
- Muscular
  - Initial flaccid paralysis (E) for the duration of spinal shock (4–6 weeks)
  - Spastic paralysis ensues after the initial period of spinal shock
- Gastrointestinal
  - 2–3 weeks of paralytic ileus and delayed gastric emptying
  - Gastric stress ulcers
  - Constipation
- Metabolic
  - Hypothermia due to vasodilation
  - Hyperglycaemia due to the stress response

18. A True

B False

C True

D False

E True

Post-operative nausea and vomiting occurs in about 25% of adults and is associated with increased morbidity. The causes can be divided into patient factors, surgical factors and anaesthetic factors (**Table 5.3**).

Table 5.3 Causes of post-operative nausea and vomiting		
Patient	**Surgical**	**Anaesthetic**
Female	Gynaecological	Nitrous oxide
Obesity	Gastrointestinal	Inhalational agents
Previous post-operative nausea and vomiting	Laparoscopic	Opioids
Non-smoker	ENT	Etomidate, thiopentone
Prolonged fasting	Testicular	Hypoxia
History of motion sickness	Ophthalmic (especially squint correction)	Hypotension
History of migraine	Prolonged surgery	Gastric insufflation
Menstrual cycle		Anticholinesterases

19. A False

B False

C True

D True

E False

Parathyroid hormone (PTH) increases the number and activity of osteoclasts. It has the opposite effects to calcitonin (A). Therefore, PTH causes the increased breakdown of the bone matrix (i.e. it increases bone resorption), which releases more calcium and phosphate into the blood.

PTH also has various effects on the kidneys. It increases the renal reabsorption of magnesium and calcium from the urine and returns it to the bloodstream. It also causes more phosphate to be lost in the urine by decreasing its renal reabsorption. The overall effect is to decrease phosphate levels, as more is excreted in the urine than is generated by bone resorption.

The overall effects of PTH are to increase Ca^{2+} and Mg^{2+} levels and decrease HPO_4^{2-} levels (B, C).

PTH promotes the kidneys to form calcitriol (D), which is the active form of vitamin D. Calcitriol increases the absorption of calcium, phosphate and magnesium from the gastrointestinal tract.

PTH exhibits a negative feedback control system which does not involve the pituitary gland (E). When blood calcium levels fall, PTH is released and when calcium levels rise, less PTH is secreted (but more calcitonin is secreted).

20. **A** True

B True

C False

D True

E False

Blood storage solutions are designed to maintain viability of red blood cells for an extended time period to allow safe transfusion. This is achieved using preservatives and storage at 2–6°C (**Table 5.4**).

Table 5.4 Properties of different blood storage solutions	
SAG-M	Saline 140 mmol/L
	Adenine 1.5 mmol/L
	Glucose 50 mmol/L
	Mannitol 30 mmol/L
	Resuspends after removal from CPD
	Reduced haemolysis with mannitol added
	Red cell survival of 35 days
CPD	Citrate, phosphate, dextrose
	Red cell survival of 28 days
CPD-A	Citrate, phosphate, dextrose, adenine
	Adenine increases ATP levels and thus red cell survival to 35 days
BAGPM	Bicarbonate, added glucose, phosphate, mannitol
	Red cell survival of 35 days

21. A False

   B True

   C False

   D True

   E True

Table 5.5 Pharmacological properties of intravenous anaesthetic agents

Property	Propofol	Thiopentone	Ketamine	Etomidate	Methohexitone
Heart rate	–/0	+	+	0	+
Blood pressure	–	–	+	0	–
Cardiac output	–	–	+	0	–
Systemic vascular resistance	–	–/+	0	0	–/+
Respiratory rate	–	–	+	–	–
Intracranial pressure	–	–	+	0	–
Intraocular pressure	–	–	+	0	–
Emetogenic	Antiemetic	No	Yes	Yes	No
Painful injection	Yes	No	No	Yes	Yes

'–' Signifies a decrease, '+' signifies an increase and '0' signifies no effect.

22. A True

   B True

   C False

   D False

   E True

Midazolam is a benzodiazepine commonly used as a hypnotic, anxiolytic and anticonvulsant. Its structure is dependent on the surrounding pH. At an acidic pH of 3.5, its ring structure is open and this makes the molecule ionised (A) and water soluble. At a relatively more alkaline pH of 4, the ring structure closes, making it unionised and therefore more lipid soluble. At physiological pH, it is mostly in the unionised form, therefore rapidly crosses cell membranes.

Midazolam can be given intravenously, intramuscularly, intranasally or orally. The oral bioavailability is approximately 40% (B).

Midazolam is metabolised by hepatic P450 isoenzymes, which also metabolise alfentanil, so when administered together, their effects are prolonged. Midazolam does not prolong the effect of fentanyl (C).

Midazolam is metabolised in the liver (E) by hydroxylation to mostly inactive metabolites which are excreted in the urine as glucuronide conjugates, but a small proportion is converted to oxazepam, an active metabolite (D).

23. **A** True

    B False

    C True

    D True

    E False

The minimum alveolar concentration (MAC) is defined as the minimum concentration of inhalational agent required to prevent movement in response to a standard surgical stimulus in 50% of subjects. It is defined in terms of per cent of an atmosphere and is unaffected by altitude. However, MAC can be affected by a number of factors (**Table 5.6**).

Table 5.6 Factors affecting MAC	
Factors increasing MAC	**Factors decreasing MAC**
Infancy	Increasing age
Hyperthermia	Hypothermia
Hyperthyroidism	Hypothyroidism
Hypernatraemia	Pregnancy
Catecholamines	Hypotension
Chronic opioid abuse	Acute opioid abuse
Chronic alcohol intake	Acute alcohol intake
	Lithium
	α_2 agonists
	Sedatives

24. **A** False

    B False

    C False

    D False

    E True

Non-steroidal anti-inflammatory drugs (NSAIDs) inhibit the enzyme cyclo-oxygenase (COX); therefore, they prevent the production of prostaglandins and thromboxanes from membrane phospholipids (see **Figure 4.10**). They do not inhibit phospholipase A2 (A) or lipoxygenase (B). Steroids inhibit phospholipase A2.

Cyclo-oxygenase exists as two isoenzymes, called COX-1 and COX-2 (C).

COX-1 is responsible for producing prostaglandins that control renal blood flow (D), haemostatic function and form the protective mucosal barrier of the stomach. COX-2 facilitates the inflammatory response after tissue damage.

Inhibition of COX-1 is largely responsible for the side effects of the NSAIDs (E), but COX-2 is involved in the production of prostaglandins in the presence of *Helicobacter pylori*. The main effects of COX-2 inhibition are anti-inflammatory, antipyretic and analgesic.

25. **A** True

    B False

    C True

    D False

    E True

Diamorphine is a diacetylated morphine derivative with no affinity for the opioid receptors. It is actually a prodrug whose active metabolites are responsible for its pharmacological effects. Compared with morphine, it is approximately twice as potent. It is highly lipid soluble and well absorbed from the gut, but undergoes extensive first-pass metabolism; it is approximately 40% plasma protein bound and is metabolised in the liver and plasma by ester hydrolysis (A) to the active metabolites morphine and 6-monoacetylmorphine.

Fentanyl is a synthetic phenylpiperidine derivative. It is not a prodrug (B) and has similar effects to morphine. It has a more rapid onset of action, larger volume of distribution and is more lipid soluble than morphine. It has poor oral bioavailability due to high first-pass metabolism.

Pethidine is a synthetic phenylpiperidine derivative and has anti-cholinergic actions (C); therefore it can cause mydriasis, dry mouth and tachycardia. It is more lipid soluble than morphine and has an oral bioavailablilty of 50%. It is metabolised in the liver to the active norpethidine and the inactive pethidinic acid. Norpethidine is eliminated by the kidneys so can accumulate in renal failure.

Codeine is a 3-methoxymorphine (D). It has a methyl group which reduces the hepatic conjugation, thereby giving it an oral bioavailability of approximately 50%. It is mostly metabolised to inactive metabolites, but about 10% is metabolised to morphine.

Papaveretum is a mixture of the anhydrous hydrochlorides of the alkaloids of opium. It contains morphine, codeine and papaverine (E).

26. **A** True

    B False

    C True

    D True

    E False

Nitrates provide an exogenous source of nitric oxide (C), a very short-lived free radical which has a potent vasodilator effect (A). It induces coronary vasodilatation, even if the endogenous production of nitric oxide is impaired by coronary artery disease.

The chronic use of nitrates produces tolerance (D), which can be a significant problem.

Nitrates preferentially dilate coronary arteries (E) and arterioles. This redistributes blood flow along collateral channels and from epicardial to endocardial regions. It also relieves coronary artery spasm and dynamic stenosis, especially at epicardial sites which have been constricted as a result of exercise. This explains why nitrates are effective vasodilators for angina.

Nitrates dilate the venous capacitance vessels that reduce venous return to the heart (B).

27. A True

   B False

   C False

   D True

   E False

β-blockers have inhibitory effects on the sinoatrial node, atrioventricular node and myocardial contraction. These result in negative chronotropic (heart rate) (A), dromotropic (conduction) (B) and inotropic (contractility) (E) effects. The inhibitory effect on the atrioventricular node is especially useful in the management of myocardial ischaemia, as these effects decrease myocardial oxygen demand.

The inhibitory effect on the atrioventricular node is used in the therapy of supraventricular tachycardias and when controlling the ventricular response rate in atrial fibrillation.

β-blockers reduce afterload (C) and therefore reduce the oxygen demand of the heart. They also increase diastolic perfusion (D) by increasing diastolic filling time. This is achieved by decreasing the heart rate and cardiac output.

28. A True

   B True

   C False

   D False

   E False

Calcium channel blockers act largely by peripheral arterial dilatation, with a lesser diuretic effect. They also evoke counter-regulatory mechanisms, dependent on stimulation of renin and formation of angiotensin, as well as the reflex release of noradrenaline. They also inhibit the release of aldosterone (B).

In addition to lowering blood pressure, β-blockers can also cause a loss of insulin sensitivity with resultant increased risk of diabetes, raise plasma triglyceride levels (C), reduce levels of high-density lipoprotein and increase body weight.

For the treatment of hypertension, a β-blocker plus calcium channel blocker works well, although heart rate, atrioventricular conduction and left ventricular function may sometimes be adversely affected. In practice, β-blockers and calcium channel blockers can be safely combined (D) in the treatment of angina or hypertension.

Angiotensin-converting enzyme inhibitors (see **Figure 5.5**) combine well with thiazide diuretics (E). In hypertension diuretics must provide enough natriuresis (A) to achieve some persistent volume depletion; they also work as vasodilators.

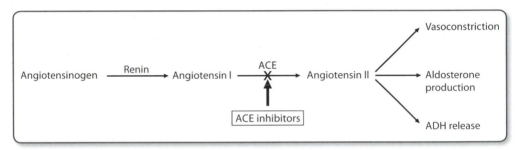

Figure 5.5 Mechanism of action of angiotensin-converting enzyme inhibitors.

29. **A** False

 B True

 C True

 D False

 E False

For clearance by haemodialysis or haemofiltration, drugs should have low molecular weight, low volume of distribution and low plasma protein binding. This includes vancomycin, theophylline (C), tazocin (piperacillin with tazobactam), sotalol, morphine, metoprolol, metronidazole, methanol (B), mannitol, meropenem, ethylene glycol, gentamicin, co-amoxiclav, cephalosporins, atenolol and aspirin. Paracetamol (A), digoxin (D) and tramadol (E) are not cleared.

30. **A** True

 B True

 C True

 D True

 E True

Context-sensitive half-time is defined as the time taken for the plasma concentration of a drug to fall by half after stopping an infusion that has been designed to maintain a steady plasma concentration (D), the 'context' being the duration of the infusion. When a steady state is reached, there is equilibrium between all compartments, and elimination from the plasma is equal to drug infusion rate. Upon cessation of administration, drug metabolism (E) from the plasma decreases plasma concentration, causing redistribution of drug from other compartments.

Remifentanil is described as having a context-'insensitive' half-time because it is rapidly metabolised, and has a small volume of distribution and a high clearance, thus has a relatively constant half-time (B) (see **Table 5.7**).

Table 5.7 Context-sensitive half-time (CSHT) for common drugs		
Drug	**CSHT after 2-hour infusion (minutes)**	**CSHT after 8-hour infusion (minutes)**
Alfentanil	50	65
Fentanyl	50	280
Propofol	15	40
Remifentanil	4	9
Thiopentone	90	110

31. **A** False

B False

C True

D False

E False

A chiral centre is a central atom, usually carbon or nitrogen, bound by four dissimilar groups, generating a potential mirror image that is not superimposable. It is responsible for generation of optical isomers and is classified by the arrangement of atomic numbers of the four atoms. If the atomic numbers descend clockwise around the chiral centre, this is the rectus, *R*, arrangement. If the atomic numbers descend in an anticlockwise fashion, this is a sinister, *S*, arrangement. Ketamine contains a chiral centre (C), and can be presented as either *R*-ketamine or *S*-ketamine, the latter demonstrating a more favourable pharmacodynamic profile.

Morphine does not contain a chiral centre, but it does demonstrate isomerism in the keto-enol form (B). Enflurane demonstrates structural isomerism, with isoflurane being an isomer (D). Prednisolone and aldosterone are structural isomers, not optical isomers (E). Propofol does not demonstrate isomerism (A).

32. **A** True

B False

C False

D False

E True

Rocuronium is a rapidly acting aminosteroid taken up by the liver and excreted predominantly (95%) unchanged in the bile. Less than 5% is metabolised (A) to 17-deacetylrocuronium which is 20 times less potent than rocuronium.

Diclofenac is a phenylacetate that is significantly hydroxylated in the liver (B) followed by conjugation to glucuronide and sulphate metabolites. It undergoes significant first-pass metabolism, and is excreted in urine and bile.

Fentanyl is a synthetic phenylpiperidine that undergoes significant first-pass metabolism when given orally. It is *N*-demethylated to norfentanyl and may also undergo hydroxylation and amide hydrolysis to inactive metabolites (C).

Mivacurium is a short-acting non-depolarising muscle relaxant that undergoes ester hydrolysis (D) by plasma cholinesterase, producing inactive quaternary alcohols and monoesters.

Ephedrine is minimally metabolised in the liver (E), with 90% of the administered dose being excreted unchanged in the urine.

33. **A** True

    B False

    C True

    D False

    E True

Rocuronium is a rapid-acting monoquaternary aminosteroid that is very similar in structure to vecuronium (A). Because of its low potency (D), it must be administered at high doses to demonstrate clinical effects. A larger number of molecules are delivered to the plasma, making a greater concentration gradient between the plasma and the neuromuscular junction, thus reducing onset time. It has an intermediate duration of action, with pancuronium having a prolonged duration (E). Rocuronium is 10–30% protein bound (B), with a volume of distribution of 0.2 L/kg, and is minimally metabolised before elimination in the bile (60%) and the urine (40%). As with other neuromuscular blocking drugs, duration of action is prolonged in the presence of hypothermia, hypocalcaemia (C), hypokalaemia and hypermagnesaemia (see Table 3.8).

34. **A** False

    B False

    C True

    D True

    E True

Flumazenil is a competitive antagonist (A) of central benzodiazepine activity that is given intravenously at an initial dose of 100 µg (B). Although it is well absorbed orally (C), it undergoes extensive hepatic first-pass metabolism, rendering it less useful via this route. It is 50% plasma protein bound and has a volume of distribution of 1 L/kg. It undergoes hepatic metabolism (D) to inactive metabolites that are excreted renally. It may precipitate hypertension, arrhythmias, nausea, vomiting, anxiety, headache and convulsions (E), particularly in epileptics.

35. A False

   B False

   C True

   D True

   E False

Drugs that increase cholinergic or parasympathetic tone will aid the 'rest and digest' physiological response. Amitriptyline has significant anticholinergic effects due to inhibition of muscarinic acetylcholine receptors, thus reducing parasympathetic tone and reducing gastric motility (A).

Hyoscine, an antimuscarinic related to atropine, acts similarly to antagonise muscarinic M3 receptors to reduce gastric motility (B) and lower oesophageal sphincter tone.

Domperidone is an antiemetic and prokinetic, inhibiting D2 dopaminergic receptors and increasing gastric motility (C).

Neostigmine is an acetylcholinesterase inhibitor, increasing gut motility (D) by increasing acetylcholine availability.

Alfentanil, as with other opioids, acts on μ-opioid receptors in the myenteric plexus to delay gastric transit time and reduce motility (E).

36. A True

   B True

   C False

   D True

   E False

Placental transfer of drugs depends on ionisation and pKa, protein binding, lipid solubility and molecular weight.

Atropine is a tertiary charged anticholinergic agent, thus it crosses the placenta readily (A). Glycopyrrolate is a quaternary charged structure therefore does not.

Ephedrine is a naturally occurring sympathomimetic that crosses the placental barrier readily (B), as does phenylephrine.

Because of its large, highly protein bound, polar structure, heparin does not cross the placenta significantly (C), whereas warfarin does cross easily.

Non-steroidal anti-inflammatory drugs such as diclofenac easily cross the placenta (D), potentially having adverse effects on fetal renal development and premature closure of the ductus arteriosus beyond 32 weeks' gestation.

The anticholinesterase agents neostigmine, pyridostigmine and edrophonium are quaternary charged structures that do not cross the placenta significantly (E); however, physostigmine is a tertiary amine and therefore crosses with greater ease.

37. **A** True

　B True

　C False

　D False

　E False

Heparins are acid mucopolysaccharides that are found naturally (D) in hepatocytes and mast cells. They can be unfractionated (molecular weight 8000–25,000 Da) (C) or low molecular weight (2000–8000 Da). Unfractionated heparins bind reversibly to antithrombin III (B), promoting inhibition of factors Xa as well as factors IXa, XIa, XIIa and XIIIa. They may also reduce platelet aggregation at higher doses, further augmenting their anticoagulant effect. The most important side effects include bleeding, osteoporosis and aldosterone suppression. Heparin-induced thrombocytopenia can either be type I, with no immune basis (A) and minimal clinical significance, or type II which is immune mediated and associated with significant platelet aggregation, thrombocytopenia and thrombosis.

Because of their highly polar acidic nature, they are highly protein bound to albumin (70%) (E) and antithrombin III (30%), are poorly lipid soluble thus do not cross the placenta or blood–brain barrier. They are desulphated and depolymerised by heparinises and excreted in the urine. Protamine is an effective reversal agent; however, it is ineffective against low molecular weight heparin.

38. **A** True

　B False

　C True

　D True

　E False

Antimicrobial agents kill or suppress the growth of micro-organisms and this includes antiviral drugs (A).

Aciclovir inhibits nucleic acid synthesis (B). Rapid intravenous injection may cause renal impairment (C) and the dose of aciclovir should be reduced in renal failure. Aciclovir is highly irritant when administered intravenously and can cause thrombophlebitis (D). Aciclovir also causes central nervous system side effects such as tremors and seizures, but it is not known to cause anaemia or neutropenia (E).

39. **A** True

　B False

　C True

D True

E False

Thiazide diuretics are moderately potent diuretics that act on the distal convoluted tubule by inhibiting the reabsorption of Na^+ and Cl^- (A) which leads to increased excretion of water. They are used in heart failure and hypertension.

Thiazide diuretics can cause hypokalaemic, hypochloraemic alkalosis (B). This occurs as a result of the increased Na^+ load reaching the distal tubules, which is exchanged for K^+ and H^+ and thus causing the alkalosis (see Table 3.9).

They reduce the activity of the enzyme carbonic anhydrase which results in an increase in the excretion of bicarbonate (C).

Thiazides have many metabolic effects; they increase serum triglyceride and cholesterol levels (D) and increase plasma glucose levels in diabetic patients by reducing glycogenesis, increasing glycogenolysis (E) and reducing insulin secretion.

40. A True

B True

C False

D True

E False

Malignant hyperthermia is an autosomal-dominant condition characterised by dysfunctional skeletal muscle ryanodine receptors (RYR1) that are activated by triggers causing uncontrolled release of calcium (Ca^{2+}) into muscle cytoplasm. This leads to the clinical features of skeletal muscle rigidity, masseter muscle spasm, increased O_2 consumption and hypoxia, increased CO_2 production, tachycardia and metabolic acidosis. Increasing temperature is a late sign but can be very rapid (>0.5°C every 5–10 minutes). Triggering agents include all the volatile anaesthetic agents (C) and suxamethonium (E). Once diagnosed, all triggering agents must be stopped and a clean, volatile-free anaesthetic circuit must be introduced, with anaesthesia being maintained with intravenous anaesthetic agents. Patients should be hyperventilated with 100% O_2 and prompt treatment with dantrolene has been shown to significantly reduce mortality. Drugs that are safe to use in patients with malignant hyperthermia include propofol, thiopentone, etomidate, ketamine (B), midazolam, local anaesthetics, opioids (D) and nitrous oxide (A).

41. A True

B False

C False

D True

E False

The following are electrical units:

- Volt (V) – measure of potential difference, units of watts/amps (W/A)

- Ohm (Ω) – measure of resistance, units of volts/amps (V/A) (D)
- Coulomb (C) – measure of charge, units of amperes × seconds (A.s)
- Farad (F) – measure of capacitance, units of coulombs/volts (C/V) (A)

The watt (W) is the unit of power and is measured in joules/second (J/s) (B). The joule (J) is the unit of energy, with units of Newtons × metres (N.m) (C). The candela (cd) is a measure of luminous intensity (E).

42. A False

  B False

  C True

  D True

  E False

There are four principal mechanisms by which heat is lost from the body in humans: radiation, convection, evaporation and conduction. Small amounts of heat are lost in the expired air, urine and faeces (A).

Radiation is the transfer of heat from a warmer body to a cooler one (B), without direct contact. It can occur through air or a vacuum and depends on surface area and the temperature difference between the surfaces.

Convection is the warming of air situated next to the skin (E); this warm air then rises and is replaced by cooler air and with greater air flow there is greater heat loss.

Conduction is the transfer of heat from one object to another with which it is in contact (C); the rate of heat transfer depends on the conducting properties of the objects and the temperature difference between the two. Within the body, conduction is not an important method of heat transfer and not much heat is lost by this method.

In temperate climates radiation can account for up to 60% of heat lost (D) from the body, but typical contributions to heat loss are:

- Radiation   40%
- Convection   30%
- Evaporation   20%
- Respiration   8%
- Conduction   2%

Surface evaporative heat loss is the loss of latent heat of vaporization of moisture from the skin's surface. This is increased by sweating.

43. A False

  B True

  C True

  D False

  E True

Latent heat is the heat required to change a substance from a liquid to a vapour or from a solid to a liquid, at a constant temperature (A). If the change is from liquid to vapour, then it is known as the latent heat of vaporization, and if it is from solid to liquid, then it is known as the latent heat of fusion. The latent heat of crystallisation is associated with solids dissolving in a liquid (B) or crystallising out of a liquid.

The critical temperature is the temperature above which a gas cannot be liquefied, regardless of the amount of pressure applied (C). Above this point, distinct liquid and gas phases do not exist and at this temperature the substance changes spontaneously from liquid to vapour without the supply of any external energy (E). Above its critical temperature, a substance cannot exist as a liquid (D).

44. A True

    B False

    C True

    D False

    E True

There are three different modes of ultrasound scanning: A, B and M. C-mode is not a function of ultrasound scanning (D).

A-mode is the most basic type (A) and simply displays the reflected ultrasound pulses from a single line scan on a time axis. It can accurately give the time difference between reflected pulses and the acoustic attenuation of the tissue layers (indicated by the amplitude of the pulses). In anaesthesia, this mode is not clinically useful (B).

B-mode is the most widely used in anaesthesia and is a two-dimensional version (C) of the A-mode. Ultrasound beams are passed through a slice of tissue and the reflected pulse is displayed which correlates with the anatomical cross section. High amplitude reflections produce a bright or white appearance on the monitor.

M-mode is used to detect movement of reflecting surfaces along a single scan line (E), it is used in conjunction with B-mode. M-mode is used by cardiologists and cardiac anaesthetists to evaluate the movement of heart valves.

45. A False

    B False

    C True

    D False

    E True

Fick's law states that the rate of diffusion is directly proportional to the membrane surface area and inversely proportional to the thickness (A, B). It also states that the greater the concentration difference, the greater the rate of diffusion, from high concentration to low.

Graham's law states that the rate of diffusion of a gas is inversely proportional to the square root of its density or molecular weight (C). Thus, the larger the molecules of a gas, the slower the diffusion across a membrane.

If a concentration gradient exists between two gases or liquids across a membrane, then diffusion can still occur even in the absence of a pressure gradient being present (D).

Carbon monoxide is used to test the diffusion capacity of the lungs (E). This is because the rate-limiting step for its diffusion across the alveolar–capillary membrane is the uptake of carbon monoxide.

46. A True

B False

C False

D False

E True

Modern automated devices such as the Device for Indirect Non-Invasive Automatic Mean Arterial Pressure (DINAMAP) use the principle of oscillometry to give non-invasive blood pressure readings. The systolic blood pressure is interpreted as the point at which the rate of increase in pulsations is at a maximum (A) and not when they start to appear. The diastolic pressure is when the rate of decrease is at a maximum (B) and not when they disappear. The mean arterial pressure is read when the cuff oscillations are at a maximum (C).

Inaccuracies using this method occur during rapid blood pressure changes (E), excessive cuff movement and arrhythmias (D).

47. A True

B True

C True

D False

E False

Oxygen concentrators are efficient, portable and reliable devices used to supply oxygen to individual patients or through a pipeline (C). Air is taken into the device, filtered and compressed to 137 kPa then transferred to one of two cylinders containing zeolite granules (D). Zeolite absorbs nitrogen from the air delivered. The air supply switches between each cylinder every 20–30 seconds under control of solenoid valves (A) to allow release of nitrogen and regeneration of zeolite, thus ensuring a constant supply of oxygen. The oxygen is then transferred to a reservoir before being available for use.

A concentration of up to 95% oxygen can be produced (B) with flow rates of up to 5 L/minute, and up to 5% argon is generated but has no known toxic effects (E).

48. A False

B False

C True

D False

E True

Pressure regulators are devices used to protect the anaesthetic machine against damage due to high pressures, serving no patient protection (D). They act by reducing variably high inlet pressures from cylinders to a constant lower pressure of 400 kPa (A, C), thus regulating gas flow (B). They are gas specific, are placed between cylinders and the anaesthetic machine and have relief valves downstream (E) that open at 700 kPa in the event of pressure regulator failure.

49. A True

B True

C False

D False

E False

Soda lime is most commonly utilised within a circle breathing system to absorb exhaled carbon dioxide, although it can be used in a Mapleson C (E) system as a 'Waters canister'. Soda lime allows use of low fresh gas flows and reduces pollution. It is composed of 94% calcium hydroxide, 5% sodium hydroxide and 0.1% potassium hydroxide. The granules are of 4–8 mesh size (A), meaning 4–8 granules can pass through a mesh with holes of 1 inch square. Dye within the granules provides an indicator of granule exhaustion:

- Blue, pink or red to white
- White or green to violet (B)

Soda lime canisters are positioned in the expiratory limb of circle breathing systems and 1 kg of soda lime may absorb up to 120 L of carbon dioxide (C). The lower the fresh gas flows used, the more quickly the soda lime is exhausted (D) as a larger proportion of exhaled gases pass through the soda lime canister.

50. A False

B False

C True

D True

E False

The Humphrey ADE is a breathing system that essentially allows shifts between Mapleson A, D and E systems. It may be used in a parallel or coaxial arrangement. The block sits at the machine end of the circuit (A) and comprises:

- Non-corrugated 15 mm tubing to and from the patient

- Reservoir bag (C)
- APL valve
- Ventilator port
- Pressure relief valve opening at 60 cmH$_2$O (B)
- Soda lime
- Lever, selecting spontaneous (Mapleson A) or controlled (Mapleson D) ventilation modes (D)

The block is suitable for paediatric use in children weighing less than 25 kg (E) in both spontaneous and controlled ventilation modes.

51. A True

B True

C False

D True

E False

Carbon dioxide can be measured directly with a Severinghaus electrode using a modified pH mechanism, or indirectly using:

- Campbell and Howell rebreathing techniques
- Gas chromatography (A)
- Haldane apparatus (D)
- Infrared absorption
- Interferometers
- Mass spectrometry
- Siggaard-Andersen nomogram
- Transcutaneous electrodes (B)
- Van Slyke apparatus

Piezoelectric resonance is utilised for measurement of volatile anaesthetic agents (E), while polarography is the principle used in the Clark electrode (C).

52. A False

B False

C False

D True

E True

Blood gas analysers assess heparinised samples of blood using oxygen polarographic electrodes, pH electrodes and carbon dioxide (Severinghaus) electrodes. Thus, the only directly measured parameters are the Pao_2, $Paco_2$ (D) and the pH via the hydrogen ion concentration (E). Other parameters including bicarbonate (B), oxygen saturation (A) and base excess (C) can be derived using mathematical equations and nomograms.

53. A True

B True

C False

D False

E False

The probe is inserted through the mouth and the tip should sit at the point where the aorta is closest to the oesophagus, usually at T5–6 (A). Using the Doppler principle, the device measures flow in the descending aorta, with the cross-sectional area being derived (D) from nomograms, with various indices being calculated on a beat-to-beat basis:

Flow time corrected (FTc): Systolic aortic blood flow time corrected to a heart rate of 60 beats per minute. This is normally 330–360 ms and is inversely proportional to the afterload (C).

Peak velocity (PV): The peak velocity of blood flow in the systolic phase, and is used as a marker of contractility (B). It varies with age, but increases with exercise and inotropes, while it decreases with β-blockers and left ventricular failure.

Stroke volume (SV): The volume of blood ejected during systole and is usually between 60 and 90 mL.

Cardiac output (CO): The volume of blood ejected from the heart per minute.

Cardiac index (CI): The cardiac output indexed to body surface area (BSA), CO/BSA (E), and is normally 2.6–4.2 L/min/m².

54. A False

B True

C True

D False

E False

In the UK intravenous cannulae have flow rates determined by a British Standard method, whereby distilled water at 22°C is placed under a constant pressure of 10 kPa and connected via 110 cm tubing to the cannula and maximum flow rates are determined (**Table 5.8**).

Table 5.8 Characteristics of different sized cannulae			
Gauge ('G')	Colour	Internal diameter (mm)	Flow rates (mL/min)
14 G	Orange	1.7 mm	250–360 (D)
16 G	Grey	1.3 mm	130–220
18 G	Green	0.9 mm	75–120
20 G	Pink	0.8 mm	40–80(A)
22 G	Blue	0.6 mm	25–45
24 G	Yellow (B)	0.5 mm	10–30

Central venous catheters (CVC) have lumens of a maximum of 1.3 mm internal diameter; however, they have a longer length; thus, by the principles of the Hagen–Poiseuille equation flow rates are lower (C). Hartmann's solution has a lower viscosity than blood; therefore, flow rates are higher (E) if all other variables are unchanged.

$$\text{Flow} = \frac{\Delta P \pi r^4}{8 \eta l}$$

where η is fluid viscosity, l is length of the tube, ΔP is pressure gradient along the tube.

55. A False

B False

C True

D False

E False

Chest drains are inserted to remove air, blood or fluid from the interpleural space and can be inserted using the Seldinger technique or with blunt dissection. The drain is usually inserted into the 'safe triangle' bordered anteriorly by the pectoralis major muscle, posteriorly by the latissimus dorsi muscle, inferiorly by the line of the nipple and superiorly by the axilla. The 5th intercostal space, mid-axillary line is usually chosen (A).

The drain (see **Figure 5.6**) should have a drainage tube (tube 1) of low resistance and large diameter and whose volume is more than half the patients' maximum inspiratory capacity (C). This reduces the risk of water being drawn from the drainage bottle into the pleural space during inspiration.

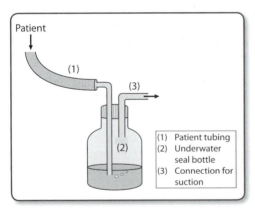

Figure 5.6 Chest drain bottle system.

Patient

(1)

(3)

(2)

(1) Patient tubing
(2) Underwater seal bottle
(3) Connection for suction

Within the bottle, the tubing (tube 2) should be no more than 5 cm (D) below the surface of the water to avoid high resistance to patient expiration. The drain bottle should be more than 45 cm (B) below the patient at all times, and clamping tube 1 should precede any reduction in height. Suction may be employed to tube 3 of up to 20 cmH$_2$O (E), although this is usually used in specific circumstances and should not be routinely employed.

56. A True

   B True

   C False

   D True

   E False

Fuses act as circuit breakers. They use the principle that increasing flow of current will cause an increase the production of heat (A). If the current exceeds the rating of a fuse, the wire contained within it will rapidly overheat and melt (B), thus breaking the circuit and stopping the flow of excessive current. The rating of a fuse is varied by changing the diameter (C) of the wire within the fuse. Fuses are placed in electrical circuits to prevent the flow of higher than expected currents, thereby improving the safety of electrical equipment (D). Fuses are conductors and act as circuit breakers; they are not capacitors (E).

57. A True

   B False

   C False

   D False

   E True

Modern diathermy machines have outputs that are isolated from earth (C) to minimise leakage currents from the diathermy circuit to earth. Capacitors (A) allow the flow of alternating current, the higher the frequency of the current, the lower the resistance of the capacitor. Incorporating a capacitor into the circuit minimises the flow of dangerous low-frequency currents. The passive electrode is the diathermy plate which has to be securely attached to the patient and burns can arise if this pad has a small surface area (B) or is poorly attached due to high current density present at the pad.

Stray currents can burn a patient by completing an alternative circuit. With increasing frequency, the risk of stray currents is greater (D) and this is the reason modern isolated systems operate at a lower frequency range, about 500 kHz.

Alarms are installed in the diathermy equipment to warn users that the device is active. They also warn of faulty electrode connections and of high stray leakage currents (E).

58. A True

   B True

   C False

   D False

   E True

The use of lasers in the theatre setting can be hazardous for staff and patients and safety precautions must be taken to minimise the risk of accidental injury.

- All staff should be appropriately trained (A) in the use of laser equipment
- All exposed surfaces should be matt-finished
- All instruments should be matt-finished
- Remove all shiny/reflective surfaces from the theatre
- No flammable material should be near the patient
- Theatre door should be locked (E)
- Signs should be put up indicating the use of laser
- All theatre staff should wear appropriate eye protection (B)
- The patient's eyes and exposed skin should be covered with damp swabs (C)
- Laser-resistant endotracheal tubes should be used
- Inspired oxygen should be kept at low as possible, preferably below 35% (D)

59. A False

  B False

  C True

  D False

  E True

Paramagnetic substances are those that are attracted to magnetic fields, usually due to the presence of unpaired electrons in their outer shells. The two most common examples of this are oxygen (C) and nitric oxide (E). The principle of paramagnetism is used in Pauling oxygen gas analysers that are rapid and highly accurate.

Most gases, including nitrogen (B), carbon dioxide (D) and nitrous oxide (A), are diamagnetic, meaning they are repelled by a magnetic field.

60. A False

  B True

  C True

  D True

  E False

Parametric tests are statistical tests that make a number of assumptions regarding the data:

- All observations made are independent
- The population follows a normal (Gaussian) distribution (C)
- The variance between observations are the same

Parametric tests allow many conclusions to be drawn and are more powerful than non-parametric tests but are affected by outliers. The central measure is the mean, which in a normal distribution should equal the median and the mode (B) (see **Figure 5.7**). Non-parametric data uses the median as the measure of central tendency and can assess either normal or non-normally distributed data.

Parametric statistical tests include Student's t-test or ANOVA (analysis of variance), each of which can be paired or unpaired (D) and assess quantitative (E) numerical data. The Mann–Whitney U test (A) is sued for ordinal unpaired data (see **Table 5.9**).

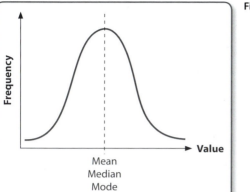

Figure 5.7 Normal distribution.

Table 5.9 Classification of statistical tests		
Data type	**Two groups**	**More than two groups**
Qualitative (categorical)	Contingency tables (χ^2)	Contingency tables (χ^2)
Non-parametric (including ordinal)	Unpaired: Mann–Whitney	Unpaired: Kruskal–Wallis
	Paired: Wilcoxon rank	Paired: Friedman
Continuous parametric	Unpaired: Student's *t*-test	Unpaired: ANOVA*
	Paired: Student's *t*-test	Paired: ANOVA
*ANOVA, analysis of variance.		

Answers: SBAs

61. D Hypovolaemia

In this scenario, the blood gas suggests the patient has a mixed respiratory and metabolic acidosis that is probably due to hypovolaemia. The discrepancy between end-tidal CO_2 (ET_{CO_2}) and arterial CO_2 (Pa_{CO_2}) is most likely due to increased dead space ventilation because expired gas from areas of dead space is not involved in gas exchange, thus diluting the CO_2 from lung areas that are involved in gas exchange.

Basal atelectasis would most likely cause hypoxia as well as hypercapnia, whereas hypoventilation would lead to an increased ET_{CO_2} as well as an increased Pa_{CO_2}. CO_2 absorption from the pneumoperitoneum would also cause an elevated ET_{CO_2}. Pulmonary shunt would lead to hypoxia without an increase in the Pa_{CO_2}.

Tautz TJ, Urwyler A, Antognini JF, Riou B. Case scenario: increased end-tidal carbon dioxide: a diagnostic dilemma. Anesthesiology 2010; 112:440–446.

62. B Apply high-flow oxygen to the face and tracheostomy

If the patient is trying to breathe through the tracheostomy, but is struggling to do so, then the most appropriate first step is to apply high-flow oxygen to the face and over the tracheostomy. This must be followed by assessment of tracheostomy patency. This can be done by removing the speaking valve if present or removing the inner tube, which may have been blocked by dry secretions. Try to pass a suction catheter to determine if the tracheostomy tube is patent, if not then deflate the cuff and assess whether the patient is able to breathe.

63. C Regional anaesthesia instead of general anaesthesia

The four pathological mechanisms underlying nerve injuries are:

- Stretch
- Compression
- Generalised ischaemia
- Metabolic derangement

Nerve injuries can present up to a few days after the initial injury, and the theory that nerve injuries can be prevented by avoiding general anaesthesia is not true; this is supported by a prospective study comparing the incidence of ulnar nerve neuropathy in patients undergoing general anaesthesia, regional anaesthesia and sedation. They found that there was no difference in the incidence of ulnar neuropathy between the groups.

Knight DJW, Mahajan RP. Patient positioning in anaesthesia. Contin Educ Anaesth Crit Care Pain 2004; 4.

64. B Metoclopramide

The chemoreceptor trigger zone is located in the area postrema of the medulla, on the lateral wall of the fourth ventricle and lies outside the blood–brain barrier. Its cells are stimulated by noradrenaline, dopamine, acetylcholine, and opioid receptor agonists.

Metoclopramide is a dopamine receptor antagonist that acts on the chemoreceptor trigger zone.

The other class of antiemetics that acts on the chemoreceptor trigger zone are the cholinergic (muscarinic) antagonists, such as hyoscine and atropine.

Histamine receptor antagonists (e.g. cyclizine) and serotonin ($5HT_3$) receptor antagonists (e.g. ondansetron) do not act on the chemoreceptor trigger zone.

Pierre S, Whelan R. Nausea and vomiting after surgery. Contin Educ Anaesth Crit Care Pain 2013; 13(1):28–32.

65. E There are no vessels or nerves penetrating it

The cricothyroid membrane is situated at the level of the 6th cervical vertebra and lies between the cricoid and thyroid cartilages. It is easier to locate in men as they have a prominent thyroid cartilage, and the cricothyroid membrane is located just below this. There are no vessels or nerves penetrating it whereas the thyroid ligament has the superior laryngeal nerve and artery penetrating it.

Patel B, Frerk C. Large-bore cricothyroidotomy devices. Contin Educ Anaesth Crit Care Pain 2008; 8:157–160.

66. B Hyperglycaemia

This patient has a body temperature of below 35°C; therefore, he is suffering from mild hypothermia (between 32°C and 35°C). Moderate hypothermia is between 28°C and 32°C and severe hypothermia is less than 28°C. The physiological responses to preserve heat include sympathetic nervous system excitation; therefore, clinical features such as shivering, hypertension, tachycardia, tachypnea and vasoconstriction occur. As the core temperature drops, the rate of metabolism increases by adrenergic stimulation in order to generate heat.

Hyperglycaemia may occur because glucose consumption by cells and insulin secretion both decrease and sympathetic activation releases glucose from the liver.

Sullivan G, Edmondson C. Heat and temperature. Contin Educ Anaesth Crit Care Pain 2008; 8:104–107.

67. A Fentanyl

This patient is suffering from moderate renal impairment.

- Mild: glomerular filtration rate (GFR) 20–50 mL/minute
- Moderate: GFR 10–20 mL/minute
- Severe: GFR <10 mL/minute

Patients with a GFR above 50 mL/minute do not usually require dosage adjustment.

Fentanyl is a synthetic phenylpiperidine derivative with a rapid onset of action. It is a μ-receptor agonist and shares many of the properties of morphine, but it has a much lower propensity to release histamine when administered intravenously and has a high hepatic first-pass metabolism where it is N-demethylated to norfentanyl which is further hydroxylated to inactive metabolites excreted in the urine. For this reason, a dose adjustment is not necessary in moderate renal impairment.

All of the other drugs are renally excreted so they will need to have dose adjustments when administered, even in moderate renal impairment.

Milner Q. Pathophysiology of chronic renal failure. BJA CEPD Reviews 2003; 3:130–133.

68. E Hepatitis

In prehepatic jaundice, bilirubin production is increased and the liver is unable to form enough bilirubin conjugates as the enzyme glucuronyl transferase is saturated; therefore, there is an excess of unconjugated bilirubin in the plasma. This is water insoluble so does not enter the urine, which therefore does not become brown in colour.

Intrahepatic jaundice can occur due to:

- damage to liver cells by inflammation (hepatitis); here the transport and conjugation of bilirubin is impaired; therefore, the amount of water-soluble conjugated bilirubin in the urine is elevated (hence brown colouration)
- a deficiency of glucuronyl transferase (Gilbert's syndrome)
- inhibition of glucuronyl transferase by steroids
- inhibition of bilirubin secretion into the bile canaliculi (by drugs)

With intrahepatic jaundice, the stool colour remains brown as bilirubin does enter the intestine to serve as a source of stercobilinogen.

Posthepatic jaundice is as a result of obstruction to the bile ducts by stones or tumour. This causes conjugated bilirubin to enter the bloodstream, and as it is water soluble it enters the urine and discolours it; it is also unable to enter the intestine due to the obstruction which is why the stools become pale (no conjugated bilirubin present to form stercobilinogen, which gives the stool its brown colour)

As this patient has dark brown discoloured urine and normal coloured stools, the most likely cause for her jaundice is hepatitis.

Vaja R, McNicol L, Sisley I. Anaesthesia for patients with liver disease. Contin Educ Anaesth Crit Care Pain 2010; 10:15–19.
Lai WK, Murphy N. Management of acute liver failure. Contin Educ Anaesth Crit Care Pain 2004; 4:40–43.

69. A Elevated blood sugar level

The main stimulus for insulin release is an elevated blood sugar level. There are other processes which also promote the release of insulin such as the hormones glucagon, insulin releasing peptide and somatostatin.

Certain amino acids such as lysine, arginine and leucine also cause an increase in insulin release.

Adrenaline and noradrenaline actually slow down the release of insulin via α-receptors in order to increase the amount of glucose available.

The normal insulin content of the pancreas is about 6–10 mg, of which 2 mg is released daily. The half-life of insulin is between 10 and 30 minutes and it is mainly broken down in the liver and kidney.

Nicholson G, Hall GM. Diabetes and adult surgical inpatients. Contin Educ Anaesth Crit Care Pain 2011; 11:234–238.

70. D Nimodipine

Cerebral vasospasm is a potentially life-threatening complication of subarachnoid haemorrhage. It is prevented and treated with nimodipine 60 mg four times a day. Nimodipine, like the other dihydropyridine calcium channel blockers nifedipine and amlodipine, acts on peripheral 'slow' calcium channels to reduce vascular tone. Nimodipine, however, is more lipid soluble, and therefore penetrates the blood–brain barrier more effectively than the other dihydropyridine calcium channel blockers. It can increase cerebral blood flow by up to 18% in patients with subarachnoid haemorrhage, and its use is associated with reduced morbidity and mortality.

Nimodipine is also used in the treatment of migraine, acute cerebrovascular accidents and epilepsy.

Keyrouz SG, Diringer MN. Clinical review: Prevention and therapy of vasospasm in subarachnoid hemorrhage. Crit Care 2007; 11:220.

71. D Reduced acetylcholine transmission

The most common cause of hypotension following spinal anaesthesia is pharmacological sympathectomy. Local anaesthetic agents block sympathetic outflow from the sympathetic chain, thereby preventing preganglionic transmission via acetylcholine. This leads to a reduction in vascular smooth muscle tone and both arterial and venous dilatation, reducing venous return and thus blood pressure. A reflex tachycardia takes place to compensate for the reduced preload (cardiac output = stroke volume × heart rate), and this increases the cardiac sodium channel activity, so does not contribute to hypotension.

As the patient is first on the list, intravascular hypovolaemia is less likely to be the cause of her acute hypotension.

The underlying cause is inadequate sympathetic outflow at the level of the sympathetic chain, thus a reduction in adrenaline is less likely to be the underlying pathogenesis. A reduction in sympathetic activation of peripheral vasculature leads to a reduction in smooth muscle intracellular calcium concentrations causing the vasodilatation.

New York School of Regional Anesthesia. http://www.nysora.com/regional_anesthesia/neuraxial_ techniques/3119-spinal_anesthesia.html (Last accessed 01/10/2012)

72. C Increased glycogenolysis

The physiological changes occurring in starvation depend on the duration of starvation. There is an initial attempt to meet glucose requirements followed by a shift within body organs to utilise other fuels.

First 24 hours

- Reduced insulin secretion, increased glucagon secretion
- Increased glycogenolysis; glycogen stores last for 24 hours
- Glucose is produced from pyruvate and lactate via the Cori cycle
- Increased fatty acid utilisation by muscles due to reduced glucose uptake and low insulin

24–72 hours

- Hepatic conversion of acetyl-CoA to ketone bodies (ketogenesis)
- Brain and heart begin to utilise ketones for energy
- Start of proteolysis and lipolysis as an energy source

>72 hours

- Ketones are the main source of energy for the brain
- Further proteolysis and lipolysis
- Gluconeogenesis is reduced as ketoadaptation ensues

Campbell I. Starvation, exercise, injury and obesity. Anaesth Intensive Care Med 2007;7:299–303.

73. E Increased intracellular cyclic guanosine monophosphate (GMP)

Glyceryl trinitrate (GTN) is an organic nitrate that is used in the treatment of cardiac failure, angina and following cardiac surgery. It acts predominantly on veins rather than arterioles, and exerts its action by being denitrated to produce nitric oxide, activating guanylate cyclase to generate cyclic GMP. This reduces intracellular calcium influx, reducing cytoplasmic calcium concentrations and leads to a reduced availability of calcium for smooth muscle contraction, therefore causing smooth muscle relaxation. The overall result is a reduced preload, venous return and left ventricular end-diastolic pressure, reduced myocardial oxygen demand and increased myocardial oxygen supply.

Marsh N, Marsh A. A short history of nitroglycerine and nitric oxide in pharmacology and physiology. Clin Exp Pharmacol Physiol 2000; 27:313–319.

74. B Molecular weight

The two most important factors determining transfer of drug across the blood–brain barrier (BBB) are the drug lipophilicity and the molecular weight of the substance. The lipophilicity only plays a role if the molecular weight is less than 600 Da, above which any transfer across the BBB is extremely limited. Although protein binding and drug concentration play a role, they do not influence the individual drug unit transfer across the barrier.

Lawther KB, Kumar S, Krovvidi H. Blood–brain barrier. Contin Educ Anaesth Crit Care Pain 2011; 11:128–132.

75. E Bronchial veins

This question refers to physiological shunt. The alveolar Po_2 (P_{AO_2}) can be calculated from the alveolar gas equation:

$$P_{AO_2} = P_{IO_2} - \frac{P_{aCO_2}}{R}$$

where P_{IO_2} is the inspired partial pressure of oxygen,

$$P_{IO_2} = F_{IO_2} \times (\text{Atmospheric pressure} - \text{Humidification})$$

P_{aCO_2} is the arterial partial pressure of carbon dioxide, R is the respiratory quotient and is normally approximately 0.8.

Thus:

$$P_{AO_2} = 19.8 - \frac{5.3}{0.8} = 13.2 \text{ kPa}$$

The alveolar–arterial oxygen gradient may be contributed to by physiological shunt and is normally less than 2.0 kPa (1.1 kPa in this patient). The contribution to physiological shunt, also known as venous admixture, is from Thebesian and bronchial veins and causes a ventilation/perfusion mismatch.

This patient is not hypoxic and does not have any evidence of increased dead space ventilation as would be seen with asthma. A pulmonary embolism would demonstrate hypoxia, as would pneumonia and atelectasis. Therefore, venous admixture is the most likely explanation in this patient.

Armstrong JAM, Guleria A, Girling K. Evaluation of gas exchange deficit in the critically ill. Contin Educ Anaesth Crit Care Pain 2007; 7:131–134.

Ng A, Swanevelder J. Hypoxaemia during one-lung anaesthesia. Contin Educ Anaesth Crit Care Pain 2010; 10:117–122.

76. C Histamine

Reversal of flow through an atrial septal defect (ASD) is caused by disturbance to the balance between pulmonary vascular resistance (PVR) and systemic vascular resistance (SVR). An increase in PVR would increase right-sided pressures, while a reduction in SVR would reduce left-sided pressures, either or both of which could potentially cause blood to flow from the right atrium to the left atrium through the ASD. Thus, any cause for increased PVR could be responsible as shown in Table 3.2.

As well as increasing PVR, histamine also has the effect of reducing SVR, thus potentially tipping the balance in favour of reversal of flow.

Vigorito C, Russo P, Picotti GB et al. Cardiovascular effects of histamine infusion in man. J Cardiovasc Pharmacol 1983; 5:531–537.

77. B Reduced cerebral blood flow

Propofol has a number of neurological effects other than anaesthetic and antiemetic effects. It causes a reduction in cerebral blood flow and cerebral perfusion pressure, while reducing the intracranial pressure as a consequence. In addition, intraocular pressure is reduced. Although epileptiform movements can be seen with propofol administration, there is no evidence for epileptic electroencephalogram activity, in fact propofol has been successfully used to terminate seizures. Because of its anaesthetic affect, cerebral oxygen consumption is reduced. This leads to a reduction in offloading of oxygen from haemoglobin, thus the jugular bulb saturations will be increased rather than decreased.

Mishra LD, Rajkumar N, Hancock SM. Current controversies in neuroanaesthesia, head injury management and neuro critical care. Contin Educ Anaesth Crit Care Pain 2006; 6:79–82.

78. C 3400L

Size J oxygen cylinders contain 6800 L of oxygen when full, at which point the gauge pressure in the cylinder is 13,700 kPa (137 bar). Because oxygen is stored as a gas in cylinders, the reduction in gauge pressure is directly proportional to the volume remaining within the cylinder. Therefore, a reduction of 50% in the gauge pressure to 6850 kPa indicates a proportional reduction in the volume remaining to 3400 L.

Al-Shaikh B, Stacey S. Essentials of anaesthetic equipment, 3rd edn. Edinburgh: Churchill Livingstone; 2007.

79. E No changes are required

The minimum alveolar concentration of volatile agents is a percentage of the ambient pressure that is usually calibrated at 1 atmosphere (101.325 kPa). However, it is the partial pressure delivered that is responsible for the clinical effect, and as saturated vapour pressure is independent of ambient pressure, it remains unchanged at different pressures. As vaporizers are calibrated at 1 atmosphere, the delivered concentration varies proportionally, but the actual partial pressure remains unchanged.

2.5% sevoflurane delivered at 1 atmosphere:

$$2.5\% \times 101.325 \text{ kPa} = 2.53 \text{ kPa}$$

2.5% sevoflurane delivered at 2 atmospheres:

$$2.5\% \times \frac{101.325 \text{ kPa}}{202.65 \text{ kPa}} = 1.25\% \text{ of 2 atmospheres}$$

Thus, the partial pressure of sevoflurane is 1.25% of 202.65 kPa, which is 2.53 kPa. Therefore, no changes will need to be made to maintain appropriate delivery of sevoflurane in hyperbaric conditions.

Magee P, Tooley M. The physics, clinical measurement and equipment of anaesthetic practice for the FRCA, 2nd edn. Oxford: Oxford University Press; 2011.

80. C 5.6 L/minute

The Magill (Mapleson A) breathing system is the most efficient for spontaneously ventilating patients, requiring fresh gas flow rates of 70 mL/kg/minute to prevent rebreathing. Therefore, in pre-oxygenating this patient:

$$70 \text{ mL/kg/min} \times 80 \text{ kg} = 5600 \text{ mL/min} = 5.6 \text{ L/min}$$

The more commonly used Bain (Mapleson D) system requires two to three times the minute ventilation, which is likely to require flow rates of 10–12 L/minute of oxygen to prevent rebreathing.

Magee P, Tooley M. The physics, clinical measurement and equipment of anaesthetic practice for the FRCA, 2nd edn. Oxford: Oxford University Press; 2011.

81. B Myocardial infarction

The end-tidal carbon dioxide (ET_{CO_2}) gives an indication of alveolar ventilation, ventilation/perfusion mismatching, carbon dioxide production or delivery and equipment errors (**Table 5.10**).

Table 5.10 Causes of altered ET_{CO_2}

Increased ET_{CO_2}		Decreased ET_{CO_2}	
↓ Alveolar ventilation	↑ Dead space	↑ Alveolar ventilation	↓ Dead space
	↓ Minute ventilation		↑ Minute ventilation
↑ CO_2 production	Sepsis	↓ CO_2 production	↓ Temperature
	↑ Temperature		Hypothyroidism
	Thyrotoxicosis		↓ Metabolism
	Malignant hyperthermia	↑ Alveolar dead space	Pulmonary embolism
	Phaeochromocytoma		↓ Cardiac output
	Neuroleptic malignant syndrome		Hypovolaemia
Equipment	Rebreathing	Equipment	Sampling line errors
	Exhausted soda lime		Low tidal volumes
	Pneumoperitoneum		

Bhavani-Shankar K, Moseley H, Kumar AY et al. Capnometry and anaesthesia. Can J Anaesth 1992; 39:617–632.

82. E $O_2 + 4 \cdot \text{(electrons)} + 2 \cdot H_2O \rightarrow 4 \cdot OH^-$

The galvanic fuel cell is similar to the oxygen electrode but generates a power-independent current that is proportional to oxygen partial pressures. It is composed of a gold mesh cathode, a lead anode, a potassium chloride solution, an oxygen permeable membrane, a thermistor and a galvanometer (see **Figure 5.8**). At the lead anode, electrons are liberated:

$$Pb + 2OH^- \rightarrow PbO + H_2O + 2 \cdot \text{(electrons)}$$

while at the gold mesh cathode, the electrons react with oxygen:

$$O_2 + 4 \cdot \text{(electrons)} + 2 \cdot H_2O \rightarrow 4 \cdot OH^-$$

This generates an electrical current that is demonstrated on the galvanometer. The device is affected by temperature and thus contains a thermistor for temperature

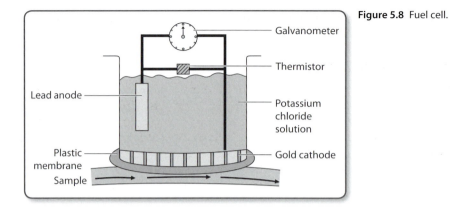

Figure 5.8 Fuel cell.

compensation. In addition, it is affected by nitrous oxide and has a relatively slow response time of 20–30 seconds.

Al-Shaikh B, Stacey S. Essentials of anaesthetic equipment. 3rd edn. Edinburgh: Churchill Livingstone; 2007.
Magee P, Tooley M. The physics, clinical measurement and equipment of anaesthetic practice for the FRCA, 2nd edn. Oxford: Oxford University Press; 2011.

83. D Reduces the onset time of the block

Speed of onset for local anaesthetic agents is related to the pKa and surrounding pH. The higher the pH, the more unionised the drug will be and thus the onset time will be reduced. By adding bicarbonate to the solution, the pH in the epidural space will increase causing more levobupivacaine to become unionised and therefore active, thereby providing a faster block. This is utilised in situations where time is of the essence, such as in emergency caesarean sections.

Milner QJW, Guard BC, Allen FG. Alkalinization of amide local anaesthetics by addition of 1% sodium bicarbonate solution. Eur J Anaesthesiol 2000; 17:38–42.

84. A Increased activity of vasoactive amines

Phenelzine is a non-selective, irreversible monoamine oxidase inhibitor (MAOI) that acts on both MAO_A and MAO_B. It causes central nervous system toxicity, anticholinergic effects and hepatotoxicity. In addition, it has numerous interactions with various drugs. The most dangerous is the co-administration of indirect-acting sympathomimetics such as ephedrine or metaraminol, which may precipitate an exaggerated hypertensive crisis as seen here, the mechanism of which is thought to involve increased activity of vasoactive amines. This is most effectively treated with phentolamine, an α-adrenergic receptor antagonist. For this reason, only direct-acting sympathomimetics should be used, and with great caution.

MAOIs may also interact with piperidine-derived opiates, including pethidine and fentanyl, causing agitation, hyperpyrexia, tachycardia and hypertension. This is thought to be due to increased release of serotonin.

MAOIs should be omitted for 2 weeks prior to a general anaesthetic, although this may not be possible in emergency situations.

Rennick RA, Jewesson P, Ford RW. Monoamine oxidase inhibitors and general anaesthesia: a reevaluation. Convulsive Ther 1987; 3:196–203.

85. B Prochlorperazine

Parkinson's disease is a degenerative condition of the substantia nigra in the basal ganglia due to loss of dopaminergic neurones. It is characterised by rigidity, akinesia, tremors and autonomic dysfunction. An imbalance between dopaminergic and cholinergic neurones leads to the features seen, and treatment aims to increase dopaminergic transmission. Drugs with antidopaminergic effects, particularly phenothiazines such as prochlorperazine or butyrophenones such as droperidol, may exacerbate symptoms significantly causing extra-pyramidal crises.

Nicholson G, Pereira AC, Hall GM. Parkinson's disease and anaesthesia. Br J Anaesth 2002; 89:904–916.

86. B Vomiting

Atropine is a tertiary anticholinergic in a racemic mixture, where the L-form is active. It is used to treat bradycardias, e.g. due to the oculocardiac reflex, as well as being an anti-sialogogue. Cardiovascular effects include an initial bradycardia due to the Bezold–Jarisch reflex, followed by tachycardia. It produces bronchodilatation and an increase in physiological dead space with a reduction in secretions. Sedation, agitation, confusion, hallucinations and dysarthria may occur, and atropine has antiemetic properties. Mydriasis, raised intraocular pressure and a reduction in sweating may also occur, with hyperthermia manifesting particularly in children.

87. A Bronchoconstriction

Neostigmine is a quaternary amine that carbamylates the esteratic site of the acetylcholinesterase enzyme, thereby deactivating it. This will increase availability of acetylcholine, leading to cholinergic effects systemically. This includes bradycardia, reduced cardiac output and hypotension. Increased bronchial secretions and bronchoconstriction may occur, particularly in asthmatics, together with nausea and vomiting and an increase in gastrointestinal secretions and motility. Urinary incontinence and an increase in peristalsis may be seen, while sweating, miosis and blurred vision also occur. In low doses (0.05–0.07 mg/kg), neostigmine can cause muscle contraction; however, at higher doses flooding of the neuromuscular junction with acetylcholine may paradoxically block neuromuscular transmission potentially leading to weakness.

Sasada M, Smith S. Drugs in anaesthesia and intensive care, 4th edn. Oxford: Oxford University Press; 2011.

88. A Warfarin

Plasma protein binding is dependent on the pharmacology of individual drugs. Basic drugs bind to globulins, particularly α_1-glycoprotein (α_1-acid glycoprotein), while acidic or neutral drugs bind to albumin (see **Table 5.11**).

Table 5.11 Protein binding of common drugs			
Bound to albumin		**Bound to α₁-glycoprotein**	
Drug	Protein binding (%)	Drug	Protein binding (%)
Warfarin	99	Bupivacaine	95
Propofol	98	Ropivacaine	94
Diazepam	97	Alfentanil	90
Phenytoin	95	Fentanyl	83
Thiopentone	80	Morphine	35
		Pancuronium	30
		Rocuronium	30

Calvey N. Bonding, binding and isomerism. Anaesth Intensive Care Med 2004; 5:345–347.

89. E Amitriptyline

Amitriptyline is a tricyclic antidepressant that inhibits uptake 1 in monoaminergic neurones, increasing synaptic noradrenaline and serotonin. It also antagonises muscarinic acetylcholine receptors, H1 histaminergic receptors and α-adrenergic receptors. Typically, an amitriptyline overdose presents with anticholinergic effects, sedation and postural hypotension. Sinus tachycardia, hyperthermia, mydriasis, coma, hyperreflexia, convulsions and hypotension all are features. Electrocardiogram changes include right bundle branch block, prolonged QT interval with a wide QRS complex of more than 120 ms.

Moclobemide is a reversible selective monoamine oxidase A inhibitor, with a relatively safe profile in overdose, although serotonin syndrome may rarely occur.

Lithium has a narrow therapeutic index, and overdose may cause nausea and vomiting, abdominal pain, diarrhoea, visual changes, tremor, arrhythmias, hyperreflexia and convulsions.

Phenelzine is a non-selective irreversible monoamine oxidase inhibitor and toxicity usually manifests as serotonin syndrome, which may be delayed up to 36 hours.

Fluoxetine is a selective serotonin re-uptake inhibitor that manifests as serotonin syndrome in overdose, with minimal anticholinergic effects or sedation.

Ward C, Sair M. Oral poisoning: An update. Contin Educ Anaesth Crit Care Pain 2010; 10:6–11.

90. C Paired Student's *t*-test

To decide what statistical test is ideal for each set of data, four questions must be answered:

- Is the data quantitative or qualitative?
- Is the data normally distributed or not normally distributed?
- Is the data paired or unpaired?
- Are there more than two groups of data?

Quantitative data can be continuous such as height, weight, blood pressure or biochemical markers. Alternatively, it can be ordinal such as numerical rating scales or scoring systems. Qualitative (categorical) data expresses characteristics in a non-numerical manner, such as blood group, eye colour or ASA score.

Continuous data can be normally distributed, following a Gaussian or bell-shaped distribution where the mean, median and mode are all equal and is parametric, or non-normally distributed where there is skewing or bimodality of the data and is non-parametric.

Paired data generally looks at data that comes from a single patient such as before/after treatment, while unpaired data comes from different patients or patient groups (see **Table 5.9**).

Campbell MJ, Swinscow TDV. Statistics at square one, 11th edn. BMJ Books. Oxford: Wiley-Blackwell; 2009.

Index

Note: Page numbers in **bold** or *italic* refer to tables or figures respectively.